Skill-mix Innovation, Effe
and Implementation

What are skill-mix innovations and why are they relevant? This systemic analysis of health workforce skill-mix innovations provides an overview of the evidence and lessons for implementation across multiple countries. The authors focus on six core segments of health systems: health promotion and prevention, acute care, chronic care, long-term and palliative care, as well as access for vulnerable groups and people living in underserved areas. In addition, the book analyses the roles of educational systems, workforce planning and policy, and financing within individual countries' healthcare organisations from a cross-country perspective. Although implementing skill-mix changes may be prone to stakeholder opposition or other barriers, this book helps identify ways to steer the process. The authors ultimately determine what skill-mix innovations exist, who may benefit from the changes and how to implement these changes within health systems. This Open Access title is the sixth book in Cambridge's European Observatory on Health Systems and Policies series.

Claudia B. Maier is Senior Researcher at the Berlin University of Technology.

Marieke Kroezen is Senior Researcher at the Netherlands Institute of Mental Health and Addiction.

Reinhard Busse is a Professor and Director at the Berlin University of Technology.

Matthias Wismar is a Programme Manager at the European Observatory of Health Systems and Policies.

European Observatory on Health Systems and Policies

The volumes in this series focus on topical issues around the transformation of health systems in Europe, a process being driven by a changing environment, increasing pressures and evolving needs.

Drawing on available evidence, existing experience and conceptual thinking, these studies aim to provide both practical and policy-relevant information and lessons on how to implement change to make health systems more equitable, effective and efficient. They are designed to promote and support evidence-informed policy-making in the health sector and will be a valuable resource for all those involved in developing, assessing or analyzing health systems and policies.

In addition to policy-makers, stakeholders and researchers in the field of health policy, key audiences outside the health sector will also find this series invaluable for understanding the complex choices and challenges that health systems face today.

List of Titles

Challenges to Tackling Antimicrobial Resistance: Economic and Policy Responses
Edited by Michael Anderson, Michele Cecchini, Elias Mossialos

Achieving Person-Centred Health Systems: Evidence, Strategies and Challenges
Edited by Ellen Nolte, Sherry Merkur, Anders Anell

The Changing Role of the Hospital in European Health Systems
Edited by Martin McKee, Sherry Merkur, Nigel Edwards, Ellen Nolte

Private Health Insurance: History, Politics and Performance
Edited by Sarah Thomson, Anna Sagan, Elias Mossialos

Ageing and Health: The Politics of Better Policies
Scott L. Greer, Julia Lynch, Aaron Reeves, Michelle Falkenbach, Jane Gingrich, Jonathan Cylus, Clare Bambra

Series Editors

Skill-mix Innovation, Effectiveness and Implementation

Improving Primary and Chronic Care

Edited By

CLAUDIA B. MAIER
Berlin University of Technology

MARIEKE KROEZEN
Netherlands Institute of Mental Health and Addiction (Trimbos Institute)

REINHARD BUSSE
Berlin University of Technology

MATTHIAS WISMAR
European Observatory on Health Systems and Policies

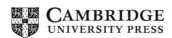
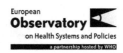

CAMBRIDGE
UNIVERSITY PRESS

University Printing House, Cambridge CB2 8BS, United Kingdom

One Liberty Plaza, 20th Floor, New York, NY 10006, USA

477 Williamstown Road, Port Melbourne, VIC 3207, Australia

314–321, 3rd Floor, Plot 3, Splendor Forum, Jasola District Centre, New Delhi – 110025, India

103 Penang Road, #05–06/07, Visioncrest Commercial, Singapore 238467

Cambridge University Press is part of the University of Cambridge.

It furthers the University's mission by disseminating knowledge in the pursuit of education, learning, and research at the highest international levels of excellence.

www.cambridge.org
Information on this title: www.cambridge.org/9781009013758
DOI: 10.1017/9781009031929

© World Health Organization 2022

First published 2022

A catalogue record for this publication is available from the British Library.

Library of Congress Cataloging-in-Publication Data
Names: Maier, Claudia, author.
Title: Skill-mix innovation, effectiveness and implementation : improving primary and chronic care / Claudia B. Maier.
Description: New York : Cambridge University Press, 2022. | Series: European observatory on health systems and policies | Includes index.
Identifiers: LCCN 2021032811 (print) | LCCN 2021032812 (ebook) | ISBN 9781009013758 (paperback) | ISBN 9781009031929 (ebook)
Subjects: LCSH: Public health personnel--Education. | Public health--Study and teaching.
Classification: LCC RA440.8 .M35 2021 (print) | LCC RA440.8 (ebook) | DDC 362.1071--dc23
LC record available at https://lccn.loc.gov/2021032811
LC ebook record available at https://lccn.loc.gov/2021032812

ISBN 978-1-009-01375-8 Paperback

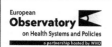

European
Observatory
on Health Systems and Policies
a partnership hosted by WHO

European Observatory
on Health Systems
and Policies

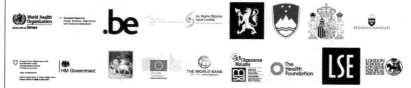

The European Observatory on Health Systems and Policies supports and promotes evidence-based health policy-making through comprehensive and rigorous analysis of health systems in Europe. It brings together a wide range of policy-makers, academics and practitioners to analyse trends in health reform, drawing on experience from across Europe to illuminate policy issues.

The European Observatory on Health Systems and Policies is a partnership hosted by the World Health Organization Regional Office for Europe, which includes the Governments of Austria, Belgium, Finland, Ireland, Norway, Slovenia, Spain, Sweden, Switzerland, the United Kingdom, and the Veneto Region of Italy; the European Commission; the World Bank; UNCAM (French National Union of Health Insurance Funds); the Health Foundation; the London School of Economics and Political Science; and the London School of Hygiene & Tropical Medicine. The Observatory has a secretariat in Brussels and it has hubs in London (at LSE and LSHTM) and at the Berlin University of Technology.

Contents

Figures

Tables

Boxes

Contributors

Mathilde S. Akeroyd, Research Assistant, University of
    Gothenburg, Sweden
Ramona Backhaus, Postdoctoral Researcher, Maastricht
    University, the Netherlands
Ronald Batenburg, Professor, Radboud University Nijmegen
    & Programme Coordinator, Nivel, the Netherlands
Elke Berger, Research Fellow, Berlin University of Technology,
    Germany
Pauline Boeckxstaens, Researcher, Ghent University, Belgium
Christine Bond, Professor, University of Aberdeen, United Kingdom
Ivy Bourgeault, Professor, University of Ottawa, Canada
Hannah Budde, Research Assistant, Berlin University of
    Technology, Germany
Reinhard Busse, Professor, Berlin University of Technology,
    Germany; European Observatory on Health Systems and
    Policies
Katarzyna Czabanowska, Professor, Maastricht University, the
    Netherlands
Jan De Maeseneer, Professor, Director WHOCC on Family
    Medicine and PHC, Ghent University, Belgium
Gilles Dussault, Researcher, Global Health and Tropical
    Medicine, Institute of Hygiene and Tropical Medicine, Portugal
Christian Gericke, Professor, School of Clinical Medicine,
    University of Queensland, Australia
Jan Hamers, Professor, Maastricht University, the Netherlands
Marieke Kroezen, Senior Researcher, Trimbos Institute, the
    Netherlands
Ellen Kuhlmann, Research Group Leader, Medizinische
    Hochschule Hannover, Germany
Romy Mahrer Imhof, Professor, Nursing Science & Care Ltd,
    Basel, Switzerland

Claudia B. Maier, Senior Researcher, Berlin University of
    Technology, Germany
Laura Pfirter, Research Assistant, Berlin University of
    Technology, Germany; Senior Fellow, European
    Observatory on Health Systems and Policies
Katherine Polin, Research Fellow, Berlin University of
    Technology, Germany
Peter Pype, Associate Professor, Ghent University, Belgium
Dheepa Rajan, Health Systems Adviser, Department for
    Health Systems Governance and Financing, World Health
    Organization, Geneva
Bernd Rechel, Researcher, European Observatory on Health
    Systems and Policies at the London School of Hygiene
    and Tropical Medicine, United Kingdom
Erica Richardson, Researcher, European Observatory on
    Health Systems and Policies at the London School of
    Hygiene and Tropical Medicine, United Kingdom
Mieke Rijken, Professor, Senior Researcher, Nivel, the
    Netherlands, University of Eastern Finland, Finland
Giada Scarpetti, Research Fellow, Berlin University of
    Technology, Germany
Walter Sermeus, Professor, KU Leuven, Belgium
Stephan Van den Broucke, Professor, Université Catholique de
    Louvain, Belgium
Juliane Winkelmann, Research Fellow, Berlin University of
    Technology, Germany
Gemma A. Williams, Research Fellow, European Observatory
    on Health Systems and Policies, United Kingdom
Matthias Wismar, Programme Manager, European
    Observatory on Health Systems and Policies, Belgium

Abbreviations

ACT	Asthma Control Test
ANF	National Association of Pharmacies (Portugal)
APN	advanced practice nurse
BMI	body mass index
CHC	community health centre
CHD	coronary heart disease
CHW	community health worker
CI	confidence interval
CKD	chronic kidney disease
CMHT	community mental health team
CNCM	community nurse case manager
COPD	chronic obstructive pulmonary disease
COVID-19	coronavirus disease 2019
CPD	continuing professional development
CVD	cardiovascular disease
DMP	disease management programme
ESP	extended scope-of-practice
ESTICOM	European Surveys and Training to Improve MSM Community Health
EU	European Union
GP	general practitioner
HbA1c	glycated haemoglobin
HNCM	hospital nurse care manager
ILO	International Labour Organization
IPE	interprofessional education
ISCO	International Standard Classification of Occupations
LTC	long-term care
MARS	Medication Adherence Report Scale
MD	mean difference
MSM	men who have sex with men

NCD	noncommunicable disease
NHS	National Health Service
NMS	New Medicines Service
NOSM	Northern Ontario School of Medicine
NP	nurse practitioner
n/r	not reported
OECD	Organization for Economic Co-operation and Development
OR	odds ratio
PA	physician assistant
PC	palliative care
PMAS	pharmacy-based minor ailment schemes
PN	patient navigator
QoL	quality of life
RCT	randomized controlled trial
RR	relative risk
SDG	Sustainable Development Goal
SEPEN	Support for the health workforce planning and forecasting expert network
SMD	standard mean deviation
TB	tuberculosis
WHO	World Health Organization

Foreword

Health systems all over the world rely on their health workers, their skills and education, as well as commitment and dedication to improve population health and treat individual patients. Achieving or maintaining universal health coverage is closely linked to a sufficient number of health workers with the right skills and knowledge to perform high-quality care. Yet, the health workforce in many countries across Europe is undergoing rapid changes in the education, scope-of-practice and ways of collaboration in teams.

These changes are exemplified by the COVID-19 pandemic. Health workers were at the frontline to respond quickly to public health emergencies and crises. The COVID-19 pandemic has affected virtually all countries worldwide – albeit to different extents – and has shown the public what contribution doctors, nurses, public health professionals, health care assistants and other health professionals make to treat patients. Across Europe and globally, the flexibility, commitment and motivation of health professionals to treat patients were remarkable. New skills and knowledge had to be acquired in limited time, new teams had to be formed and tasks had to be transferred from one profession to another. Many of these factors had to be implemented in limited time and under constraint contexts. There was limited evidence on what worked and with which outcomes.

The topic of the book on skill-mix innovations in primary care and for patients with chronic conditions could therefore not be more timely. Although it does not cover skill-mix changes during the COVID-19 pandemic – partly because it remains too early to evaluate results – the book addresses what we know from the scientific evidence on skill-mix and outcomes on individuals, population groups and health systems. The book provides an overview on skill-mix models, what additional, new roles (for example, patient navigators, case managers) can mean for patients and their outcomes, which tasks can be shifted to which profession(s) and for which patient groups, and what team configurations and ways of collaboration mean in practice.

The year 2020 was not only instrumental in raising the public's awareness of the contribution of health workers to patients' health during the COVID-19 pandemic, but was also timely, as the International Year of Nurses and Midwives. WHO has organized a number of events to celebrate the contribution of nurses and midwives and raise public awareness of these two important professions globally. As the book shows, many of the innovations in skill-mix are related to nurses who are now working in expanded roles in many functions, partly due to substantial changes to their education across Europe over the past decade.

In addition, WHO Regional Office for Europe has established several priorities to strengthen health professionals across the European region. The priorities link closely with the education, skills, teams and work conditions under which health workers work. The priorities are as follows:

- Formulate national strategies for modernizing the working conditions and modus operandi of the existing workforce and for aligning the production of the future workforce with the requirements of post-COVID-19 recovery.
- Convene a supranational consortium to develop in-service training programmes to reorient and requalify the existing workforce towards people-centred care in the post-COVID-19 context.
- Build consensus around regional and subregional policies for a fairer distribution of the health workforce: monitoring of mobility and migration; shared strategies to mitigate push factors (including deskilling, burnout and demotivation); and actions to foster a relationship of trust between health workers and health authorities.[1]

Skill-mix towards people-centred, high-quality health services is instrumental to ensure that health systems continue to be resilient and sustainable. Analysing and evaluating what skill-mix models exist for different population and patient groups, and with which outcome(s), is therefore a first step to understand what might work in what context and for which

---

[1] WHO Europe: European Programme of Work; https://apps.who.int/iris/bitstream/handle/10665/333908/70wd11e-rev4-EPW-200673.pdf?sequence=1&isAllowed=y

groups. The book makes an important contribution on this topic, it is the first of its kind to synthesize the evidence in a systematic manner.

Second, implementation is key. This is also addressed by the book. Analysing the policy context – that is, the role that policy, regulation and payment models can have on new professional roles, new tasks and division of work in teams – is critical for practice uptake. This also applies to the health care organization in which health workers work. Strategies are required not only at the policy level, but also by health care managers to strategically plan and implement change management, which takes account of the individual workers needs and concerns. Effective implementation can therefore be a strategic way for countries towards building a flexible, well-performing health workforce with the right skill-sets and competencies to provide timely, high-quality care.

Dr Hans Henri P. Kluge, WHO Regional Director for Europe

Acknowledgements

We are most grateful to Marius Ungureanu and Christiane Wiskow for their critical and constructive review of the entire volume. Jim Buchan, Gilles Dussault and Anita Charlesworth have reviewed several chapters and provided most relevant and valuable feedback. In addition, we thank Giorgio Cometto for his top-level comments and advice with regard to skill-mix and primary care. The external reviews were valuable for the development of the book. A big thank you is due to to Josep Figueras for his strategic advice in shaping the volume.

We thank the research assistants Hannah Budde and Laura Pfirter for continuous dedication and support for the entire book. Mathilde Akeroyd was instrumental in the finalization of the volume and in the drafting and shaping of selected abstracts. Theresa Meier has read all chapters and provided comments and edits. Maxim Hjortland and Kimberly Hartl have provided support for individual chapters, in particular by extracting research evidence or editing text.

The authors would like to thank Lesley Simon for the copy-editing, and Jonathan North for overseeing the publication process.

Input by experts on selected country examples (for example, 'mini case studies')

France: Anne Depaigne-Loth, Agence Nationale du Développement Professionnel Continu, France

France: Yann Bourgueil, Research Director, IRDES, France

Finland: Johanna Heikkilä, Senior Advisor, JAMK University of Applied Sciences, School of Health and Social Studies, Jyväskylä, Finland

Switzerland: Luc Besançon, Adviser, Swiss association of pharmacists / Société Suisse des Pharmaciens

Funder

The financial contribution by the UK Health Foundation is gratefully acknowledged. The funder had no role in the design of the study, the analysis or interpretation of the results, nor in the write-up phase of the chapters.

1 Skill-mix for primary and chronic care: definitions, conceptual framework and relevance for policy and practice

CLAUDIA B. MAIER, GEMMA A. WILLIAMS,
HANNAH BUDDE, LAURA PFIRTER, REINHARD
BUSSE, MATTHIAS WISMAR

1.1 Introduction: why skill-mix?

Access to and the quality of health services are closely linked to the density and skill-mix of a country's health workforce (OECD, 2016; World Health Organization, 2006, 2016). High rates of chronic conditions and multimorbidity, new treatment options, and technological advances and economic pressure have led to fundamental changes to health systems and have impacted on the daily work of health professionals. Many countries worldwide are experiencing a shortage of primary care providers, particularly in rural or socially deprived urban areas (OECD, 2016; World Health Organization, 2013). Primary care systems face the challenge of ensuring a sustainable workforce to allow timely access to services, high-quality care and person-centred services (Kringos et al., 2015a, 2015b). Against this backdrop, the skills and composition of the workforce have changed in many countries and settings to meet the increasing and diversifying demands of patients (Dubois & Singh, 2009; Freund et al., 2015). At the same time, health promotion and prevention are gaining increasing attention among primary care providers to ensure that all people can live in good health. Moreover, the global coronavirus disease 2019 (COVID-19) pandemic has brought to the forefront the necessity of having a well-qualified health workforce that has surge capacity, competencies and flexibility to react to short-term crises (WHO Regional Office for Europe, 2020). The pandemic has not only attracted more policy interest in strengthening the health workforce, it has also triggered a change in the public's view of the value and importance of health professionals and their contribution to the health of individuals and patients.

1

In a context where health care needs, demands and resources are rapidly changing, policy-makers aim to better understand which skill-mix reforms and strategies are effective. Global debates have in the past frequently focused on the required density and distribution of specific health professions to ensure universal access to and coverage of health services (for example, the number of physicians, nurses or other professions per population) (Campbell et al., 2013). There has been limited attention on identifying the right composition and skill-mix of the health workforce. This has changed over the past decade, with the World Health Organization (WHO), Organization for Economic Co-operation and Development (OECD) and European Commission moving skill-mix higher up the political agenda. The notion that the education, skills and competencies of health professions are essential for high-quality care and efficiency has been increasingly recognized. For instance, the OECD report "right skills, right jobs, right places" took an integrated approach covering the density, distribution and skill-mix of health professions (OECD, 2016). The WHO has published several reports on the health workforce including skill-mix or task shifting specifically (World Health Organization, 2007, 2008, 2016).

Yet, there has been a lack of common understanding of what skill-mix is, what professions are involved and what models exist in different care contexts. This knowledge is critical for identifying the effects of skill-mix on outcomes for patients, population groups and health systems. It is likewise important to identify lessons for implementation. Previous research has primarily focused on skill-mix among individual professions or between two professions, with less evidence available covering multiple professions. One skill-mix example that has been the subject of a considerable amount of research is the changing roles of nurses at the interface to the medical profession (Maier, 2015; Maier & Aiken, 2016; Maier, Aiken & Busse, 2017; Maier et al., 2016; Martínez-González et al., 2014a, 2014b, 2015a, 2015b; Morilla-Herrera et al., 2016; Swan et al., 2015). Fewer studies have analysed skill-mix changes covering multiple professions (Dubois & Singh, 2009; Freund et al., 2015; Sibbald, Shen & McBride, 2004; Tsiachristas et al., 2015). One cross-country analysis focused on a description of "typical" primary care teams in six countries (the United States of America, Canada, Australia, England, Germany and the Netherlands) (Freund et al., 2015). It found that general practitioners (GPs) and nurses were the main professions providing primary care in all countries, but they performed considerably different tasks and roles. Moreover, the number and contributions of medical assistants and other support workers varied considerably within practices. According to an international study on primary care systems in Europe, the organizational structures of primary care providers also vary, ranging from primarily solo practices to health centres (Kringos et al., 2015a, 2015b). These cross-country variations in the composition and roles of the health workforce and health systems are critical to identify as important contextual factors, which will be described in Section 1.5. A systematic review (Tsiachristas et al., 2015) analysed the effects of new professional roles on a variety of outcome parameters, including all professions. It identified primarily studies on nurses and a few studies on new professional roles among other professions. The review included all care sectors, including hospital settings. It did not differentiate by care sectors, conditions or care contexts and concluded that more research on the optimal skill-mix is required (Tsiachristas et al., 2015).

1.2 Aims of this skill-mix volume

Given the general paucity of systematic reviews on skill-mix covering multiple professions and a break-down by patient groups, this volume seeks to provide a synthesis of skill-mix in primary care and ambulatory care and outcomes in individuals and health systems. The volume therefore addresses skill-mix changes aimed at different population or patient groups, ranging from prevention to long-term and palliative care. Moreover, this volume aims to identify country reforms, common developments and lessons for implementation.

This volume has two overarching aims:

- First, to identify skill-mix changes, and in particular skill-mix innovations and the evidence on outcomes in patients and health systems. Within health systems, the role of health care professionals is critical, so a particular emphasis was given on outcomes for health professionals.
- Second, to identify lessons for implementation in different contexts and countries. The volume will analyse what the common barriers and enablers are that have been shown to influence the uptake of new skill-mix reforms in practice. It will address if and how education, regulation, financing and payment policies impact on the timely implementation of skill-mix reforms. Based on the evidence from

country experiences, it will suggest lessons to overcome barriers in practice. Moreover, it will analyse what factors and strategies exist to implement skill-mix changes in health care organizations.

How are skill-mix innovations defined for the purpose of this study? Skill-mix innovations are examples of changes to the skills, roles or clinical activities involving at least two professions, and characterized by three parameters: first, (perceived as) new in a country-specific context (novelty); second, discontinuous with previous practice (disruptive); and third, aimed at improving at least one health outcome (aimed at value), for example, with positive effects on access, quality, patient experience, coordination of care and/or costs (Greenhalgh et al., 2004).

This volume was written before the COVID-19 pandemic; therefore the book does not cover the literature on skill-mix changes that originated during the pandemic. Moreover, as the pandemic is still ongoing, it is premature to analyse what effects changes to the roles, tasks and competencies of specific health professionals have had on patient or health system outcomes.

1.3   Policy relevance: why now?

The notion that the health workforce is instrumental for improving access to health services as well as the quality of care has been recognized for decades, most notably with the publication of the *The World Health Report 2006: working together for health* (World Health Organization, 2006). Investing in the health workforce has received renewed policy attention recently during the COVID-19 pandemic (WHO Regional Office for Europe, 2020), in addition to previously ongoing WHO action on strengthening the health workforce (Campbell et al., 2013; Cometto et al., 2013). Achieving universal health coverage and other health-related sustainable development goals (SDGs) is dependent on a multitude of investments and reforms, including a sufficiently educated health workforce with the right skills and competencies (Cometto et al., 2013; World Health Organization, 2016). There is increasing evidence that strengthening the health workforce can not only have positive effects on health (for example, maternal and child health, among many others) (World Health Organization, 2006), but can also positively impact on other sectors beyond health. Effects beyond health include multiple potential spill-over effects on the economy, women's participation and societal well-being (World Health Organization, 2018). Yet, globally, health worker shortages, skill-mix imbalances, maldistribution and barriers to interprofessional collaboration prevail and are among the main obstacles preventing countries from reaching universal health coverage (Cometto et al., 2013).

The Global Burden of Disease study suggested that the health worker density would need to increase from a global average of 5.9 physicians, nurses and midwives per 1000 population in 2015 to 10.9 in 2030 (Global Burden of Disease 2017 SDG Collaborators, 2018). The study recognized the limitation of not covering other health professions, nor taking account of team composition and skill-mix requirements in reaching the SDGs. From an international perspective, there is little research evidence available that goes beyond density levels per profession and covers teams, the composition and the specific division of roles and tasks in practice. This is of relevance for all health systems and all care sectors, including primary care. Primary care is the care sector that has been estimated to determine to a large extent whether the goals of achieving universal health coverage and the SDGs can be met (Campbell et al., 2013; Cometto et al., 2013), yet, it is often less financed and not as attractive to health professionals compared with the secondary and tertiary care sectors.

The year 2016 was a landmark year with the creation of the United Nation's High Level Commission of Health Employment and Economic Growth (United Nations, 2016). The commission increased policy attention and commitment internationally on the necessity of strengthening the health workforce towards achieving the SDGs. The commission brought together heads of state and government, health and finance ministers and a wide research and practice community to demonstrate the evidence and create awareness of the link between strengthening the health workforce, economic growth and gender equality, which mutually reinforce each other on the quest towards the SDGs. There is increased recognition now that investment in a strong health workforce is required to reach the SDGs. The Commission developed a *Five year action plan for health employment and inclusive economic growth* led by the WHO, OECD and the International Labour Organization (ILO) in 2018 (World Health Organization, 2018). The action plan aims to strengthen the health and social care workforce globally as an important means to achieve the SDGs. The plan lists ten recommendations and five immediate actions, including actions to improve the education, skills and jobs of all health professionals, but with a particular focus on those countries with the largest shortage of health professionals in low- and middle-income countries. The action plan recommends the assessment of skill-mix shortages and suggests strategies to overcome these shortages. At the same time, the action plan is directed at all countries, including high-income countries. The reason is that many countries worldwide are facing challenges in ensuring a sustainable health workforce, particularly in primary care, long-term and palliative care and in underserved regions. The plan identifies interprofessional education and multiprofessional service provision, including the identification of skills and competencies as critical to achieve integrated people-centred care (World Health Organization, 2018, p. 15).

Moreover, in 2016, the WHO published the *Global strategy on human resources for health: Workforce 2030* (World Health Organization, 2016). Its main aim is to reach universal health coverage via a new global strategy for human resources for health. The strategy paper recommends the implementation of "health-care delivery models with an appropriate and sustainable skills mix in order to meet population health needs equitably" (World Health Organization, 2016). According to the WHO, the skill-mix should be community-based and include a variety of different health professions from different educational levels and backgrounds, including mid-level health workers in interprofessional primary care teams. There is limited additional guidance and evidence for what an appropriate and sustainable skill-mix entails, particularly for high-income countries and different care sectors.

For strengthening primary health care, the 2018 Astana declaration was critical to reach a renewed commitment among policymakers, 30 years after the 1978 Alma Ata declaration (World Health Organization/UNICEF, 2018). The declaration highlighted the importance of knowledge and capacity-building and strengthened capacity in human resources for health in primary health care, alongside the use of new technologies and financing. Through governmental, intersectoral action and a coordinated governance strategy, the aim is to build capacity for a high-quality, well-performing health workforce with an effective skill-set to provide high-quality, safe, comprehensive, integrated, accessible, available and affordable care (World Health Organization/UNICEF, 2018).

At the European Union (EU) level, several initiatives have been introduced, including the *Support for the health workforce planning and forecasting expert network* (SEPEN) (SEPEN, 2019). SEPEN was a follow-up network emanating from the Joint Action on Health Workforce Planning and Forecasting to foster exchange of knowledge, capacity and good practice in the field of European health workforce planning. The aims of the network are to encourage and sustain cross-country collaboration, to provide support to Member States and improve countries' health workforce planning processes and policy (SEPEN, 2019). The network has suggested capacity building so that the workforce can effectively work in multiprofessional teams, has access to high-quality knowledge and evidence about policies, regulations and planning. One major focus is on the mobility and migration of health professionals in the EU's single market and how countries can react and plan for inflows and outflows. Moreover, in 2019 the European Commission's Expert Panel on effective ways of investing in Health published an expert opinion on task shifting and health system design (European Commission, 2019). The publication of an opinion on this topic demonstrated the timeliness of skill-mix and health workforce themes at EU level. The opinion focused on one element of skill-mix (see definitions below, Table 1.1), namely task shifting; from one health professional to another, to patients or caregivers or to machines, hence including digital transformation. It did not, however, analyse other skill-mix changes, for instance the add-on of new roles and tasks (supplementation) or changes to multiprofessional teamwork.

The section below provides an overview of the definitions on skill-mix as an umbrella term and different typologies that fall within the definition.

1.4   Skill-mix and the health workforce: definitions

Before addressing what is meant by skill-mix, it is necessary to provide clarity on what is meant by the health workforce. The WHO defines the health workforce as "all people engaged in actions whose primary intent is to enhance health" (World Health Organization, 2006). This broad definition encompasses in its widest meaning also lay health workers, for example, community health workers, peers or family carers. To distinguish between the formally qualified and unqualified members of the health workforce, this volume will refer to health professionals as those with formal education (physicians, nurses, midwives, pharmacists, physiotherapists) and to health workers as those with no or

Table 1.1 *Definitions: skill-mix and its typologies*

Term	Definitions and examples
Skill-mix	Changes to the skills, competencies, roles or tasks within and across health professionals and health workers (including community-based workers, peers, informal caregivers) and/or teams
Skill-mix typologies	
1. Re-allocating tasks	Task-shifting (other terms: delegation, substitution) between physicians, nurses, pharmacists and other providers. Examples include: nonmedical prescribing of medicines, diagnosis performed by advanced practice providers, screening performed by nurses or pharmacists
2. Adding new tasks/ roles	Supplementation of tasks or add-on of new roles that did not previously exist or were not routinely provided. Examples include care coordination role, patient navigator, eHealth monitoring, health promotion role
3. Introducing or changing teamwork	Changes to the (way) of collaboration between at least two professions or more. Examples include shared care provided jointly by physicians and nurses and multiprofessional collaboration

Source: Based on and modified from the following sources (Buchan & Dal Poz, 2002; Friedman et al., 2014; Laurant et al., 2005; Sibbald, Shen & McBride, 2004).

very limited health-related education (lay, informal, community-based or peer workers). A similar approach is taken by the International Standard Classification of Occupations (ISCO) (International Labour Organization (ILO), 2010a), which has classified the health workforce into three major functions: health professionals, health associate professionals and (personal care) workers. For example, GPs, nurses and physiotherapists are covered under health professionals; whereas nurse assistants and medical technicians are summarized under health associate professionals. Home-based personal care workers subsume a large number of diverse, primarily lay workers with considerable contribution to individual health, particularly in long-term care. This volume covers all health professions working in primary and ambulatory care settings or at the interface to hospital care, and also includes lay workers, such as peers, community-based workers and family caregivers as long as they are covered by skill-mix changes and reforms.

What is skill-mix?

Several definitions of the term skill-mix exist in the literature with different focus, levels of breadth and depth (Buchan & Dal Poz, 2002; Dubois & Singh, 2009). Terms used commonly are skill-mix as an overarching term, but also changing roles, task shifting, task sharing, task supplementation, delegation and substitution, among others. For the purpose of this study and informed by two definitions (Buchan & Dal Poz, 2002; Sibbald, Shen & McBride, 2004), the following working definition was developed: skill-mix is defined as "directly changing the skills, competencies, attitudes, roles or tasks within and across individuals and teams". This definition was chosen deliberately with a broad remit to cover all changes that directly and purposefully change the roles of individual health professionals or teams in primary and ambulatory care settings. Differentiating between skill-mix change and a skill-mix innovation, the following additional three criteria were applied to qualify as an innovation: novelty of skill-mix changes (in its widest sense), being of disruptive nature (changing the status quo) and aimed at improving at least one health or health system outcome (Greenhalgh et al., 2004).

Further, to grasp the range and type of changes in the health workforce a modified typology of skill-mix innovations has been used for the study (Laurant et al., 2005; Friedman et al., 2014) (Table 1.1).

The first typology addresses re-allocating tasks between two professions. Commonly the term task shifting, or sometimes task sharing, has been used, although the latter term often lacks clarity over which tasks are shifted and which ones are being shared and by whom. Task shifting has also been referred to as substitution or delegation. While substitution refers to tasks being entirely shifted to a new profession, delegation is frequently referred to as the transfer of tasks to nonmedical professions such as nurses, but with physicians maintaining ultimate responsibility (Laurant et al., 2005; Sibbald, Shen & McBride, 2004). The two terms are sometimes also used simultaneously when it comes to questions of oversight and jurisdictional responsibility. This typology refers to a new division of work between at least two professions and the team in which they work.

The second typology concerns the addition of new tasks or roles, also referred to as task supplementation, such as care coordination, use of new technologies or eHealth monitoring. Adapted from Laurant et al. (2005), this typology refers to health professionals expanding their roles and performing new functions that were previously not or not routinely performed. Hence, this typology refers to expansions of the skills set and roles of an individual and the team.

The third typology covers the introduction of teamwork and collaboration for at least two professions, for instance shared care of physicians and nurses. The use of the term teamwork across this volume is based on changes to at least two professions directly affecting their method of collaboration. This also touches upon interventions to improve cooperation and collaboration such as teamwork effectiveness or interprofessional education (Friedman et al., 2014; Laurant et al., 2005).

In some cases, skill-mix changes result directly or indirectly in response to changes in service delivery models, which change the interface of care provision. A transfer of care from hospital to ambulatory or community care (such as community-based treatment and testing, for example, for HIV/AIDS, which would previously have been provided in hospitals or clinics) has major implications for the composition of teams providing this service and is also influenced by new technologies, treatment options and laboratory testing devices. Liaison functions are skill-mix changes aimed at improving the care across care settings to provide a smooth, continuous provision of services. This also applies to the relocation of care, which comprises a shift of entire service delivery models (for example, hospital-at-home). These models are more complex and although they may result in skill-mix changes, they are larger service delivery reforms of which skill-mix is only one important element among others. Hence, the evaluation of these models is more complex and attribution of causality is limited compared with the typologies 1–3 listed in Table 1.1.

1.5   The diversity and skill-mix of health professions in Europe: a snapshot

Strengthening primary care to meet the health and social care needs of an ageing population is prompting many countries in Europe to make far-reaching changes to the primary care workforce. The traditional primary care model of small, solo general practices is becoming increasingly unsustainable and unable to manage growing workloads, work intensity and work complexity, especially with many countries facing escalating GP shortages and economic constraints. As a result, these traditional ways of working are gradually being replaced by new models of primary care practice, centred on collaborative, multiprofessional teams (Groenewegen et al., 2015; Kuhlmann et al., 2018). To support these new ways of working and the delivery of more complex care and procedures, many countries have enhanced the scope of practice and skills of established health professionals such as nurses or pharmacists, reoriented professions such as paramedics or social workers that traditionally worked elsewhere in the health system into primary care settings or introduced new professions entirely such as physician assistants.

The scale and pace of these changes has, however, not been unified across Europe and considerable variation in the composition of the health workforce across the region exists (Groenewegen et al., 2015; Kringos et al., 2015a). Although some countries (for example, the United Kingdom, Iceland, Lithuania, Spain, Sweden) have introduced health centres or larger practices with multiprofessional teams incorporating a range of health professionals such as physicians, nurses, medical assistants, health care assistants, psychologists, physiotherapists and social workers, other countries (for example, Austria, Belgium, Czech Republic, Germany and Romania) still rely primarily on smaller primary care practices where GPs work alone or with one or two other professionals, usually a nurse or medical assistant (Groenewegen et al., 2015; Kringos et al., 2015a). In addition, the scope of practice and skill-profiles of an individual profession such as advanced practice nurses differs considerable from one country to the next (Maier & Aiken, 2016; Maier, Aiken & Busse, 2017; Maier, Koppen & Busse, 2018). Even within the same country, ways of working and responsibilities of different professions often vary between practices and settings, depending on patients' needs, individual competencies, professional boundaries and the division of work.

International definitions of health professionals

In light of the variations of teams and skill-mix within and across countries, it is important to have an understanding of how a physician, a nurse or a pharmacist is defined in different country contexts and internationally. Although there are clear variations across countries, there are also attempts at the international level to define health professions, their core tasks and clinical roles. Core definitions are provided in the Appendix, for instance based on International Standard

Classification of Occupations (ISCO)-08 codes that have been developed by the International Labour Organization (ILO) (International Labour Organization (ILO), 2010a, 2010b) or by standard definitions from other sources.

Hence, ISCO classifications provide a common understanding of the definition of different health professions and their scope of practice. For example, among other tasks, generalist medical practitioners or GPs are defined as carrying out clinical examinations of patients to assess, diagnose and monitor a patient's condition and provide continuing medical care for patients including prescribing, administering, counselling on and monitoring of curative treatments and preventive measures (modified from: ILO: ISCO 2211). Nursing professionals, including specialist nurses, plan and provide personal care, treatments and therapies; develop and implement care plans for biological, social and psychological treatment and provide information about prevention of ill-health, treatment and care "for people who are in need of nursing care due to the effects of ageing, injury, illness or other physical or mental impairment, or potential risks to health" (ILO: ISCO 2221). Pharmacists meanwhile are professionals that "store, preserve, compound and dispense medicinal products and counsel on the proper use and adverse effects of drugs and medicines following prescriptions issued by medical doctors and other health professionals" (ILO: ISCO 2262). ISCO does not cover all health professions; new professions that have emerged more recently and have a comparatively younger tradition in many countries are often missing. Some examples are Nurse Practitioners/ Advanced Practice Nurses and Physician Assistants, or dental hygienists. For these professions, standard definitions by other sources were used (see Appendix). Moreover, there are a multitude of other health professionals working in primary care, ambulatory care settings or at the interface between inpatient and outpatient care. Further details on these professions, their definitions and common tasks for other health professionals can be found in the Appendix.

Although international definitions are helpful to have a common, minimum understanding of the role and tasks of certain health professions, the definitions need to be seen in the country-specific contexts, which include the minimum level education of these professions, their scopes-of-practice, which comprises the clinical activities and tasks that these professions are officially authorized to perform, and the clinical practice settings.

The EU's free movement zone: minimum qualification of health professionals

In 2005 the Council of the EU adopted Directive 2005/36/EC on the recognition of professional qualifications in practice, with the Directive modernized in 2013 (European Union, 2013). The legally binding Directive aims to support the policy of freedom of movement by granting automatic and mutual recognition of professional qualifications between Member States and other countries belonging to the EU's free movement zone (for example, Norway, Switzerland). The Directive covers five regulated health professions: physicians (including GPs and specialists), nurses, midwives, dental practitioners and pharmacists. The Directive provides a legal definition of minimum education qualifications and medical training that must be achieved in order to practice and has led to a process of minimum harmonization of education and training requirements across the EU, although variations remain across countries.

For physicians, basic medical education must consist of 5500 hours of practical and theoretical training over a minimum of 5 years. General practice is a distinct postgraduate qualification separate from other medical specialities, with mandatory postgraduate training defined as: (i) a full-time course of a minimum of 3 years; (ii) at least 6 months in an approved hospital or clinic and at least 6 months in an approved GP practice or centre where doctors provide primary care. Although specialist training is a mandatory prerequisite for becoming a GP in the EU/EEA, subjects studied and the duration of training vary markedly from 3 years (for example, Belgium, Bulgaria, Italy, Latvia, Malta, the Netherlands and the United Kingdom) to 6 years (Finland) (European Academy of Teachers in General Practice/Family Medicine (EURACT), 2020).

Following the Directive and reforms under the Bologna process, qualification as a registered nurse across the EU is now primarily achieved through obtaining a Bachelor-level degree (Lahtinen, Leino-Kilpi & Salminen, 2014). Few countries (for example, Austria and Germany) still have a co-existence of educational pathways, consisting of Bachelor programmes and vocational trainings at nursing schools. Advanced practice nurses (including nurse practitioners) are generally educated to at least Master's level (Maier, Aiken & Busse, 2017). According to the Directive, pharmacists must complete "training of at least five years' duration, including at least: (i) four years of full-time theoretical and practical training at a university or at a higher institute of a level recognised as equivalent, or under the supervision of a university; (ii) six-month traineeship in a pharmacy". In France, completion of a 5- or 6-year Doctor of Pharmacy degree is necessary to become a licensed pharmacist. In a small number of countries (for example, England), specific education and training programmes are also available to support pharmacists working in primary care (Middleton, Howard & Wright, 2019).

Role developments and scope-of-practice variations across Europe

The roles and tasks undertaken by health professionals have expanded in scope and complexity in recent years in a number of countries (Dubois & Singh, 2009; Freund et al., 2015; Kringos et al., 2015a). In primary care, GPs are now increasingly expected to provide more complex, all-round care to patients, including those with multimorbidity or long-term chronic conditions and to work as part of multiprofessional teams. Kringos et al. (2015a, b) have grouped the range of services provided by GPs into five broad categories: first-contact care and triage; diagnostic services, treatment and follow-up care; medical technical procedures; prevention and health promotion; and mother, child and reproductive health care. However, an assessment of services provided by GPs in 13 case study countries found GP involvement in treatment and follow up was generally high but involvement in preventive care was limited. GP involvement in first-contact care was highest in countries with stronger and well-developed primary care services such as France, the Netherlands and the United Kingdom (Kringos et al., 2015b).

The move towards a broader skill-mix in primary care has allowed physicians to relinquish several clinical and non-clinical tasks to other professions such as to Advanced Practice Nurses/Nurse Practitioners with a Master's degree or other postgraduate qualifications (for example, Finland, Ireland, the Netherlands, the United Kingdom) or nurses with additional education but not at the Master's level (for example, Cyprus, Denmark, Estonia, Poland, Spain), to community pharmacists (for example, Switzerland, the United Kingdom), health care assistants (for example, in Spain and the United Kingdom), physician assistants (for example, in the Netherlands and the United Kingdom) or medical assistants (for example, in Austria, Germany and Switzerland) (Freund et al., 2015;

Maier, Aiken & Busse, 2017; Wismar, Glinos & Sagan, forthcoming). This task shifting, which has resulted in an expanded scopes-of-practice and a new division of work among teams, has been facilitated by reforms to the education and training of these professions in Europe.

Examples of the changing roles of health professionals are multi-faceted and highly context-specific. An overview of in-depth country reforms and developments is provided in the European Observatory on Health Systems and Policies skill-mix case study companion volume (Wismar, Glinos & Sagan, forthcoming).

In this section, we provide a snapshot of trends with regard to two professions: nurses and pharmacists, for which a large number of reforms and developments have occurred in Europe. One notable example is the introduction of Advanced Practice Nurses/Nurse Practitioners roles, facilitated by reforms in line with the Bologna process and the move of nursing education to Bachelor's degree, followed by Master's programmes (Lahtinen, Leino-Kilpi & Salminen, 2014; Praxmarer-Fernandes et al., 2017). An analysis in 39 countries found that within Europe, Finland, Ireland, the Netherlands and the United Kingdom have expanded the scopes-of-practice of Advanced Practice Nurses/Nurse Practitioners considerably, authorizing them to perform a complex set of clinical activities. These include being responsible for a panel of patients, performing diagnoses/clinical assessments, ordering medical tests, deciding on certain treatments, prescribing certain medications, acting as first-point-of-contact and referring patients to other providers or settings (Maier & Aiken, 2016; Maier, Aiken & Busse, 2017). Another related trend across Europe is country reforms on nurse prescribing. As of 2019, 13 countries in Europe had adopted laws to grant nurses with additional qualifications certain prescribing rights, thereby expanding their official scopes-of-practice. These countries are Cyprus, Denmark, Estonia, Finland, France, Ireland, the Netherlands, Norway, Poland, Spain, Sweden, the United Kingdom and the canton of Vaud, in Switzerland. Of these, eight countries adopted new laws in the last decade, demonstrating the novelty of the skill-mix change (Maier, 2019).

In a similar way to changes in the role of nurses, several countries have expanded the role of pharmacists in primary care (for example, Belgium, Denmark, France, Italy, Portugal and the United Kingdom), leading to a substantial increase in the range of services provided by the profession (Pharmaceutical Group of the European Union, 2019).

Pharmacists now increasingly take on a more patient-focused role and work as part of a multidisciplinary team. Pharmacists are seen as key professionals to assess and treat patients and assist with medication management, in particular for older people and those with chronic conditions and complex polypharmacy. According to the European Pharmacists Forum, pharmacist services now include work in five key areas (European Pharmacists Forum, 2015): (i) medicine adherence, (ii) administering vaccines in pharmacies, (iii) pharmacist-provided screenings, (iv) supporting patients and the public in self-care, (v) disease prevention and support in individual behaviour change (European Pharmacists Forum, 2015).

In sum, the scope of practice, education and training of health professionals differs markedly across Europe. Many countries have implemented or started implementing reforms. This inevitably influences not only the roles and responsibilities that individual professions can undertake, but methods of working within the various ambulatory and primary care settings and the composition of multidisciplinary teams.

Yet, to date, there has been no systematic, cross-country synthesis of the evidence on the implications of skill-mix changes on individual and population health outcomes or health system outcomes, including on the professions themselves, which is the overarching aim of this study.

In the following section, the conceptual framework that guided the study is described.

1.6   Conceptual framework of the skill-mix study

This volume is based on a conceptual health workforce framework that illustrates the interrelated factors that can lead to skill-mix changes (Fig. 1.1). The major two objectives are to analyse the evidence of skill-mix changes on (i) outcomes and (ii) factors that influence the implementation process. The changes to skill-mix are influenced by the status quo of a workforce often triggered by health worker shortages (for example, in rural areas), skill gaps (for example, in providing health promotion or prevention or social care), and other health workforce challenges. Health workforce challenges are often influenced by changing patient needs as well as drivers at the macro level – mutually influencing each other, for example, new financing mechanisms or cost containment strategies.

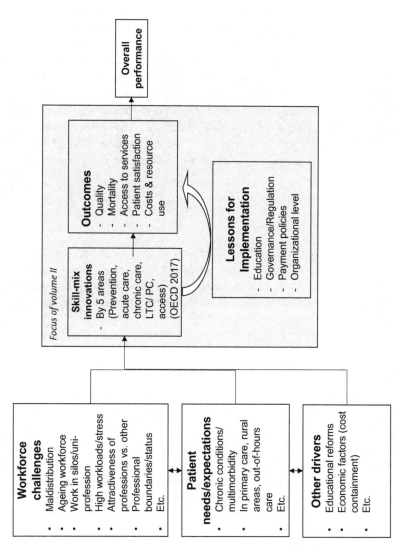

Figure 1.1 Conceptual framework

Abbreviations: LTC: long-term care; PC: palliative care.

Source: Authors.

Specifically, this volume – which complements and builds upon its companion volume, consisting of in-depth country case studies (Wismar, Glinos & Sagan, forthcoming) – performs a systematic synthesis of the evidence on skill-mix changes with a focus on skill-mix innovations and outcomes. It focuses on five core care segments of relevance to any health system: health promotion and prevention, acute care, chronic care and multimorbidity, long-term and palliative care, and access to services in rural and socially deprived areas. Chapters 4 to 8 synthesize the current evidence on the effect of skill-mix innovations according to the five domains. Education, regulation, payment policies and organizational strategies present core elements of the implementation of skill-mix innovations and reforms. Hence, chapters 9 to 11 focus on lessons for implementation, including facilitators and barriers and possible outcomes.

1.7   Methods

The volume is based on a systematic review of the literature ("overview of reviews"), which analyses all relevant systematic reviews on skill-mix and outcomes in a systematic manner, and additional, complementary evidence on implementation and country-specific information on reforms and implementation.

Overview of reviews

An overview of reviews ("umbrella review") was conducted, summarizing all systematic reviews either on skill-mix and outcomes or on implementation. A protocol was developed a priori, which includes further information about the methodology (Maier et al., 2018b). All patients and population groups in primary care and all ambulatory care were covered. Excluded were inpatient settings and emergency care (for example, hospitals, long-term care institutions, hospice if inpatient), except for skill-mix interventions across several sectors including inpatient and ambulatory care (for example, coordination across sectors, liaison roles). The intervention was defined as changes to skill-mix (see definition in Table 1.1) over status quo/compared with standard-of-care. The comparator consisted of status quo (no changes to skill-mix), and/or as standard-of-care (traditional service provision) at the time of the individual study. Systematic reviews covering only low- and middle-income countries were excluded.

Search strategy

The search for eligible reviews was carried out in the following databases: Embase, MEDLINE in Ovid, Cochrane CENTRAL, Web of Science Core Collection, CINAHL, PsycINFO Ovid; in addition, a search in Google Scholar was conducted in January 2018. Search terms were developed together with the core team of researchers and a medical librarian. The full list of search terms is available in the addendum of the protocol (Maier et al., 2018a). For the search, no restrictions were applied regarding the year of publication, whereas in the screening process only articles with publication dates from January 2010 to January 2018 were taken into account. The reasons were twofold: first, for feasibility reasons as the screening showed a high number of relevant systematic reviews published in the time period, and second, the focus was on skill-mix innovations, hence the element of novelty also played a role in the decision to focus on more recent evidence instead of reviews published before 2010. Furthermore, snowballing was performed to identify additional relevant reviews.

Data collection and analysis

The data management was executed with Rayyan QCRI, which is online software specifically designed for screening of articles for systematic reviews. The search in the databases produced a total of 8300 hits. The snowballing produced an additional 323 possibly eligible reviews. After several pilot phases to ensure consistency of the screening phase, the titles and abstracts of the first 100 hits were reviewed by three reviewers according to the inclusion and exclusion criteria. From these search results, interrater agreement for the first 100 hits scored >0.8 using an extended version of Cohen's k coefficient, suitable for three reviewers (Zapf et al., 2016). As a high interrater agreement was reached, the remaining hits were divided among the three reviewers for both the screening of titles and abstracts, and then the screening of full-text versions. Authors were contacted if the full-text version was not available or if additional information was needed. Data analysis was based on a narrative synthesis on the main outcome measures by each of the five care segments [see conceptual framework (OECD, 2017)]. The form used was informed by previous overviews of reviews (Thomson et al., 2010) and covered the following elements: country, study design, methods, participants, intervention, health profession, comparator, outcomes, care settings and context. Meta-analysis was not a priori excluded, but because of the type of review (overview of reviews) and the coverage of a broad topic (skill-mix), the outcome measures were too heterogeneous to perform meta-analyses.

Additional evidence on implementation and country reforms

In addition to the overview of reviews, evidence from other sources was included in this volume, particularly with a focus on the implementation of skill-mix changes and the identification of country reforms. To this end, each author team from each of the chapters performed additional literature searches to identify relevant material: the material included additional studies, reports, policy documents as well as other grey literature (for example, from health-related international organizations such as WHO, OECD, European Commission). In addition, country experiences were summarized with a particular focus on the implementation of reforms and outcomes, as available. To this end, the author teams identified suitable countries to be covered as mini case studies in the chapters, based on the authors' collective expertise in their field. Information on suitable country case studies was also supplemented from the companion volume on skill-mix, which includes in-depth country case studies in 17 countries in Europe and other regions (Wismar, Glinos & Sagan, forthcoming). The material together was synthesized for each chapter focused on country-specific policy reforms and barriers/facilitators to implementation.

1.8   Overview of this volume

The volume is divided into three parts (see Fig. 1.2). The volume begins with a general part arranged in three chapters (Part I) on the rationale, definitions and conceptual framework of the book and the skill-mix situation in Europe (Chapter 1), a synthesis of the evidence on skill-mix changes and relevant outcome measures on patients, health systems and professions (Chapter 2) and lessons for implementation (Chapter 3).

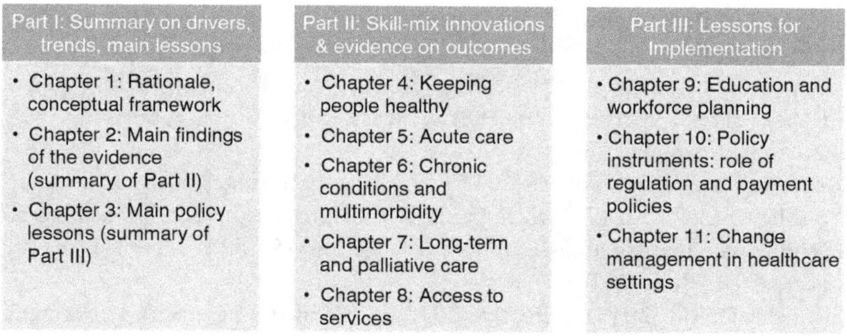

Part I: Summary on drivers, trends, main lessons	Part II: Skill-mix innovations & evidence on outcomes	Part III: Lessons for Implementation
• Chapter 1: Rationale, conceptual framework • Chapter 2: Main findings of the evidence (summary of Part II) • Chapter 3: Main policy lessons (summary of Part III)	• Chapter 4: Keeping people healthy • Chapter 5: Acute care • Chapter 6: Chronic conditions and multimorbidity • Chapter 7: Long-term and palliative care • Chapter 8: Access to services	• Chapter 9: Education and workforce planning • Chapter 10: Policy instruments: role of regulation and payment policies • Chapter 11: Change management in healthcare settings

Figure 1.2 Structure of the skill-mix volume (Volume II)

Source: Authors.

The second part consists of five chapters that present the evidence on outcomes as well as major country developments and trends. These are categorized into five areas of relevance to health systems and primary care, identified by and modified from OECD classifications: Keeping people healthy, acute care, chronic conditions and multimorbidity, long-term and palliative care, and access to services (OECD, 2017). The last part (Part III) consists of three chapters covering the implementation and lessons for uptake in policy and practice, with a focus on education and workforce planning (Chapter 9), the policy level (Chapter 10) and organizational change (Chapter 11).

References

Buchan J, Dal Poz MR (2002). Skill mix in the health care workforce: reviewing the evidence. Bull World Health Organ, 80:575–580.

Campbell J, Dussault G, Buchan J et al. (2013). A universal truth: no health without a workforce. Forum Report, Third Global Forum on Human Resources for Health. Recife, Brazil. Geneva: Global Health Workforce Alliance and World Health Organization.

Cometto G, Boerma T, Campbell J et al. (2013). The Third Global Forum: framing the health workforce agenda for universal health coverage. Lancet Glob Health, 1:e324–e325.

Dubois C-A, Singh D (2009). From staff-mix to skill-mix and beyond: towards a systemic approach to health workforce management. Hum Resour Health, 7:87.

European Academy of Teachers in General Practice/Family Medicine (EURACT) (2020). Dynamic Interactive Database of Specialist Training

in General Practice/Family Medicine [Online]. (https://euract.woncaeurope
.org/specialist-training-database, accessed 13 July 2020).

European Commission (2019). Task Shifting and Health System Design.
Report of the Expert Panel on effective ways of investing in Health (EXPH).
Brussels: European Union.

European Pharmacists Forum (2015). The role of pharmacy in supporting the
public's health. An EPF white paper and call to action. [Online]. (https://
ec.europa.eu/eip/ageing/sites/eipaha/files/library/54f835f311f93_EPF.pdf,
accessed 12 June 2020).

European Union (2013). Directive 2013/55/EU of the European Parliament
and of the Council amending Directive 2005/36/EC on the recognition
of professional qualifications and Regulation (EU) No 1024/2012 on
administrative cooperation through the Internal Market Information System
('the IMI Regulation'). Text with EEA relevance. Official Journal of the
European Union, L 354/132.

Freund T, Everett C, Griffiths P et al. (2015). Skill mix, roles and remuneration
in the primary care workforce: Who are the healthcare professionals in the
primary care teams across the world? Int J Nurs Stud, 52:727–743.

Friedman A, Hahn KA, Etz R et al. (2014). A typology of primary care
workforce innovations in the United States since 2000. Med Care, 52:101–
111.

Global Burden of Disease 2017 SDG COLLABORATORS (2018). Measuring
progress from 1990 to 2017 and projecting attainment to 2030 of the health-
related Sustainable Development Goals for 195 countries and territories: a
systematic analysis for the Global Burden of Disease Study 2017. Lancet,
392:2091–2138.

Greenhalgh T, Robert G, Macfarlane F et al. (2004). Diffusion of innovations
in service organizations: systematic review and recommendations. Milbank
Q, 82:581–629.

Groenewegen P, Heinemann S, Greß S et al. (2015). Primary care practice
composition in 34 countries. Health Policy, 119:1576–1583.

Hooker RS, Cawley JF, Asprey DP (2010). Physician Assistant:Policy and
Practice, 3rd edn. Philadelphia, PA, F. A. Davis Company.

International Council of Nurses (ICN) (2019). Definition and characteristics
of the role [internet]. (https://international.aanp.org/Practice/APNRoles,
accessed 12 May 2020).

International Labour Organisation (ILO) (2010a). International Standard
Classification of Occupations (ISCO). ISCO-08 [Online]. Geneva, ILO.
(http://www.ilo.org/public/english/bureau/stat/isco/, accessed 6 December
2019).

International Labour Organisation (ILO) (2010b). International Standard
Classification of Occupations (ISCO). ISCO-08. Part III. Definitions of

major groups, sub-major groups, minor groups and unit groups [Online]. Geneva, ILO. (http://www.ilo.org/public/english/bureau/stat/isco/docs/ groupdefn08.pdf, accessed 12 June 2020).

Kringos DS, Boerma WGW, Hutchinson A et al. (2015a). Building primary care in a changing Europe. Geneva, World Health Organization 2015 (acting as the host organization for, and secretariat of, the European Observatory on Health Systems and Policies).

Kringos DS, Boerma WGW, Hutchinson A et al. (2015b). Building primary care in a changing Europe. Case studies. Geneva, World Health Organization 2015 (acting as the host organization for, and secretariat of, the European Observatory on Health Systems and Policies).

Kuhlmann E, Groenewegen PP, Bond C et al. (2018). Primary care workforce development in Europe: an overview of health system responses and stakeholder views. Health Policy, 122:1055–1062.

Lahtinen P, Leino-Kilpi H, Salminen L (2014). Nursing education in the European higher education area - variations in implementation. Nurse Educ Today, 34:1040–1047.

Laurant M, Reeves D, Hermens R et al. (2005). Substitution of doctors by nurses in primary care. Cochrane Database of Systematic Reviews, 2:CD001271.

Maier CB (2015). The role of governance in implementing task-shifting from physicians to nurses in advanced roles in Europe, U.S., Canada, New Zealand and Australia. Health Policy, 119:1627–1635.

Maier CB (2019). Nurse prescribing of medicines in 13 European countries. Hum Resour Health, 17:95.

Maier CB, Aiken LH (2016). Task shifting from physicians to nurses in primary care in 39 countries: a cross-country comparative study. Eur J Public Health, 26:927–934.

Maier CB, Barnes H, Aiken LH et al. (2016). Descriptive, cross-country analysis of the nurse practitioner workforce in six countries: size, growth, physician substitution potential. BMJ Open, 6:e011901.

Maier CB, Aiken LH, Busse R (2017). Nurses in advanced roles: policy levers to implementation. OECD Health Working Paper. Paris, OECD.

Maier CB, Koppen J, Busse R (2018). Task shifting between physicians and nurses in acute care hospitals: cross-sectional study in nine countries. Hum Resour Health, 16:24.

Maier CB, Kroezen M, Hartl K et al. (2018a). Overview of systematic reviews: outcomes of health workforce skill-mix changes in primary and ambulatory care. Search strategy and terms. Supplement. *PROSPERO* [Online], CRD42018090272. (https://www.crd.york .ac.uk/PROSPEROFILES/90272_STRATEGY_20180315.pdf, accessed 12 June 2020).

Maier CB, Kroezen M, Hartl K et al. (2018b). Overview of systematic reviews: outcomes of health workforce skill-mix changes in primary and ambulatory care. PROSPERO, CRD42018090272. (https://www.crd.york.ac.uk/PROSPEROFILES/90272_STRATEGY_20180315.pdf, accessed 12 June 2020).

Martínez-González NA, Djalali S, Tandjung R et al. (2014a). Substitution of physicians by nurses in primary care: a systematic review and meta-analysis. BMC Health Serv Res, 14:214.

Martínez-González NA, Tandjung R, Djalali S et al. (2014b). Effects of physician-nurse substitution on clinical parameters: a systematic review and meta-analysis. PLoS One, 9:e89181.

Martínez-González NA, Rosemann T, Djalali S et al. (2015a). Task-shifting from physicians to nurses in primary care and its impact on resource utilization: a systematic review and meta-analysis of randomized controlled trials. Med Care Res Rev, 72:395–418.

Martínez-González NA, Tandjung R, Djalali S et al. (2015b). The impact of physician-nurse task shifting in primary care on the course of disease: a systematic review. Hum Resour Health, 13:55.

Middleton H, Howard D, Wright E (2019). Clinical pharmacists in general practice education. Pathway handbook. Manchester, Centre for Pharmacy Postgraduate Education.

Morilla-Herrera JC, Garcia-Mayor S, Martin-Santos FJ et al. (2016). A systematic review of the effectiveness and roles of advanced practice nursing in older people. Int J Nurs Stud, 53:290–307.

OECD (2016). Health Workforce Policies in OECD Countries: Right Jobs, Right Skills, Right Places. OECD Health Policy Studies. Paris, Organisation for Economic Co-operation and Development (OECD).

OECD (2017). *Data for Measuring Health Care Quality and Outcomes* [Online]. OECD. (http://www.oecd.org/els/health-systems/health-care-quality-indicators.htm, accessed 12 June 2020).

Pharmaceutical Group of The European Union (2019). Pharmacy 2030: A Vision for Community Pharmacy in Europe. Position Paper. 2019. (https://www.pgeu.eu/wp-content/uploads/2019/04/Pharmacy-2030_-A-Vision-for-Community-Pharmacy-in-Europe.pdf, accessed 12 June 2020).

Praxmarer-Fernandes S, Maier CB, Oikarainen A et al. (2017). Levels of education offered in nursing and midwifery education in the WHO European region: multicountry baseline assessment. Public Health Panorama, 3:419–430.

SEPEN (2019), Support for the health workforce planning and forecasting expert network (SEPEN) [Online]. (http://healthworkforce.eu/, accessed 8 December 2019).

Sibbald B, Shen J, McBride A (2004). Changing the skill-mix of the health care workforce. J Health Serv Res Policy, 9:28–38.

Swan M, Ferguson S, Chang A et al. (2015). Quality of primary care by advanced practice nurses: a systematic review. Int J Qual Health Care, 27:396–404.

Thomson D, Russell K, Becker L et al. (2010). The evolution of a new publication type: Steps and challenges of producing overviews of reviews. Research Synthesis Methods, 1:198–211.

Tsiachristas A, Wallenburg I, Bond CM et al. (2015). Costs and effects of new professional roles: Evidence from a literature review. Health Policy, 119:1176–1187.

United Nations (2016). Secretary-General Appoints Commission on Health Employment and Economic Growth [Online]. New York: United Nations. (http://www.un.org/press/en/2016/sga1639.doc.htm, accessed 12 June 2020).

WHO Regional Office for Europe (2020). Strengthening the health system response to COVID-19: Maintaining the delivery of essential health care services while mobilizing the health workforce for the COVID-19 response. Technical working guidance #1. Copenhagen, WHO Regional Office for Europe on behalf of the European Observatory on Health Systems and Policies.

WHO/UNICEF (2018). Declaration of Astana. Global Conference on Primary Health Care From Alma-Ata towards universal health coverage and the Sustainable Development Goals Astana, Kazakhstan, 25 and 26 October 2018. (https://www.who.int/docs/default-source/primary-health/declaration/gcphc-declaration.pdf).

Wismar M, Glinos I, Sagan A (forthcoming). Skill-mix innovation in primary and chronic care. Mobilizing patients, peers, professionals. Copenhagen, WHO Regional Office for Europe on behalf of the European Observatory on Health Systems and Policies.

World Federation of Occupational Therapists (2012). About Occupational Therapy [Online]. (https://www.wfot.org/about/about-occupational-therapy; accessed 13 July 2020).

World Health Organization (2006). The world health report 2006: working together for health. Geneva, World Health Organization.

World Health Organization (2007). Task shifting to tackle health worker shortages. WHO/HSS/2007, 03, 1-12. Geneva, World Health Organization.

World Health Organization (2008). Task shifting: rational redistribution of tasks among health workforce teams: global recommendations and guidelines. Geneva, World Health Organization.

World Health Organization (2013). A universal truth: no health without a workforce. Third Global Forum on Human Resources for Health Report. Geneva, Global Health Workforce Alliance and World Health Organization.

World Health Organization (2016). Global strategy on human resources for health: Workforce 2030. (http://apps.who.int/iris/bitstream/10665/250368/1/9789241511131-eng.pdf?ua=1, accessed 12 June 2020).

World Health Organization (2018). Five-year action plan for health employment and inclusive economic growth (2017–2021). Geneva, World Health Organization.

Zapf A, Castell S, Morawietz L et al. (2016). Measuring inter-rater reliability for nominal data - which coefficients and confidence intervals are appropriate? BMC Med Res Methodol 16:93.

Appendix *Overview of international definitions of selected health professions working in primary and ambulatory care*

Health professions	Definitions	Common roles and tasks	Included professions
Physician	"(...) study, diagnose, treat and prevent illness, disease, injury and other physical and mental impairments in humans through the application of the principles and procedures of modern medicine." (ILO: ISCO 221)	• Conduct physical examinations • Determine patients' health status • Order and analyse diagnostic tests • Prescribe and administer curative treatments and preventive measures • Perform surgery and clinical procedures • Plan and manage referral plans (modified from: ILO: ISCO 221))	Specialist and generalist physicians

(cont.)

Health professions	Definitions	Common roles and tasks	Included professions
Generalist medical practitioner	" (…) Generalist medical practitioners diagnose, treat and prevent illness, disease, injury, and other physical and mental impairments in humans through application of the principles and procedures of modern medicine. They do not limit their practice to certain disease categories or methods of treatment, and may assume responsibility for the provision of continuing and comprehensive medical care to, and the maintenance of general health of, individuals, families and communities…" (ILO: ISCO 2211)	• Conduct clinical examinations of patients to assess, diagnose and monitor a patient's condition • Order, carry out and interpret tests within the surgery to assist with diagnosis • Provide continuing medical care for patients including prescribing, administering, counselling on and monitoring curative treatments and preventive measures (modified from: ILO: ISCO 221)	• District medical doctor • Family medical practitioner/ General practitioner • Medical doctor/ Officer (general)
Dentist	"(…) diagnose, treat and prevent diseases, injuries and abnormalities of the teeth, mouth, jaws and associated tissues by applying the principles and procedures of modern dentistry." (ILO: ISCO 2261)	• Diagnose diseases, injuries, irregularities and malformations of teeth and associated structures in the mouth and jaw • Provide restorative oral care such as implants, crowns and orthodontics, and repair damaged teeth • Provide surgical treatments • Design, make, and fit prosthodontic appliances or write fabrication instructions or prescriptions for them	• Dental practitioner • Dental surgeon • Endodontist • Oral and maxillofacial surgeon

Term	Definition	Tasks	Examples
		• Diagnose general diseases having oral manifestations • Provide preventive oral health care (adapted from: ILO: ISCO 2261)	• Nurse anaesthetist • Nurse practitioner • Public health nurse • Specialist nurse • Clinical nurse
Nurse practitioner/ advanced practice nurse	A Nurse practitioner/advanced practice nurse "is a registered nurse who has acquired the expert knowledge base, complex decision-making skills and clinical competencies for expanded practice, the characteristics of which are shaped by the context and/or country in which s/he is credentialed to practice." (ICN, 2019)	• Integrate research, education, practice and management • Case management and take on own cases • Assess and diagnose health status • Carry out advanced clinical competencies • Consult other health providers • Plan, implement and evaluate care programmes • Act as the first point of contact for patients and families (modified from: Kringos et al., 2015a, b)	
Nursing professionals	"(...) provide treatment, support and care services for people who are in need of nursing care due to the effects of ageing, injury, illness or other physical or mental impairment, or potential risks to health." (ILO: ISCO 2221)	• Plan and provide personal care, treatments and therapies • Develop and implement care plans for the biological, social and psychological treatment of patients • Clean wounds, apply surgical dressings and bandages • Monitor and alleviate pain and discomfort of patients • Answer questions from patients or families and provide information about prevention of ill-health, treatment and care (modified from: ILO: ISCO 2221)	• Registered nurse • Specialist nurse • Clinical nurse consultant • District nurse

Health professions	Definitions	Common roles and tasks	Included professions
Midwife	"(…) plan, manage, provide and evaluate midwifery care services before, during and after pregnancy and childbirth. They provide delivery care for reducing health risks to women and newborn children, working autonomously or in teams with other health care providers." (ILO: ISCO 2222)	• Plan, provide and evaluate care and support services for women and babies before, during and after pregnancy • Assess progress during pregnancy and monitor the health status of neonates, manage complications and recognize required referral to specialized doctors • Monitor and alleviate pain experienced by women • Provide advice and conduct community education (modified from: ILO: ISCO 2222)	• Professional midwife
Nursing associate professional	"(…) provide nursing and personal care for people who are physically or mentally ill, disabled or infirm, in support of implementation of health care, treatment and referral plans usually established by medical, nursing and other health professionals They usually work under the direction of nursing or other health professionals and perform tasks of more limited range and complexity than nursing professionals." (ILO: ISCO 3221)	• Assess, plan and provide personal and nursing care, treatment and advice to the sick, injured, disabled within a defined scope-of-practice • Administer medications and other treatments and monitoring responses • Clean wounds and apply surgical dressings under the guidance of professional nurses or medical doctors • Monitor and observe patients' condition and maintain a record of observations and treatment • Assist in planning and managing the care of individual patients • Assist in giving first-aid treatment in emergencies (modified from: ILO: ISCO 3221)	• Associate professional nurse • Assistant nurse • Enrolled nurse • Practical nurse

Health care assistant	"(...) provide direct personal care and assistance with activities of daily living to patients and residents in a variety of care settings such as hospitals, clinics and residential nursing care facilities. They generally work in implementation of established care plans and practices, and under the direct supervision of medical, nursing or other health professionals or associate professionals." (ILO: ISCO 5321)	• Assisting patients with personal and therapeutic care needs such as personal hygiene, feeding, dressing, physical mobility and exercise, communication, taking oral medication and changing dressings • Maintaining patient's environmental hygiene standards • Observing patients' condition, responses and behaviour and reporting changes to a professional	• Health care assistant (clinic or hospital) • Nursing aide (clinic or hospital) • Psychiatric aide
Physician assistant	"(...) health care professionals trained within the medical model and licensed to practice medicine under the supervision of a licensed doctor" (Hooker, 2010)	• Conduct physical examination, diagnose and treat illnesses • Order and interpret medical tests • Write prescriptions • See patients with undifferentiated diagnoses or long-term chronic conditions • Provide preventive health care services • Formulate differential diagnoses and management plans (modified from (Hooker, Cawley & Asprey, 2010))	• Physician assistant • Physician associate • Anaesthesia Associates

(cont.)

Health professions	Definitions	Common roles and tasks	Included professions
Medical assistant	"(…) Medical assistants perform basic clinical and administrative tasks to support patient care under the direct supervision of a medical practitioner or other health professional. They perform routine tasks and procedures such as measuring patients' vital signs, administering medications and injections, recording information in medical records keeping systems, preparing and handling medical instruments and supplies, and collecting and preparing specimens of bodily fluids and tissues for laboratory testing." (ILO: ISCO 3256)	• Interview patients to obtain medical information and measure their vital signs, weight and height • Show patients to examination rooms and prepare them for examination • Collect blood, tissue or other laboratory specimens, logging the specimens, and prepare them for testing • Explain treatment procedures, medications, diets and physicians' instructions to patients • Prepare treatment rooms for patient examinations, keep the rooms neat and clean, sterilize instruments and dispose of contaminated supplies • Arrange and schedule appointments and prepare documentation required for billing, reporting and insurance (adapted from: ILO: ISCO 3256)	• Clinical assistant • Medical assistant • Ophthalmic assistant
Pharmacist	"(…) store, preserve, compound and dispense medicinal products and counsel on the proper use and adverse effects of drugs and medicines following prescriptions issued by medical doctors and other health professionals." (ILO: ISCO 2262)	• Receive prescriptions for medicinal products from health professionals, check patients' medicine histories, and ensure proper dosage administration and drug compatibility before dispensing • Provide information and advice to prescribers and clients regarding drug interactions or incompatibility, side-effects, dosage and proper medication storage (adapted from: ILO: ISCO 2262)	• Dispensing chemist • Hospital pharmacist • Industrial pharmacist • Retail pharmacist

| Psychologist | "(…) research into and study the mental processes and behaviour of human beings as individuals or in groups, and apply this knowledge to promote personal, social, educational or occupational adjustment and development." (ILO: ISCO 2634) | • Plan and carry out tests to measure mental, physical and other characteristics such as intelligence, abilities, aptitudes, potentialities, etc.
• Analyse the effect of heredity, social, occupational and other factors on individual thought and behaviour
• Conduct counselling or therapeutic interviews with individuals and groups, and provide follow-up services
• Maintain required contacts, such as those with family members, educational authorities or employers, and recommend possible solutions to, and treatment of, problems
• Study psychological factors in the diagnosis, treatment and prevention of mental illnesses and emotional or personality disorders, and conferring with related professionals (adapted from: ILO: ISCO 2634) | • Clinical psychologist
• Educational psychologist
• Organizational psychologist
• Psychotherapist
• Sports psychologist |

(cont.)

Health professions	Definitions	Common roles and tasks	Included professions
Social worker and counselling professional	"(...) provide advice and guidance to individuals, families, groups, communities and organizations in response to social and personal difficulties. They assist clients to develop skills and access resources and support services needed to respond to issues arising from unemployment, poverty, disability, addiction, criminal and delinquent behaviour, marital and other problems." (ILO: ISCO 2635)	• Interview clients individually, in families, or in groups, to assess their situation and problems and determine the types of services required • Maintain contact with other social service agencies, educational institutions and health care providers involved with clients • Compile case records or reports for courts and other legal proceedings • Provide counselling, therapy and mediation services and facilitate group sessions to assist clients to deal with and resolve their social and personal problems • Plan and implement programmes of assistance including crisis intervention and referral to agencies that provide financial assistance, legal aid, housing, medical treatment and other services	• Addictions counsellor • Bereavement counsellor • Child and youth counsellor • Family counsellor • Marriage counsellor • Parole officer • Probation officer • Social worker • Women's welfare organizer

Dental assistants and therapists	"(…) provide basic dental care services for the prevention and treatment of diseases and disorders of the teeth and mouth, as per care plans and procedures established by a dentist or other oral health professional. They examine patients' mouths, teeth and related structures to assess oral health status; provide advice on dental hygiene; perform basic or routine clinical dental procedures; and assisting dentists during complex dental procedures." (ILO: ISCO 3251)	• Provide dental health education about tooth care and diet • Remove plaque and calculus by scaling and polishing teeth • Take impressions and/or dental radiographs of teeth • Apply prophylactic/antibacterial materials, fissure sealants and topical fluorides to help prevent tooth decay • Carry out screening and monitoring procedures • Treat and help to prevent gum disease	• Dental assistant, • Dental hygienist • Dental therapist
Paramedical practitioner	"(…) provide advisory, diagnostic, curative and preventive medical services more limited in scope and complexity than those carried out by medical doctors. They work autonomously or with limited supervision of medical doctors, and perform clinical, therapeutic and surgical procedures for treating and preventing diseases, injuries, and other physical or mental impairments common to specific communities." Source: (ILO: ISCO 2240)	• Conduct medical examinations and question patients to determine the nature of disorders or illnesses • Prescribe and administer treatments, medications and other remedial measures of a more restricted scope and complexity than medical doctors • Perform therapeutic procedures, such as injections, immunizations, suturing and wound care, and infection management • Refer complex or unusual cases to medical doctors, hospitals or other health workers if necessary. (adapted from: ILO: ISCO 2240)	• Clinical officer • Primary care paramedic • Advanced care paramedic • Surgical technician • Feldsher

(cont.)

Health professions	Definitions	Common roles and tasks	Included professions
Physiotherapist	"(…) assess, plan and implement rehabilitative programmes that improve or restore human motor functions, maximize movement ability, relieve pain syndromes, and treat or prevent physical challenges associated with injuries, diseases and other impairments." (ILO: ISCO 2264)	• Administer muscle, nerve, joint functional ability and other tests to identify physical problems of patients • Develop, implement and monitor programmes or treatments using the therapeutic properties of exercise, heat, cold, massage, manipulation, hydrotherapy, electrotherapy, ultraviolet or infrared light and ultrasound • Instruct patients or families in procedures to continue outside clinical setting (adapted from: ILO: ISCO 2264)	• Geriatric physical therapist • Manipulative therapist • Orthopaedic physical therapist • Paediatric physical therapist • Physical therapist • Physiotherapist

Dietician and nutritionist	"(...) dieticians and nutritionists assess, plan and implement programmes to enhance the impact of food and nutrition on human health. They may conduct research, assessments and education to improve nutritional levels among individuals and communities." (ILO: ISCO 2265)	• Instruct individuals, families and communities on nutrition, the planning of diets and preparation of food • Plan diets and menus, supervise the preparation and serving of meals, and monitor food intake and quality to provide nutritional care in settings • Compile and assess data relating to health and nutritional status of individuals, groups and communities • Develop and evaluate food and nutrition products to meet nutritional requirements • Conduct research on nutrition and disseminate findings (adapted from: ILO: ISCO 2265)	• Clinical dietician • Food service dietician • Public health nutritionist • Sports nutritionist
Audiologist and speech therapist	"(...) evaluate, manage and treat physical disorders affecting human hearing, speech communication and swallowing. They prescribe corrective devices or rehabilitative therapies for hearing loss, speech disorders, and related sensory and neural problems. They plan hearing screening programs and provide counselling on hearing safety and communication performance." (ILO: ISCO 2266)	• Evaluate hearing and speech/language disorders to determine diagnoses and courses of treatment, required assistive devices and referrals • Administer hearing or speech/language evaluations, tests or examinations using specialized instruments and electronic equipment • Interpret audiometric test results alongside other medical, social and behavioural diagnostic data • Counsel and guide hearing and/or language-handicapped individuals, their families, teachers and employers (adapted from: ILO: ISCO 2266)	• Audiologist • Language therapist • Speech therapist, • Speech pathologist

(cont.)

Health professions	Definitions	Common roles and tasks	Included professions
Occupational therapist	"(...) client-centred health profession concerned with promoting health and well-being through occupation. The primary goal of occupational therapy is to enable people to participate in the activities of everyday life. Occupational therapists achieve this outcome by working with people and communities to enhance their ability to engage in the occupations they want to, need to, or are expected to do, or by modifying the occupation or the environment to better support their occupational engagement (World Federation of Occupational Therapists, 2012).	• Assess patients or clients to determine the nature of the disorder, illness or problem • Develop and implement treatment plans and evaluate and document patients' progress • Assess functional limitations of people resulting from illnesses and disabilities • Assess clients' functional potential in their home, leisure, work and school environments, and recommend environmental adaptations to maximize their performance	• Occupational therapists

Sources: Provided in the table.

2 Skill-mix changes: what evidence on patient outcomes and health systems?

CLAUDIA B. MAIER, HANNAH BUDDE, LAURA PFIRTER, MARIEKE KROEZEN

2.1 Overview of the evidence: skill-mix interventions, professions, care sectors

Worldwide, countries are seeking strategies to strengthen their health workforce to ensure health systems are sustainable and resilient and to reach universal health coverage (World Health Organization, 2016). In Europe, a 2019 expert opinion focused on task shifting, which is one – among several – examples of skill-mix innovations (European Commission, 2019). However, to date, a systematic analysis of skill-mix innovations and their effects on outcomes has been missing. Skill-mix changes have been suggested to be of high relevance to respond to changing patient needs (for example, for patients with chronic conditions and multimorbidity), unequal access to services (for example, for vulnerable groups), skill gaps (for example, in long-term and palliative care) and changes among the health workforce (shortages and maldistribution) (see Chapter 1).

This chapter will synthesize the evidence on skill-mix changes and outcomes for individual patients and populations, health systems and health professionals. Hence, for the purpose of this book, an overview of reviews was conducted on the outcomes of skill-mix changes, and mini case studies were written on country-specific and setting-specific developments. The methods of the overview of reviews are described in Box 2.1. More details on the methodology as well as the mini case studies are provided in Chapter 1.

The overview of reviews resulted in a total of 187 systematic reviews, of which 171 focused on skill-mix in (at least) one of the five care segments and included at least one outcome measure on patients or populations, health systems or effects on health professionals (Table 2.1). A total of 29 reviews analysed skill-mix and factors related to implementation and

Box 2.1 Methods of the overview of reviews

A short summary of the methods is provided below, for more details please refer to Chapter 1 and the protocol (PROSPERO Nr. CRD42018090272) (Maier et al., 2018).

Search strategy and screening: Systematic search conducted in six databases (Embase, MEDLINE, Cochrane CENTRAL, Web of Science, CINAHL, PsycINFO) and Google Scholar, plus snowballing. The search terms covered skill-mix using a broad definition, including all professions, lay workers and informal carers/caregivers. The search strategy was developed in cooperation with a librarian. Skill-mix was defined as changing roles, tasks and/or teamwork in primary care, ambulatory care or at the interface between hospital-ambulatory care settings. Systematic reviews on implementation of skill-mix, barriers and facilitators were also included. The protocol provides a list of all search terms (Maier et al., 2018). Titles and abstracts as well as full-text versions were screened by a team of researchers, after in-depth piloting and high levels of interrater reliability scores.

Inclusion criteria: Systematic reviews with narrative synthesis and/or meta analyses, any skill-mix intervention with patients-, health system or profession-specific outcomes or implementation, all populations or patient groups, all health professions, lay workers and informal caregivers working in primary care (including ambulatory care settings) or at the hospital–ambulatory care interface.

Exclusion criteria: Systematic reviews with no focus on skill-mix, study designs other than systematic reviews, hospital settings (inpatient), nursing homes, emergency care, non-English languages, reviews published before 2010 (because of the high number of reviews identified and the focus on skill-mix innovations, defined as a novelty).

Analysis: The analysis included the extraction of the findings and a narrative synthesis of the evidence by population group(s) and diseases, following five segments of care (modified from OECD, 2017): health promotion and prevention, acute care, chronic conditions, long-term care and palliative care; and access to health services (for vulnerable groups and in underserved areas). The findings were extracted by a core group of researchers from TU Berlin and Erasmus University into standardized excel files, after pilots and double checks by one researcher to ensure consistency.

Table 2.1 *Skill-mix and outcomes: total number and characteristics of systematic reviews included*

Areas covered	Reviews (individual studies[a] covered)	Meta-analyses	Cochrane reviews
Health promotion and prevention (Chapter 4)	35 (848 studies)	13	2
Acute care (transitional care, hospital-at-home, minor acute conditions) (Chapter 5)	28 (617 studies)	13	4
Chronic conditions and multimorbidity (Chapter 6)	78 (1560 studies)	43	10
Long-term and palliative care (Chapter 7)	17 (286 studies)	5	3
Access to health services (for vulnerable groups and in underserved areas) (Chapter 8)	13 (418 studies)	1	2

Note: [a] Total number of individual studies includes double or multiple counting if listed in more than one systematic review.

Sources: Chapters 4–8.

are summarized in the chapter on implementation and policy lessons (Chapter 3). It should be noted that 13 reviews covered skill-mix and outcomes as well as implementation, and so are covered in both this chapter and Chapter 3.

The total number of identified reviews is high, but the numbers vary between the different areas in primary care and for the patient groups covered. Especially rich is the evidence on skill-mix changes for patients with chronic conditions, which includes a total of 78 systematic reviews and is summarized in Chapter 6. Moreover, 43 reviews performed meta-analyses. Two areas that were also well researched are skill-mix changes to improve health promotion and prevention, covered by 35 reviews (Chapter 4), and for patients with acute conditions, covered by 28 reviews (Chapter 5). Two fields were less well covered: long-term and palliative care was covered by 17 reviews (Chapter 7) and skill-mix interventions to improve access to services was addressed by 13 reviews, of which only one focused specifically on rural areas (Chapter 8).

Overall, the review methods including data analysis varied. The majority of the reviews performed narrative analyses of the findings.

For skill-mix changes in chronic care, however, more than half of the reviews (43 of 78 reviews) performed meta-analyses. A total of 21 Cochrane reviews summarized skill-mix interventions and health outcomes across the five areas covered in this volume. Cochrane reviews use a highly standardized, rigorous methodology and have become the reference standard for systematic reviews.

Main topics and themes of the skill-mix interventions

A wide range of different topics and areas were covered not only across, but also within the main five care segments (Table 2.2). Within health promotion and prevention, the largest number of reviews (19 reviews) evaluated skill-mix changes related to secondary prevention for patients with risk factors, followed by 10 reviews on skill-mix aimed at improving the health of healthy populations or population groups (health promotion) and seven reviews on skill-mix and screenings (for example, patient navigator interventions to improve cancer screening uptake and nurse-delivered colorectal and skin cancer screenings) (Chapter 4).

Within acute care (which covers acute conditions, acute episodes of chronic conditions such as stroke and acute myocardial infarction, and minor illnesses), most evidence was available on skill-mix changes aimed at care transitioning between the hospital and ambulatory care interface (20 systematic reviews), followed by four reviews on hospital-at-home and four on minor acute illnesses in ambulatory care settings (Chapter 5).

Skill-mix and chronic conditions was the most researched, particularly for patients with a single chronic condition with the aim to improve the quality of care, self-management and monitoring. The interventions were primarily performed by nurses and pharmacists (20 and 18 systematic reviews, respectively). A total of 21 reviews analysed the effects of multiprofessional teams. Overall, nine reviews specifically analysed skill-mix interventions for patients with multimorbidity (Chapter 6).

On long-term care, of the 11 reviews identified, the majority covered case management for patients with dementia (eight reviews). Palliative care was less often researched, four reviews analysed skill-mix interventions directed at improving outcomes for patients with palliative care needs, whereas two focused on their caregivers (Chapter 7). Finally, 12 reviews were aimed at improving access to services for vulnerable population groups. Yet, perhaps counterintuitively, only one systematic review focused on skill-mix and access in underserved regions (Chapter 8).

Table 2.2 *Skill-mix changes in primary and chronic care: professions involved and topics of skill-mix interventions*

Areas covered	Topics of skill-mix interventions[a]	Professions involved in skill-mix changes
Health promotion and prevention	• 10 systematic reviews on skill-mix for health promotion • 19 on secondary disease prevention: 7 on skill-mix for people with CVD risk factors, 6 on nutrition-related risk factors and 6 on multiple risk factors • 7 systematic reviews on skill-mix changes and screenings[b]	• GPs/physicians, NPs, nurses, pharmacists, dieticians, midwives, physiotherapists, health counsellors, exercise professionals, health promotion specialists or trained facilitators, case-managers, mental health professionals, social workers, home visitors or lay health workers (paid or voluntary) • Working alone or in a team
Acute care (transitional care, hospital-at-home, minor conditions)	• 20 systematic reviews related to skill-mix and transitional care • 4 systematic reviews on skill-mix and relocation of care (e.g. hospital-at-home) • 4 systematic reviews on skill-mix and minor acute illnesses	• GPs/physicians, NPs, nurses, pharmacists, dieticians, physiotherapists, care coordinators, case managers, care assistants, home aide, CHWs, social workers, support workers, caregivers, volunteers, occupational or speech therapists • Working alone or in a team
Chronic conditions and multimorbidity	• 20 systematic reviews on nurse-managed care for single chronic conditions • 18 systematic reviews on pharmacist-managed interventions for single chronic conditions[c] • 13 systematic reviews delivered by other professionals[d] • 21 systematic reviews on multiprofessional teams • 9 systematic reviews on multimorbidity	• GPs/physicians, NPs, nurses, pharmacists, mental health professionals, patient navigators, transition coordinators, case managers, peers • Working alone or in a team

Table 2.2 (cont.)

Areas covered	Topics of skill-mix interventions[a]	Professions involved in skill-mix changes
Long-term and palliative care	• 11 systematic reviews on long-term care: 10 covered case management in the community (of which 8 focused on dementia) and 1 covered multidisciplinary teams • 6 systematic reviews on palliative care: 4 covered interventions focusing on patients, 2 on family caregivers	• GPs/physicians, NPs, nurses, pharmacists, dieticians, social workers, psychologists, researchers, case managers, physical; speech or occupational therapist, neurologists, support workers • Working alone or in a team.
Access to health services	• 1 systematic review on skill-mix targeting populations living in rural and remote areas • 12 systematic reviews targeting vulnerable and socially deprived populations	• GPs/physicians, NPs, nurses, pharmacists, dieticians, medical assistants, mental health professionals, social workers, CHWs, peer counsellors, home visitors or lay workers. • Working alone or in a team.

Abbreviations: CHW: community health worker; CVD: cardiovascular disease; GP: general practitioner; NP: nurse practitioner.

Notes: [a] Several reviews cover multiple skill-mix areas or several professions and are therefore listed more than once. [b] One review covers health promotion and screening. [c] One review covers pharmacist-delivered, nurse-delivered interventions and multiprofessional teams. [d] One review covers single chronic conditions and multimorbidity.

Sources: Chapters 4–8.

Professions and informal workers involved in skill-mix interventions

The changing roles of many different health professions and lay workers were evaluated in the systematic reviews. Table 2.2 shows the diversity of professions who were affected by skill-mix changes, ranging from physicians / GPs to home visitors and others, often lay workers with no or limited additional training.

However, when looking at the main providers involved in skill-mix changes, two professions stood out: the highest number of individual studies analysed skill-mix changes involving nurses and pharmacists. For instance, for patients with chronic conditions and multimorbidity, 20 reviews analysed nurse-managed care and 18 reviews analysed pharmacist-managed care (often compared with physician-managed care) for patients with chronic conditions (Table 2.2). In addition, some reviews focused on skill-mix changes targeting (primary care) physicians, physiotherapists, dieticians and physician assistants, among others.

The role of community-based workers and other lay health workers (usually with additional training) was evaluated in expanding health promotion and screenings, particularly for vulnerable population groups. Interventions often targeted the patients themselves or their caregivers, and included educational components, coaching and other measures to improve self-management and health literacy skills. This refers to reviews on health promotion (Chapter 4), including lifestyle education, but also in long-term and palliative care including caregiver and patient self-management education interventions (Chapter 7). In addition, skill-mix strategies involving peers and family caregivers were introduced and evaluated for patients with long-term care conditions and at the end-of-life (Chapter 7).

Population groups covered

Patients with chronic conditions were the main target population of skill-mix changes, which is mirrored with the high number and burden of diseases among this population group. In particular, skill-mix changes were frequently introduced and evaluated for patients with cardiovascular diseases, cancer, diabetes and mental health conditions. The population groups covered with regard to health promotion were primarily children, pregnant women, mothers and newborn infants, often with a socially or economically deprived status. Patients with acute care conditions most frequently suffered from stroke, acute myocardial infarction or other acute episodes, usually of chronic conditions. There was comparatively less research evidence on the outcomes of skill-mix interventions for patients specifically with minor acute illnesses, for example, influenza, pharyngitis, small wounds or other minor illnesses. More evidence is needed in these areas, because several countries have introduced skill-mix reforms that also focus on a new division of work, whereby physicians take care of patients with complex conditions and nurses or other professionals provide care for patients with minor conditions.

Interventions aiming at expanding access to health services were mainly targeted to vulnerable population groups, including socially or economically deprived groups. Skill-mix changes aimed at improving long-term and palliative care focused primarily on older people with dementia, Parkinson's disease, as well as patients with (end-stage) cancer and other conditions at the end of life. The majority of the reviews described the population groups, however, few exceptions existed.

Study designs and country coverage

Most systematic reviews included randomized controlled trials (RCTs), controlled before–after studies, and several also covered cross-sectional study designs, which were conducted in several countries across Europe and North America. Generally, a high number of studies were conducted in the USA and Canada and within Europe, mainly in the United Kingdom, the Netherlands, Belgium, Spain and Sweden. The wide country coverage applies to several skill-mix interventions, including advanced roles for nurses or midwives to improve maternal and child health (in 24 countries; Chapter 4), transitional care-management roles delivered by nurses and pharmacists (15 countries; Chapter 5) and skill-mix models for health screenings (Chapter 4), which has been evaluated in many countries worldwide.

Interestingly, in contrast, the role of community health workers or similar community-based workers with some, albeit limited, training was primarily studied in the USA and much less in Europe. The question arises why this group is less represented in Europe. Some countries have trained peer workers to improve access for vulnerable groups, for example in Australia, Canada, the United Kingdom and the USA. However, their roles and contribution were much less frequently evaluated. Community-based interventions to improve access and facilitate communication involving lay and qualified health workers were often limited to the USA and Canada (Chapter 8).

Summary of research evidence available

In sum, the generally high quantity of research evidence – particularly on chronic conditions and health promotion and prevention – comes at a time when the policy attention is high globally to identify effective strategies to ensure a sustainable health workforce as a prerequisite to achieve or maintain universal health coverage. The high number of systematic reviews alone and the additional research evidence identified illustrate the strong research focus and are matched with a high policy interest in this field on how to strengthen the health workforce to improve access and quality of care (United Nations, 2016; World Health Organization, 2018). Yet, there remain evidence gaps or shortcomings for some areas, including on skill-mix innovations to improve access in rural and underserved areas and in the field of palliative care.

2.2 Evidence on outcomes: what skill-mix interventions are promising?

The following section provides an overview of the main themes of the skill-mix interventions and a snapshot of the evidence on outcomes. Although a full synthesis of the evidence is provided in each of Chapters 4–8, this section will highlight those interventions of particular interest and with promising results. For a full account of all interventions, we refer the reader to the respective chapters.

The main skill-mix interventions or models emanating from the literature and country experiences were as follows (Table 2.3):

- first, new, supplementary roles for primary care providers,
- second, the re-allocation of tasks between providers (involving advanced practice for non-physician providers), and
- third, changes to multiprofessional collaboration.

The expansion of new, supplementary roles was implemented particularly to step up health promotion and prevention in primary care and to improve the care for patients with chronic conditions. Task re-allocation was most common in expanding screenings as well as for patients with acute care and chronic conditions. Changes to teamwork and multiprofessional collaboration were commonly introduced for various patient groups and care segments, but most notably for patients with chronic conditions. Moreover, several skill-mix changes were directly aimed at improving the coordination and continuity of care, models included case management roles, patient navigators and transitional care roles. Finally, some skill-mix changes were directly related to new service delivery models aimed at relocating care, for instance hospitals-at-home, requiring new, highly specialized teams.

Skill-mix changes introducing new, supplementary roles

Dedicated prevention role

New, supplementary roles have been introduced in several countries and regions worldwide with the aim of improving access, especially in the field of preventive care and health promotion. Expanding prevention roles of primary care providers has been increasingly recognized, bringing individual health promotion and prevention closer to and integrated into primary care.

Primary care providers are central in providing individual health promotion and prevention activities, this was also demonstrated by the systematic reviews. In these reviews, they took on supplementary roles to promote healthy diets and physical activity or deliver interventions targeting various risk factors. Nurses, pharmacists, dieticians and GPs performed diet-related health advice in school settings including education and counselling to school children and their parents (Bhattarai et al., 2013; Schroeder, Travers & Smaldone, 2016). Moreover, various professions performed counselling, and provided advice and motivational interviewing to increase physical activity in sedentary adults (Orrow et al., 2012), among other interventions. Dedicated prevention roles covered various skill-mix interventions across several countries, but the majority of the findings demonstrated a positive effect on prevention-related outcomes. Outcomes included significantly reduced body mass index scores for adults and children, increased

Table 2.3 *Major themes identified: skill-mix innovations*

Skill-mix changes	Aim(s)	Areas covered	Examples	Chapters in book
1 New, supplementary roles				
Dedicated prevention role in primary care	• Improve access to prevention • Health promotion • Equitable access	• Secondary and tertiary prevention • Screenings • Self-management	• Dietician/dietician-physician • School nurse • Patient navigator • Nurse-led/social worker home visits • Community-based or lay workers	4, 8
Care coordinator role	• Improve coordination • Person-centredness	• Chronic conditions • Acute conditions	• Case managers • Patient navigators • Transitional care coordinator	4–8
Patient and caregiver empowerment role	• Improve health literacy • Self-management • Person-centredness	• Coaching and goal-setting with patients • Shared decision-making	• Coaches • Community-based workers • Nurses	4–8

Table 2.3 (cont.)

Skill-mix changes	Aim(s)	Areas covered	Examples	Chapters in book
2 Re-allocation of tasks (task shifting/relocation of care)				
Advanced practice and other expanded roles	– Expand access – Workforce efficiency	• Screenings • Chronic diseases • Acute care • Community-based care	• Pharmacists- or nurse-led screenings • Immunizations • Nurse-delivered diabetes care, nurse-led transitional care • Nurse prescribing • Pharmacists	4, 5, 6
Skill-mix and relocation of care	– Patient-centredness – Resource efficiency	• Chronic conditions • Acute care	• Highly specialized, mobile teams (hospital-at-home) • Nurse-led clinics	5, 6
3 Changes to multiprofessional teamwork				
Multiprofessional teamwork and collaboration	• Improve coordination and quality of care	• Chronic conditions • Health and social care • Palliative care	• Collaboration across sectors • Transitional care teams including nurses, pharmacists, GPs, social workers	4–8

Abbreviations: GP: general practitioner.

Source: Based on Chapters 4–8.

dietary intakes of healthy food (for example, vegetables and fruits) and physical activity (Chapter 4).

Home visits were common skill-mix interventions implemented to reach out to specific groups, particularly to vulnerable populations. The professions conducting home visits ranged from qualified professions (including nurses, social workers and midwives) to lay or lower-qualified workers (including community health workers and other lay workers). The tasks performed varied considerably within and across the professions covered. Generally, higher qualified professions also performed more specialized tasks – including with a focus on clinical tasks. Lay workers provided generally no or very limited clinical tasks, but instead focused on providing general information and health advice. The home visits were often tailored to the needs of specific target populations and involved multilingual advice, counselling and referrals, and were sometimes combined with transport services or phone calls. In particular, the multicomponent approaches showed positive effects in terms of expanding access to services.

Innovative skill-mix interventions were targeted towards preventing child maltreatment and reducing health disparities and demonstrated significantly improved patient-related outcomes and significantly reduced health care utilization, such as emergency care use or hospital (re-) admissions (Chapter 4 and Chapter 8). Most studies adding supplementary roles to perform outreach and educational activities showed promising effects towards increasing the access to screening services and earlier treatment (Chapter 8). Cost savings were reported for maternity home visits to prevent child maltreatment (Dalziel & Segal, 2012), but were based on estimates and modelling; hence, require more research including costing studies and cost-effectiveness analyses to arrive at a more robust evidence base (Chapter 4).

Care coordinator roles and skills

Many countries have health systems that are fragmented and not well coordinated, particularly for people with chronic conditions and with highly complex care needs. Several skill-mix changes have been introduced establishing new roles to explicitly improve the coordination of care. Two models emerged, either new roles at the interface of hospital and ambulatory care sector, often as a one-off activity; or along the patient pathway as a supporting and coordinating role over a longer period of time. Coordinator roles have been established in many high-income countries, including virtually all European countries; however, the terms used and professions working in these roles vary considerably (care coordinator, case manager, transition coordinator).

New roles focusing on the transition, specifically from hospital to ambulatory care, were mostly referred to as transition coordinators, navigators or various terms related to discharge management. These roles were central for patients with often severe or multiple conditions who were close to discharge and they were aimed at improving the continuity of care from hospital to ambulatory care. Examples are provided in Chapter 5. Skill-mix interventions often comprised multiple components including discharge planning, patient education, medication reconciliations and sometimes home visits. These roles were primarily performed or led by nurses, including advanced practice nurses and other specialized nurses, pharmacists or sometimes social care workers. The new roles actively managed the early transitioning of care to the ambulatory setting. Introducing new roles in transitional care overall showed positive effects on at least one patient-related or health-system-related outcome. However, whereas patient satisfaction, patients' knowledge about the disease and self-management improved, findings on mortality and health-system-related outcomes, such as readmissions and service utilization, showed mixed results (Chapter 5).

To improve the coordination of care and patient centeredness over a longer period of time, new roles in care coordination – in particular case manager roles – were undertaken. These roles were most frequently performed by nurses and/or pharmacists depending on different country and care contexts. Case management roles focused on patients with chronic diseases, with major acute conditions or with long-term care needs, in particular patients with dementia. More detailed information is provided in Chapter 5 (acute care), Chapter 6 (chronic care) and Chapter 7 (long-term and palliative care). For patients with mental health problems, interdisciplinary care coordination showed significant improvements in mental health outcomes (Chapter 6).

Introducing case management in the community setting for long-term care patients and their caregivers showed some improvements, nonetheless, the evidence remains mixed for most outcome parameters (Chapter 7). Patients with dementia showed reduced feelings of isolation and embarrassment of the condition after case management roles were introduced that focused on counselling, coordinating, monitoring, assessing and educating. Yet, evidence on other outcomes such as mortality, depression and functional status remained inconclusive (Backhouse et al., 2017; Goeman, Renehan & Koch, 2016; Khanassov & Vedel, 2016; Khanassov, Vedel & Pluye, 2014; Pimouguet, Lavaud & Dartigues, 2010; Reilly et al., 2015). The reasons for these mixed, and therefore inconclusive results, are unknown and may be influenced by multiple factors: the intervention itself and differences in the intensity of the interventions, the different roles and professions involved. It may also be related to the fact that the severity of the condition (for example, dementia) has less potential for improvements in clinical outcome measures than if compared with case management skill-mix interventions for patients with acute or stable chronic conditions.

Patient navigator roles were widely implemented and researched, encompassing different tasks such as coordinating, discharge planning, educating and follow up. The patient navigator role was evaluated for cancer patients (Chapter 6), for whom the new role originally emerged. Patient navigators were also introduced for patients with acute conditions and to facilitate the access to screenings, especially for vulnerable population groups (Chapter 5 and Chapter 8). Patient navigators were shown to be health professionals with professional education, but they sometimes also involved former patients/peers, community health workers or other lay workers with some training acting as navigators through the system, particularly for vulnerable groups.

Patient navigators were particularly crucial in overcoming language barriers for vulnerable patients with limited language proficiency. Improved uptake of screenings and completion of diagnostics illustrated the positive impact of patient navigation for vulnerable patients (Chapters 4 and 8). Moreover, community health workers acting as patient navigators to improve chronic disease management showed significant positive effects regarding health outcomes for disadvantaged patients (Chapter 8).

Skill-mix to empower patients and caregivers

Empowering patients and their caregivers in the self-management of their conditions has received policy attention over the past decade as a cost-effective strategy to support self-care and person-centred care of people. Several skill-mix interventions have specifically targeted patient self-management and empowerment. Skill-mix interventions result in extended roles and new tasks, for example, providing (tailored) educational activities, motivational interviewing or coaching, consultations and self-management skills trainings. In the systematic reviews, these services were primarily provided by nurses, pharmacists or peers for patients with single chronic conditions. Overall, these interventions fostering patient autonomy in the care process showed positive effects on several health outcomes including on blood pressure and glycated haemoglobin (HbA1c) levels (Chapter 6).

Introducing peer educators was another common skill-mix intervention. Peer educators are "peers", defined as other patients usually with the same condition, often with no health profession-specific background but with extensive knowledge on the disease and having received additional, short trainings to serve as peer educators. The advantage is that they have often had a similar experience as patients in the health system. Peer educators, who have regular contact with patients, have been shown to positively impact health or peer-related outcomes (Chapter 6). For example, a peer support model for diabetes patients, which comprised face-to-face management, peer coaching and phone-based support, showed improvements in blood pressure, body mass index and physical activity, among other positive health-related outcomes (Dale, Williams & Bowyer, 2012).

For vulnerable groups, community health workers, peer counsellors or professionals with various other backgrounds emerged as a common intervention across the systematic reviews resulting in primarily positive outcomes for patients. Lay and community-based workers focused on education and navigation assistance, usually collaborating with other health professionals (Chapter 8). Interventions delivered by community health workers, who worked alongside other professionals such as nurse case managers and psychologists, showed significant improvements in the management of chronic diseases including positive effects on blood pressure levels and cardiovascular disease risk reduction (Kim et al., 2016). Similarly, lay health workers and peer counsellors assisting mothers and their children with low socioeconomic status through home visits, reminders, education and the facilitation of meetings indicated reduced child mortality and morbidity. Additionally, the interventions increased the uptake of immunization rates as well as the likelihood for women to seek care for childhood sicknesses (Lewin et al., 2010).

Interventions to support and strengthen patients and their caregivers in long-term care encompassed assessing the specific needs, planning of support interventions, monitoring, coaching and counselling (Chapter 7).

Pain management targeted at patients in palliative care and their family caregivers covering different components such as face-to-face education and follow ups demonstrated significantly improved medication adherence; yet, showed mixed results on caregivers' knowledge, for example, about pain management.

Skill-mix on re-allocation of tasks and new division of work

Many reviews analysed skill-mix and the re-allocation of tasks resulting in a new division of work between health professionals. Most prominent was the model of advanced practice providers (such as advanced practice nurses, as well as pharmacists in advanced practice roles). Other models covered the re-allocation of tasks from health professions (physicians, nurses, pharmacists) to lower qualified assistants (medical assistants, nursing assistants) or from health professionals to lay workers or patients. This new division of work usually involved task-shifting, whereby specific tasks or roles are shifted from higher to lower educated professions (European Commission, 2019). The overarching aim of task-shifting is to expand access to services, with increased workforce efficiency, work flows and/or other parameters. Task shifting covered at least two professions or workers, and usually occurred as forms of collaboration.

Advanced practice roles among nurses, pharmacists and other professions

Skill-mix models in the literature frequently analysed the effects of advanced practice roles of nurses or pharmacists, performing an expanded set of tasks, traditionally provided by physicians or other health professionals. Other professions covered were physiotherapists or dental hygienists working in expanded roles. Advanced roles ranged from introducing advanced practice providers, with a considerably expanded scope-of-practice (for example, advanced practice nurses including nurse practitioners with usually at least a Master's degree; or pharmacists) to the expansion of a limited set of additional tasks, such as for nurses or dental hygienists. This practice was found across almost all different care segments in the overview of reviews. In health promotion and prevention, advanced practice nurses (for example, nurse practitioners) or professional nurses performed screenings and skin cancer assessments and examinations.

For instance, nurses in advanced practice roles delivering skin cancer screening showed higher sensitivity to identify malignant lesions compared with physicians or general and expert dermatologists (Loescher, Harris & Curiel-Lewandrowski, 2011). Nurse-delivered colorectal cancer screenings detected higher rates of adenomas, and were shown to result in lower costs compared with physician-led services (Joseph, Vaughan & Strand, 2015). This is one example whereby nurse-led screenings were associated with reduced costs; however, to date the evidence on nurse-led screenings on costs is scarce and requires more cost-effectiveness studies (Chapter 4).

The highest number of reviews focused on task shifting and a new division of work for chronically ill patients. Nurses and pharmacists took on considerably advanced roles, which had traditionally been performed by physicians. One model was nurse-led care, defined as nurses leading the treatment and care process for a defined group of patients, like with diabetes. Nurse-led care included a wide range of different components such as prescribing of medicines, management of medication adherence, disease management or education. Models ranged from delivery either autonomously or in collaboration with other health professionals, usually with physicians. Nurse-led care for single chronic diseases indicated better or equivalent health outcomes compared with usual care (mainly physician-provided), in particular for titration and medication adherence (Parker et al., 2016; Shaw et al., 2013), yet, nurse-led care revealed insufficient evidence for health system outcomes and cost effectiveness. Inconclusive findings were demonstrated for multimorbidity (Chapter 6).

Pharmacists in expanded roles took over tasks from physicians such as health screenings, immunizations and monitoring medication adherence. Pharmacists delivering care for patients with chronic conditions were shown to positively influence cardiovascular disease outcomes such as blood pressure in several systematic reviews (Blalock et al., 2013; Cheema, Sutcliffe & Singer, 2014; Fazel et al., 2017; Greer et al., 2016; Morgado et al., 2011; Nkansah et al., 2010; Tan et al., 2014; van Eikenhorst et al., 2017). Moreover, evidence showed improvements in medication adherence for patients with hypertension (Blalock et al., 2013; Cheema, Sutcliffe & Singer, 2014; Morgado et al., 2011) and demonstrated reduced hospitalization, emergency department visits and costs for pharmacist-led chronic care (Entezari-Maleki et al., 2016; Manzoor et al., 2017).

Skill-mix interventions and task shifting practices were also identified for (minor) acute illnesses where pharmacists, physiotherapists and mid-level dental care providers had extended the scope of practices (Chapter 5). In the United Kingdom, pharmacy-based minor ailment consultations suggested less costly services than usual care delivered by GPs and an overall satisfaction among patients, GPs and pharmacists (Paudyal et al., 2013). Positive effects regarding health outcomes were also reported for mid-level dental providers such as dental hygienists delivering care (Dasanayake et al., 2012; Wright et al., 2013).

Skill-mix and relocation of care
The relocation of care settings comprised hospital-at-home, nurse-led clinics if provided in a new setting and palliative care at home interventions. Hospital-at-home services are defined as highly specialized services at patients' homes for individuals who would usually require hospitalization for their condition. Three systematic reviews including two Cochrane Reviews assessed hospital treatment at home by various health professionals in highly specialized teams (Gonçalves-Bradley et al., 2017; Qaddoura et al., 2015; Shepperd et al., 2017). One Cochrane review analysed home services delivered by a specialist respiratory nurse (Jeppesen et al., 2012). Positive or no effects were reported for mortality rates across the reviews and mixed results were shown for readmission and patient outcomes. However, no negative outcomes were reported, suggesting that hospital-at-home may be a safe model of care provision, for instance for patients with acute respiratory conditions, provided that the professions are adequately trained, possess the right skills and perform close monitoring (Chapter 5).

Nurse-led cardiac clinics suggested a positive impact on the quality of care for patients with chronic conditions. Studies demonstrated that nurse-led clinics provided equivalent or better care compared with usual care or clinics run by other health professionals. To illustrate, significant improvements were found for mortality rates and equivalent effects for self-reported mental or physical health and hospitalization episodes compared with usual care (Al-Mallah et al., 2016; Schadewaldt & Schultz, 2010). Similarly, nurse-led clinics for patients with multimorbidity indicated equivalent care compared to other clinics (Clark et al., 2011) (Chapter 6).

While the number of systematic reviews on palliative care at patients' homes was small, effects on pain management through interventions mostly delivered by teams or in collaboration showed improved pain-related outcomes. Palliative teams were composed of nurses, psychologists and researchers and targeted patients and their caregivers in palliative care. Improved caregiver satisfaction and lower caregiver burden were reported for implementing case managers and multidisciplinary collaboration models. Additionally, health system outcomes such as hospital admission and length of stay and profession-specific outcomes including communication and service relationships suggest positive impacts of palliative care delivered at patients' homes (Chapter 7).

Changing teamwork and collaboration

Skill-mix interventions involving teamwork and collaboration were identified across all care segments included in the study, ranging from health promotion, prevention to long-term and palliative care. Teamwork took various forms, for example, multiprofessional teams, shared care whereby two professionals worked closely together sharing tasks, as well as networks of care providers and multiprofessional clinics.

Skill-mix interventions involving multiprofessional teams for chronic conditions and multimorbidity evaluated different ways of collaboration such as consultation liaison, joint care coordination or shared care performed by various professions, and was compared with usual care generally provided by physicians alone (Chapter 6). For consultation liaison involving collaborative care between physicians and specialists, moderate positive effects on physical health outcomes was demonstrated (Foy et al., 2010; Mitchell et al., 2015). There was evidence that collaborative care involving mental health specialists and primary care providers improved mental health outcomes, patient satisfaction and quality of life (Archer et al., 2012; Coventry et al., 2014). Reduced utilization of inpatient care and other health care services was shown for other multiprofessional care models such as primary care provider networks (Carter et al., 2016) and multiprofessional cardiac clinics (Gandhi et al., 2017). Collaborative care targeting patients with multimorbidity showed improved adherence to medication and health outcomes; but, little or no evidence on cost savings.

Overall, the reviews suggest that multiprofessional care models can have a positive effect for patients with mental health problems and multimorbidity (Chapter 6).

Skill-mix interventions provided by multiprofessional teams were frequently reported for transitional care and early discharge planning. For instance, transitional care teams focused on care transitioning across different care settings including the inpatient/ambulatory interface and different phases of life (paediatric to adulthood). The evidence on transitional care involving various professions demonstrated positive effects on selected patients and health system outcomes; however, not all reviews and underlying studies differentiated between multiprofessional and single-profession interventions (Chapter 5)

In long-term care, multiprofessional community mental health teams and collaborative models were evaluated. Multiprofessional community mental health teams were composed of mental health nurses, social workers, psychologists, consultant psychiatrists and GPs. The mental health teams provided intensive care management and team diagnosis.

Multiprofessional collaboration models included interventions such as shared care plans and joint decision-making. Although the evidence was limited because it covered only a few studies, introducing multi-professional teams for long-term conditions such as mental health or Parkinson's disease were suggested to improve quality of life and function and mobility rates. Intensified collaboration among health professionals delivering care for patients in palliative care also demonstrated positive effects on patients and their caregivers, but was limited to few individual studies (Chapter 7).

2.3   Strength of the evidence and limitations

The overview of reviews has synthesized a considerable body of evidence on the different skill-mix interventions (for example, addition of new roles in prevention, task-shifting and new division of work in chronic care, multiprofessional teams) which have been evaluated across various countries. However, the evidence base differed across the care segments.

The outcome measures were clustered into three main categories – patient-related, health system and profession-specific. A large number of reviews reported outcomes on patients (individual health outcomes), but outcomes on health systems, costs and the professions themselves remained scarce. There was considerable heterogeneity in the outcome measures across the systematic reviews. A high number of reviews performed meta-analyses related to single chronic conditions, but in all other areas covered, the number of meta-analyses was considerably smaller and mostly narrative syntheses were performed, because of the heterogeneity of the outcome measures. The variations between outcome measures across individual studies limited their comparability. Several skill-mix interventions were multicomponent and sometimes included non-skill-mix-related changes, which limits the attribution of causality.

The study faces several limitations. First, only systematic reviews published as of 2010 were included. One reason is that the study aimed to cover skill-mix innovations, defined as a novelty in its widest sense, including the time dimension of publication. An additional reason was the feasibility of conducting the overview of reviews. It needs to be noted that there may have been systematic reviews published before 2010 on skill-mix interventions that may have been missed, although the likelihood is estimated to be low. Second, individual studies were not covered; RCTs in particular or other study designs that were recently published may have been missed. Third, although many of the included systematic reviews described the professions involved in the skill-mix interventions and how their roles changed, several reviews did not sufficiently describe the professions, their roles and tasks covered in the intervention group, particularly when it involved teams. Instead terms like "various professions", "multidisciplinary teams" or "care teams" were applied. Another limitation of the reviews and underlying studies was that the comparator groups were rarely described in detail. Therefore, professions as well as the specific roles and tasks covered often remained insufficiently reported; the comparison groups were sometimes simply referred to as "usual care". One additional limitation was that the education of the professionals was rarely described, which is essential with regards to implementation considerations.

The findings need to be interpreted in light of these limitations. However, this study is the first of its kind that synthesized the evidence of skill-mix changes on individuals, health systems and professions, covering all health professions as well as lay workers and informal caregivers in primary and ambulatory care settings. It shows that there are several promising skill-mix models to improve the quality of care and access to services.

2.4 Transferability of the findings

Some skill-mix changes work well for a defined population group, in a specific country or setting, but not in others. Assessing the transferability of a proven skill-mix intervention is therefore critical. At the same time, the question of transferability is highly complex and context specific. This volume does not suggest that an innovation can or should be easily replicated without considering how it can fit different contexts and needs. Instead, it suggests that decision-makers identify the different existing skill-mix strategies that have been identified to address a specific health need, skills gap or workforce challenge and evaluate which elements could work in the specific setting and context.

Bearing this in mind, some skill-mix models have been shown to work well in multiple contexts and been associated with positive health outcomes. This includes introducing new, dedicated prevention and health promotion roles for nurses or pharmacists in ambulatory care and community settings (Chapter 4). Expanding the roles and scope-of-practice for nurses and pharmacists to care for patients with chronic conditions (also referred to as task shifting) was found to be effective in a large number of different countries and contexts (Chapter 6). Expanding the roles for nurses, midwives or community-based workers to reach out to women and their children also shows a promising skill-mix model in several countries (Chapter 8). Introducing a care coordinator function, particularly at the hospital-to-community transitioning interface and for patients with high needs, shows promise, but it remains unclear by which profession and what level of intensity is required for which patient groups (Chapter 5). There remains insufficient evidence for which exact roles and tasks should be performed by what profession and the educational needs required to develop the new skills and roles. Finally, on effective teamwork and outcomes, the evidence remains limited.

Decision-makers can use the evidence synthesis to understand what skill-mix model involving which profession(s) and interventions has worked for what population group in which countries. Yet, when considering implementation of a skill-mix change, assessment of several transferability and implementation questions is critical:

- First, has this model been evaluated in the country, at minimum in pilots or small-scale programmes? Will new changes be externally evaluated?
- Second, are the skill sets of the concerned profession(s) available or are other professions or workers better suited to perform these roles in a specific setting? Are there sufficient professionals to ensure going to scale within the planned time period? Is additional education and training a requirement to ensure that the new roles can be performed with good quality?
- Third, what are the regulatory mechanisms and oversight requirements to ensure patient safety?
- Fourth, how is financing and payment impacting on the new roles?
- And finally, what communication strategies are effective to inform and involve patients, other health professions, managers and other key stakeholders to ensure the transfer and piloting of new skill-mix models and their evaluation.

Hence, the transfer and implementation of a specific skill-mix intervention is not only influenced by the governance and organization of a health system. Profession-specific regulatory mechanisms also play an important role, the educational system, the influence of the stakeholders involved and the political force field. These factors are critical for generating an inducive environment to support the implementation of skill-mix innovations and reforms. These factors influencing the implementation process will be addressed in Chapter 3.

2.5   Conclusions

The main skill-mix interventions identified in the overview of review focused on new, supplementary roles, new division of work (task shifting and relocation of care) and teamwork (multiprofessional teamwork and collaboration). Several examples for innovative skill-mix changes have demonstrated a positive impact on the quality of care or on the access to health services. Examples are as follows: (i) establishing a dedicated prevention role for population groups or individuals with at-risk factors; (ii) task shifting and new division of work in teams whereby nurses or pharmacists take up clinical tasks from physicians and take over certain patient groups; (iii) care coordinator roles (for example, case managers, transitional care coordinators) for patients with chronic or acute conditions and multiple needs; (iv) patient navigator roles or peers to educate, enhance health literacy and empower individuals, particularly vulnerable groups.

Although the overall body of evidence on skill-mix is remarkable, there remain several research gaps. Except for nurses and pharmacists, the evidence on other professions involved in skill-mix changes and outcomes is less well established. There is considerable evidence across many countries that task shifting between physicians and nurses or pharmacists can lead to equivalent or improved quality of care. Yet, the evidence on costs is mixed and inconclusive. There is generally a scarcity of research on skill-mix changes and effects on health systems and costs. Very limited high-quality evidence is available on the effects of skill-mix changes on the professions themselves. Evidence on teamwork and division of work is mixed. Implementation research is required to evaluate the new roles individually and as part of teams to demonstrate health outcomes, team effectiveness and satisfaction, as well as cost-effectiveness.

What can be concluded from the existing research, however, is as follows: dedicated prevention and health promotion roles performed by qualified health professionals showed promising results on patients' lifestyle, physical activity and diet. The prevention role often reached out into communities. Some models also included home visits, undertaken by health professionals themselves or in collaboration with lay health workers or peers. The evidence suggests that skill-mix changes focusing on establishing a specific, dedicated prevention role can improve health outcomes, particularly if integrated in primary health care or communities. Often the focus was on vulnerable population groups, which required tailored services. However, determining which profession should undertake this role is highly country and context specific. Countries should step up such a new role to maximize health gains for individuals and population groups and integrate these new roles in communities and health systems.

In addition, promising skill-mix changes are care coordinator roles at the hospital–ambulatory care interface for acute, high-needs patients or in ambulatory care. They were prominent for various patient groups, including for patients with single chronic conditions, multimorbidity, acute episodes of care and long-term and palliative care needs. Case management interventions yielded mixed results, due to the heterogeneity of patient groups, conditions and outcome measures. For patients with cancer or at risk of developing cancer, patient navigation interventions overall showed promising results on patients' health and access to services, particularly for socioeconomically disadvantaged individuals, migrants or other vulnerable groups. Introducing and training peers and lay health workers to empower patients and their caregivers were innovative interventions that contributed to improved patient outcomes across various care segments. Advanced roles of nurses and pharmacists were most frequently evaluated for task shifting and were found across all care segments in the systematic reviews. Additionally, extended scopes-of-practice of physiotherapists and dental mid-level providers were also among the interventions. Most of the reviews covering new division of work showed generally positive patient and health-system-related outcomes if professionals were trained and possessed the right skills.

Skill-mix interventions involving teamwork and collaboration were identified across all care sectors. The interventions were manifold and ranged from multiprofessional teams to networks of primary care providers and clinics. Models covered either various health professions within ambulatory care or across sectors. Positive results were particularly reported for multiprofessional interventions for mental health care in collaboration with primary or other health professionals.

For policy-making, the study shows that there is cross-country evidence demonstrating that skill-mix changes have been widely implemented in Europe and beyond. The trend in many countries from solo physician practices to group practices and multiprofessional health centres has also reinforced new skill-mix developments. However, instead of transferring interventions from one country context to another with no consideration given to transferability, policy-makers should identify and evaluate what skill-mix changes best suit their specific context, population or patient group and intended health aim(s). In terms of which profession(s) to perform new roles to step up prevention, care coordination and the quality of chronic condition treatment, most countries equipped nurses and/or pharmacists with additional training and responsibilities, which showed at least equivalent quality of care. For other interventions, for example for long-term care, additional health workers and caregivers were trained to perform these roles. The aim was to make better use of the skills of nurses, pharmacists and other providers, but the evidence base on other professions is less strong. Each country should consider in its specific context which profession in which team configuration is most suited to provide preventive services, care coordination or other services that can improve access and quality of care for specific patient groups. Critical for implementation is how to integrate these new roles in the communities and health systems, close to the population group(s) targeted and identify how to strengthen the professionals' capacity and training needs so as to perform these roles effectively.

References

Al-Mallah MH, Farah I, Al-Madani W et al. (2016). The impact of nurse-led clinics on the mortality and morbidity of patients with cardiovascular diseases: a systematic review and meta-analysis. J Cardiovasc Nurs, 31:89–95.

Archer J, Bower P, Gilbody S et al. (2012). Collaborative care for depression and anxiety problems. Cochrane Database Syst Rev, 10:Cd006525.

Backhouse A, Ukoumunne OC, Richards DA et al. (2017). The effectiveness of community-based coordinating interventions in dementia care: a meta-analysis and subgroup analysis of intervention components. BMC Health Services Res, 17(1):717.

Bhattarai N, Prevost AT, Wright AJ, et al. (2013). Effectiveness of interventions to promote healthy diet in primary care: systematic review and meta-analysis of randomised controlled trials. BMC Public Health, 13:1203.

Blalock SJ, Roberts AW, Lauffenburger JC et al. (2013). The effect of community pharmacy-based interventions on patient health outcomes: a systematic review. Med Care Res Rev, 70:235–266.

Carter R, Riverin B, Levesque JF et al. (2016). The impact of primary care reform on health system performance in Canada: a systematic review. BMC Health Serv Res, 16:324.

Cheema E, Sutcliffe P, Singer DR (2014). The impact of interventions by pharmacists in community pharmacies on control of hypertension: a systematic review and meta-analysis of randomized controlled trials. Br J Clin Pharmacol, 78:1238–1247.

Clark CE, Smith LF, Taylor RS, Campbell JL (2011). Nurse-led interventions used to improve control of high blood pressure in people with diabetes: a systematic review and meta-analysis. Diabet Med, 28:250–261.

Coventry PA, Hudson JL, Kontopantelis E et al. (2014). Characteristics of effective collaborative care for treatment of depression: a systematic review and meta-regression of 74 randomised controlled trials. PloS One, 9:e108114.

Dale JR, Williams SM, Bowyer V (2012). What is the effect of peer support on diabetes outcomes in adults? A systematic review. Diabet Med, 29L1361–1377.

Dalziel K, Segal L (2012). Home visiting programs for the prevention of child maltreatment: cost-effectiveness of 33 programs. Arch Dis Childhood, 97(9):787.

Dasanayake A, Brar B, Matta S et al. (2019). Are procedures performed by dental auxiliaries safe and of comparable quality? A systematic review. J Calif Dent Assoc, 40(1):65–78.

Entezari-Maleki T, Dousti S, Hamishehkar H et al. (2016). A systematic review on comparing 2 common models for management of warfarin therapy; pharmacist-led service versus usual medical care. J Clin Pharmacol, 56:24–38.

European Commission (2019). Task shifting and health system design. Report by the Expert Panel on effective ways of investing in Health (EXPH). Luxembourg: Publications Office of the European Union, 2019. (https://ec.europa.eu/health/expert_panel/sites/expertpanel/files/023_taskshifting_en.pdf, accessed 20 January 2020).

Fazel MT, Bagalagel A, Lee JK et al. (2017). Impact of diabetes care by pharmacists as part of health care team in ambulatory settings: a systematic review and meta-analysis. Ann Pharmacother, 51:890–907.

Foy R, Hempel S, Rubenstien L, Suttorp M et al. (2010). Meta-analysis: Effect of interactive communication between collaborating primary care physicians and specialists. Ann Intern Med, 152:247–258.

Gandhi S, Mosleh W, Sharma UC et al. (2017). Multidisciplinary heart failure clinics are associated with lower heart failure hospitalization and mortality: systematic review and meta-analysis. Can J Cardiol, 33:1237–1244.

Goeman D, Renehan E, Koch S (2016). What is the effectiveness of the support worker role for people with dementia and their carers? A systematic review. BMC Health Services Res 16:285.

Gonçalves-Bradley D, Iliffe S, Doll H et al. (2017). Early discharge hospital at home. Cochrane Database Syst Rev, 6(6):CD000356.

Greer N, Bolduc J, Geurkink E et al. (2016). Pharmacist-led chronic disease management: a systematic review of effectiveness and harms compared with usual care. Ann Intern Med, 165:30–40.

Jeppesen E, Brurberg KG, Vist GE et al. (2012). Hospital at home for acute exacerbations of chronic obstructive pulmonary disease. Cochrane Database Syst Rev 5: CD003573.

Joseph J, Vaughan R, Strand H (2015). Effectiveness of nurse-performed endoscopy in colorectal cancer screening: a systematic review. Gastrointest Nurs 13:26–33.

Khanassov V, Vedel I (2016). Family physician-case manager collaboration and needs of patients with dementia and their caregivers: a systematic mixed studies review. Ann Family Med, 14(2):166–177.

Khanassov V, Vedel I, Pluye P (2014): Barriers to implementation of case management for patients with dementia: a systematic mixed studies review. Ann Family Med, 12(5):S.456–465.

Kim K, Choi J, Choi E et al. (2016). Effects of community-based health worker interventions to improve chronic disease management and care among vulnerable populations: a systematic review. *Am J Public Health*, 106(4):e3–e28.

Lewin S, Munabi-Babigumira S, Glenton C et al. (2010). Lay health workers in primary and community health care for maternal and child health and the management of infectious diseases (Review). Cochrane Database Syst Rev, 3:CD004015.

Loescher LJ, Harris Jr. JM, Curiel-Lewandrowski C (2011). A systematic review of advanced practice nurses' skin cancer assessment barriers, skin lesion recognition skills, and skin cancer training activities. J Am Acad Nurse Practitioners, 23(12):667–673.

Maier CB, Kroezen M, Hartl K et al. (2018) Overview of systematic reviews: outcomes of health Workforce skill-mix changes in primary and ambulatory care. PROSPERO 2018 CRD42018090272. (https://www.crd.york.ac.uk/prospero/display_record.php?ID=CRD42018090272, accessed 30 June 2019).

Manzoor BS, Cheng WH, Lee JC et al. (2017). Quality of pharmacist-managed anticoagulation therapy in long-term ambulatory settings: a systematic review. Ann Pharmacother 51:1122–1137.

Mitchell GK, Burridge L, Zhang J et al. (2015). Systematic review of integrated models of health care delivered at the primary-secondary interface: how effective is it and what determines effectiveness? Aust J Prim Health, 21:391–408.

Morgado MP, Morgado SR, Mendes LC et al. (2011). Pharmacist interventions to enhance blood pressure control and adherence to antihypertensive therapy: review and meta-analysis. Am J Health Syst Pharm, 68:241–253.

Nkansah N, Mostovetsky O, Yu C et al. (2010). Effect of outpatient pharmacists' non-dispensing roles on patient outcomes and prescribing patterns. Cochrane Database Syst Rev, CD000336.

OECD (2017). Data for Measuring Health Care Quality and Outcomes [Online]. OECD. (http://www.oecd.org/els/health-systems/health-care-quality-indicators.htm, accessed 30 June 2019).

Orrow G, Kinmonth A-L, Sanderson S et al. (2012). Effectiveness of physical activity promotion based in primary care: systematic review and meta-analysis of randomised controlled trials. BMJ, 344:e1389.

Parker D, Maresco-Pennisi D, Clifton K et al. (2016). Practice nurse involvement in the management of adults with type 2 diabetes mellitus attending a general practice: results from a systematic review. Int J Evid Based Health, 14:41–52.

Paudyal V, Watson MC, Sach T et al. (2013). Are pharmacy-based Minor Ailment Schemes a substitute for other service providers? A systematic review. Br J GP 63(612):e472–481.

Pimouguet C, Lavaud T, Dartigues JF (2010). Dementia case management effectiveness on health care costs and resource utilization: a systematic review of randomized controlled trials. In: J Nutrition, Health & Aging 14(8):669–676.

Qaddoura A, Yazdan-Ashoori P, Kabali C et al. (2015). Efficacy of hospital at home in patients with heart failure: a systematic review and meta-analysis. PLOS One, 10(6):e0129282.

Reilly S, Miranda-Castillo C, Malouf R et al. (2015). Case management approaches to home support for people with dementia. Cochrane Database Syst Rev, 1:CD008345.

Schadewaldt V, Schultz T (2010). A systematic review on the effectiveness of nurse-led cardiac clinics for adult patients with coronary heart disease. JBI Libr Syst Rev, 8:53–89.

Schroeder K, Travers J, Smaldone A (2016). Are school nurses an overlooked resource in reducing childhood obesity? A systematic review and meta-analysis. J School Health, 86(5):309–321.

Shaw RJ, Mcduffie JR, Hendrix CC et al. (2013). Effects of nurse-managed protocols in the outpatient management of adults with chronic conditions. VA Evidence-based Synthesis Program Reports. Washington DC, Department of Veterans Affairs.

Shepperd S, Cradduck-Bamford A, Butler C et al. (2017). A multi-centre randomised trial to compare the effectiveness of geriatrician-led admission avoidance hospital at home versus inpatient admission. Trials, 18(1):491.

Tan EC, Stewart K, Elliott RA et al. (2014). Pharmacist services provided in general practice clinics: a systematic review and meta-analysis. Res Social Adm Pharm, 10:608–622.

United Nations (2016). Secretary-General Appoints Commission on Health Employment and Economic Growth [online]. New York: United Nations. (http://www.un.org/press/en/2016/sga1639.doc.htm, accessed 30 June 2019).

Van Eikenhorst L, Taxis K, Van Dijk L et al. (2017). Pharmacist-led self-management interventions to improve diabetes outcomes. A systematic literature review and meta-analysis. Front Pharmacol, 8:891.

World Health Organization (2016). Health workforce requirements for universal health coverage and the Sustainable Development Goals Human Resources for Health Observer – Issue No. 17. (https://www.who.int/hrh/resources/health-observer17/en/, accessed 30 June 2019).

World Health Organization (2018). Five-year action plan for health employment and inclusive economic growth (2017–2021). Geneva, World Health Organization.

Wright J, Graham F, Hayes C et al. (2013). A systematic review of oral health outcomes produced by dental teams incorporating midlevel providers. J Am Dent Assoc, 144(1):75–91.

3 Implementing skill-mix changes: lessons for policy and practice

CLAUDIA B. MAIER, GIADA SCARPETTI,
MARIEKE KROEZEN, MATHILDE S. AKEROYD,
HANNAH BUDDE, LAURA PFIRTER, MATTHIAS
WISMAR

3.1 Introduction

Many countries across Europe are considering implementing skill-mix strategies to better meet the needs of their patients, against the backdrop of changing service delivery models, new technologies and financing as well as payment policies. Implementing skill-mix changes in a country, region or setting is a complex intervention and impacts on the education and training of providers, multiprofessional collaboration, work flow and service provision, and ultimately, the patients and families. Skill-mix reforms are often highly controversial and prone to self-interests, influenced by various stakeholders, including different professional associations, payers, regulators or trade unions. Managing the process of implementation therefore requires a good understanding of the influencing factors, potential barriers and pitfalls involved. It also requires anticipating and actively fostering potentially facilitating factors in the process.

This chapter provides an overview of the evidence on the implementation of skill-mix changes. It identifies common barriers and facilitators at various levels, from the policy to the organizational level and summarizes the evidence from Chapter 9 (education and workforce planning), Chapter 10 (policy and financing) and Chapter 11 (organizational strategies). Workforce planning and education are key elements influencing skill-mix; they are closely intertwined and therefore covered in one distinct chapter (Chapter 9). With regard to policy, Chapter 10 covers the role of legislation, regulation and other measures as well as financing and payment policies. Chapter 11 addresses the implementation and the uptake by individual health care organizations and the influence of characteristics of the skill-mix innovation and institutional, organizational, individual and process factors.

3.2 Overview of the evidence on implementation

Based on the overview of reviews (for an overview of the methods, see Chapter 1), a total of 29 systematic reviews were identified (see Table 3.1). On implementation, the largest number, namely 21 reviews, were on the role of organization-specific factors in the implementation process (Chapter 11), whereas seven systematic reviews analysed policy-specific or finance-specific factors (Chapter 10). Only one systematic review covered education, which analysed interprofessional education and effects on outcomes (Chapter 9). Compared with the body of evidence on skill-mix changes and effects on outcomes – as shown in Chapter 2 – the number of reviews available on implementation is much lower. No review performed meta-analysis. The number of Cochrane reviews identified on implementation was very low, only one review was a Cochrane review. In sum, reviews on implementation are scarce – with the exception of reviews on implementation at the organizational level.

The systematic reviews identified covered implementation-specific factors with regard to several skill-mix typologies, including the implementation of new professions, roles or tasks for single professions, the implementation of multiprofessional teamwork and the re-allocation of tasks (Table 3.2). One systematic review analysed the outcomes of interprofessional education on a range of outcome parameters, including on teamwork and patient outcomes. Most reviews covered multiple professions, including physicians, nurses, midwives, pharmacists, social care workers and multiprofessional teamwork.

In addition to the systematic reviews, additional sources of evidence (individual studies, grey literature, mini case studies) were included. They complemented the available evidence from the overview of reviews.

Table 3.1 *Number of systematic reviews covered on implementation of skill-mix*

Implementation areas covered	Included reviews	Meta-analyses	Cochrane reviews
Education and workforce planning	1	0	1
Policy and financing	7	0	0
Organizational level	21	0	0

Sources: Based on Chapters 9–11.

Table 3.2 *Topics and professions covered by the systematic reviews on implementation*

Areas covered	Skill-mix topics	Professions covered
Education and workforce planning	• One systematic review on interprofessional education	• Health and social care professionals
Policy and financing	• Three systematic reviews on the addition of new tasks; the expansion of roles • Two systematic reviews on the introduction of teamwork • Two systematic reviews on reallocation of tasks	• NPs, pharmacists, midwives, diverse primary care providers
Organizational level	• Five systematic reviews on the addition of new tasks and expansion of roles • Twelve systematic reviews on the introduction of teamwork • Four systematic reviews on the re-allocation of tasks	• GPs, NPs, nurses, PAs, various other professions, multiprofessional teams

Abbreviations: GP: general practitioner; NP: nurse practitioner; PA: physician assistant.
Sources: Based on Chapters 9–11.

Country examples demonstrating important lessons for implementation were identified and presented as mini case studies to situate skill-mix innovations and their implementation in the specific country contexts.

3.3   Evidence synthesis: the role of education and health workforce planning and skill-mix

How can education and health workforce planning anticipate and respond to the changing skill-mix requirements in health care? The existence of skills mismatches in Europe has prompted changes and an improved responsiveness of educational systems, as well as adaptations of health workforce planning mechanisms. Simultaneously, health workforce shortages have motivated changes to health workforce planning (Kroezen et al., 2015; Schoenstein, Ono & Lafortune, 2016). Yet, there is remarkably little evidence available on either skill-mix and education, or on skill-mix and health workforce planning. The overview of reviews identified only one systematic review on education. A Cochrane systematic review by Reeves et al. (2013) focused on multiprofessional education and evidence on outcomes. No systematic review was identified on skill-mix and health workforce planning and implementation or other outcomes (Chapter 9). Additional material, such as grey literature, reports or case studies, was also available and was covered, but the availability of all evidence remained limited.

Current European professional education incorporates three noteworthy developments that can respond to the changing demand for health competencies and support skill-mix innovations, namely interprofessional education (IPE), competency-based education and the academization of health professionals.

Interprofessional education involves initiatives in health educational institutions that incorporate interactive learning between different professionals to foster collaborative practice and increase an understanding of different roles in health care (Hale, 2003). Several facilitators have been identified for the implementation and uptake of IPE: these include having a shared, open culture, support and leadership as well as strategic facilitation and planning. Barriers to IPE include practical factors, such as the coordination of different academic calendars, student timetables and determining what to teach in the IPE modules, while avoiding curriculum duplication. Education such as IPE, which deviates from didactic lectures, particularly when it uses simulations and in-practice-based learning, can increase students' positive attitudes towards interprofessional collaborative practice. However, the evidence for IPE is poor overall and where the impact was measured, it was often small (Reeves et al., 2013). More research is required to evaluate which models and intensity of IPE yield which outcomes (Chapter 9).

Competency-based education, which structures the curriculum according to relevant skills and competencies, can in theory respond well to changing population health needs and required new skills. The curriculum can break down professional silos and can be adapted to new roles and skill requirements (Gravina, 2017). An example of competency-measured basic education is CanMEDS in Canada, where competencies related to skill-mix are integrated in the stipulated values and competencies for medical experts, and physicians trained through competency-based education scored high on skill-mix-related domains such as collaboration (Charles et al., 2016). Yet, the implementation of competency-based education has been confronted with several obstacles, such as challenges to assess and measure competencies in areas of communication, collaboration or compassion (Nousiainen et al., 2016), and its effects on skill-mix innovations are largely unknown.

A further trend of particularly high relevance to skill-mix changes and innovations is the academization of some health professions, which is notably observed for the education of nurses and midwives (Lahtinen, Leino-Kilpi & Salminen, 2014). There is also an increasing trend towards moving the education of physiotherapists to higher educational institutions, for example, universities of applied science (Friedrichs & Schaub, 2011). The academization of these professions has been referred to as a stimulus to take on advanced roles (De Geest et al., 2008). Academization is seen as a driver for new roles and changes to traditional team configurations and labour markets. It remains unclear, however, to what extent it contributes overall to the implementation of skill-mix innovations.

For health professionals already in the workforce, there is a development towards postgraduate training, continuing professional development and competency based frameworks to support the uptake of skill-mix changes. Postgraduate training is often required when health professionals are faced with new tasks and assume new roles and responsibilities for which they feel inadequately prepared. In the case of professionals undertaking postgraduate training, arrangements that allow continuation of work responsibilities, such as web-enhanced courses, have been identified as key for successful engagement by participants (Kovner et al., 2012; Salyers, 2005). Continuous professional education as in-service training can provide one of the most important educational tools when implementing skill-mix in practice, if based on up-to-date knowledge and developments in health service delivery including skill-mix innovations. This trend is seen in recent French reforms, where continuing professional development is at the forefront, including skill-mix-related components such as interprofessional collaboration and shared team-based goals (Chapter 9). Lastly, competency-based education is further seen in continuing professional education, where efforts have been made to develop health workforce competencies, which are more closely related to developments in health care practice and tends to include skill-mix related domains such as teamwork.

Concurrently, health workforce planning can influence education through policies to expand or reduce student numbers and postgraduate training posts. It should also respond to changes in the health care needs of the population and challenges regarding skill-gaps in the workforce. Conventional health workforce models do not consistently cover different professions, task shifting practices or interprofessional collaboration. Of the current health workforce models, it is the needs-based models that are most suited to incorporate skill-mix innovations, but they are rarely used because of the large number of data requirements. More development is needed for all workforce planning models to account for interprofessional collaboration, changes in education and skill-mix to improve projections and estimate effects on health care delivery.

3.4 Evidence synthesis: the role of policy and financing in implementing skill-mix changes

This section provides a synthesis of the evidence on the role of policy and skill-mix implementation. It focuses on the role of legislation and regulations as well as financing and payment models and their two-way relationship with the uptake of skill-mix changes in practice. This section summarizes the evidence from Chapter 10, which was based on seven systematic reviews, plus additional material, country examples and (grey) literature.

Overall, there are a multitude of influencing factors impacting on a policy level, and therefore a macro level. They can act as either barriers or facilitators in the implementation process. Depending on how they are designed and shaped, their outcomes can contrast with each other with regard to the implementation outcomes and processes. Most of these influencing factors are amenable to change, which means that they can be modified in such a way as to alter them from a barrier to a facilitator. The following section highlights how different instruments can act as facilitators or barriers for skill-mix changes.

Regarding the impact of policy interventions on skill-mix innovation, four main themes emerged from the systematic reviews. They require particular consideration when planning or implementing a shift in the skill-mix. The first is professional role clarification, which can act as both a facilitator (if roles are clear to the relevant groups) and a barrier (if clarity is lacking) to skill-mix, depending on the context. On the one hand, increasing the understanding of the role and skills of each health professional in a team has been suggested to facilitate a smooth transition towards a new skill-mix setting. On the other hand, roles that are too narrowly delineated could limit flexibility and versatility in collaborative care models. The second theme identified was the formalization of communication, which also acts as an enabler for professional role clarification, so linking these two prominent themes that demand more attention in skill-mix policy. Along with informal communication, formalized channels of communications, such as protocols, are pivotal to improving collaboration and increasing the effectiveness of teamwork. As for the third theme, outdated regulatory and legal frameworks can create bottlenecks for skill-mix innovations but can also – if in line with recent educational developments – lay the foundations for a new skill-mix change to develop and formalize unofficial practice (for example, if new titles and/or scopes of practice are regulated by law). A lack of suitable regulation and a clear legal framework also create ambiguity concerning liability issues for skill-mix innovations. The fourth theme concerns the need for adequate training and education, which is per se closely linked with Chapter 9, which is pivotal to a successful re-orientation of health worker skill-mix. Regulation of new professional roles and their titles usually has direct impacts on education, because the curricula require a minimum level of harmonization and lead to a minimum of commonly available skills and competencies. Training is therefore also linked to the concept of professional role clarification as it allows the establishment of the role as well as understanding of the profession (see also Chapter 9).

Revisiting financing and payment mechanisms is critical to assess the impact of funding on the implementation process. Any skill-mix change, for example adding new tasks and roles or new division of work, requires adaptations to the financing, particularly in countries with primarily fee-for-service financing schemes. Countries should identify the impact of different financing models, including innovative payment schemes, such as bundled payments, on the implementation of skill-mix. Moreover, the recognition of new roles is influenced by the levels of payment and reimbursement, for example by acknowledging and supporting the need for more suitable payment mechanisms that would eventually replace those unfeasible to support change. One of the factors with potential for successful and sustainable uptake of skill-mix innovations is the appropriate funding for new or enhanced professional roles. Moreover, introducing financial incentives (or disincentives) can provide a stimulus to the implementation process, as demonstrated in Estonia (Chapter 10). While certain reimbursement models, such as bundled payments, can encourage multiple providers to work together and allow for task shifting, other mechanisms that pay individual providers separately, such as fee-for-service, can hinder effective collaboration and task shifting practices. However, as mentioned in Chapter 10, although five systematic reviews on skill-mix touched partially on health financing or payment mechanisms, no review has been identified that specifically address the impact of health financing on skill-mix.

Financing reforms are necessary, but alone not sufficient to support the creation or enhancement of roles for skill-mix implementation. Instead, the whole system of organization and governance that facilitates the success of financing reforms needs to be considered, together with individual countries' context. Although financing mechanisms represent a potential powerful lever to make a case for or against a certain skill-mix change, financing is strongly intertwined with other policy levers. Evidence from the literature indicates that organizational and regulatory structures can be a vector to either accelerate or hinder change, as demonstrated in Chapter 10.

3.5 Evidence synthesis: organizational strategies to implement skill-mix changes

This section examines barriers, facilitators and strategies for implementation of skill-mix changes at the organizational level (Chapter 11). Through the overview of reviews, 21 systematic reviews were identified. They were analysed according to the most important factors found in the literature. This chapter applies the following framework in analysing the most important factors influencing the implementation of skill-mix innovations in health care settings:

- characteristics of the skill-mix innovation, such as whether the skill-mix is perceived to be imposed or not;
- institutional factors, such as the legal framework;
- organizational factors, such as organizational structure and culture;
- individual factors, such as staff knowledge; and
- process factors, such as the planning of the skill-mix before implementation.

Institutional factors were found to represent the largest barrier through financing, also identified at the policy level (Chapters 10 and 11).

Financing acts as a barrier when there is a lack of overall funding for the skill-mix change and/or no reimbursement exists for the skill-mix innovation. This is closely linked with policy design and is shaped by laws and the financing mechanisms in place, which is highly country- and context-specific (Chapter 10). However, individual settings such as health centres and practices also have their own financing possibilities (Chapter 11), and can set up start-up funding, payment mechanisms or other financial incentives. However, the sustainability can be at risk and requires long-term planning and financing. Another institutional factor such as team-based staff training in a specific health care setting, can improve staff participation in skill-mix changes. Further enabling skill-mix changes in practice are supportive policies and regulations, which can aid organizations to initiate appropriate staff training.

Organizational factors that facilitate skill-mix innovations when addressed, are proximity of services involved in the skill-mix and established information systems. Organizational barriers are of structural nature, such as lack of time and financial resources and professional silos in individual organizations (Chapter 11). To overcome restricted financial resources for skill-mix implementation, such as insufficient start-up funding, which was identified as a strong barrier, it is suggested to analyse context-specific payment methods and identify new financing sources or newly allocated existing funding channels. One example of payment methods that are more supportive to the implementation of skill-mix innovations, such as multiprofessional teamwork, are Pay for Performance, which is seen in primary health care settings in Norway, Portugal and the United Kingdom (OECD, 2016). Pay for Performance is usually accepted by health providers, and when applied to teams, as opposed to individual providers, it may stimulate collaboration. Other payment schemes that can support skill-mix changes are bundled payments or financial incentives for multiprofessional teamwork. These can be designed at the policy level or by individual organizations, hence, there are policy options for both policy-makers and health care managers to stimulate skill-mix.

Individual barriers and facilitators were found to be interlinked and to mirror each other, where one is a barrier it can also act as a facilitator if its features are changed. Examples from Chapter 11 are (a lack of) sufficient knowledge and skills, (a lack of) good communication and (a lack of) trust and respect. Chapter 11 suggests that many individual factors are opinion-based, which are often affected by professional silos and affiliations. To overcome such individual barriers when implementing skill-mix innovations, it is effective to have cross-professional educational sessions, developing shared goals and using pilot projects for health professionals to familiarize themselves with the skill-mix change.

Characteristics of the skill-mix innovation itself can be a facilitator if health care professionals perceive a positive effect in terms of professional development or reduced workload, or by increased quality of care for patients. Whereas the opposite is true for barriers, the skill-mix innovation is received poorly if health professionals perceive their work to be overburdened or the patient relationship to be at risk.

In the process of implementing skill-mix, there are some process factors that might influence its outcome. The staff who are involved in skill-mix changes report a lack of support as an important barrier in organizations. Access to ongoing support through supervision and mentorship for staff mitigates this barrier, and acts as an enabler for implementation. Organizations can further support staff by formalizing the new roles, relationships and tasks.

3.6   Strength of the evidence and limitations

Overall, fewer systematic reviews were identified on the implementation of health workforce skill-mix changes or larger-scale reforms within and across countries, if compared with skill-mix and outcomes (Chapter 2). At the organizational level, with a total of 21 reviews, there was more evidence available (Chapter 11).

The methodology of the overview of reviews faced several limitations with regard to implementation and skill-mix. First, although a broad search was conducted in the major databases (see Chapter 1 on the methodology), relevant reviews may have been missed. The search focused on systematic reviews of the evidence and outcomes, including scoping reviews; however, unsystematic evidence summaries or syntheses (not called a systematic review) were not covered. Nevertheless, for all chapters, the systematic reviews were complemented with additional evidence from other sources, including grey material, country case studies and other material. Although this information is critical to provide an overview of the contextual side of implementation, the material was primarily a description of reforms with limited specific information on evaluations or outcomes.

In sum, there is still limited research on the implementation side of skill-mix, and high-quality studies and reviews to analyse implementation are particularly scarce. More implementation research is required, taking a systematic, cross-country comparative design. Second, context is highly relevant in implementation, but rarely taken sufficiently into account, particularly in the systematic reviews. Few countries formally evaluate the implementation of reforms, which is critical to understand why some reforms have been effectively implemented and others have been delayed or not taken off.

3.7   Policy lessons and recommendations

The implementation of skill-mix changes requires changes at various levels, including at the level of policy-making (macro), the managerial decision-making (meso) and individual providers (micro).

From a policy perspective, effective implementation requires not only strategic, multiprofessional and intersectoral workforce planning that takes into account skill-mix changes. The planning should also be linked and integrated with the educational system and requires updated curricula. Multiprofessional education has shown some positive outcomes, for example, improved collaboration, but overall has resulted in mixed findings and requires more, high-quality research on outcomes. Changes to the education and workforce planning are therefore critical to equip professionals with the new skills and project the future supply required. The research evidence base remains very weak on the interlinkage between education, workforce planning and skill-mix implementation.

Adjusting regulation and payment mechanisms is critical for skill-mix implementation. Due to the highly regulated nature of many health professionals (particularly with higher educational degrees, for example, physicians, nurses, pharmacists), a review of the respective scope-of-practice laws and regulation of the professions affected by skill-mix changes is required to identify and subsequently, remove potential regulatory barriers to practice. This concerns the regulation of specific professional titles, the scopes-of-practice, if regulated via legislation and other policies that are impacted by these professions and their daily practice. Adjusting payment mechanisms are critical to support the full implementation of skill-mix changes, but alone are not sufficient. Financial incentives may accelerate implementation.

At the organizational level, developing a clear communication strategy and related change management positively influences skill-mix uptake in practice, particularly if it involves all professions in the process and explains the (perceived) added value of the skill-mix innovation. Other factors that impact on teams and individuals are provision of sufficient information, fostering a culture of mutual trust and respect and – as required – exploring additional funding options to ensure a smooth process, full uptake and sustainability. To strengthen skill-mix implementation, the specific context should be analysed for influencing local factors, staff characteristics and organizational factors, in order to adopt the most appropriate implementation strategies for the specific context.

These are commonly cited enablers, each country and organization requires careful assessment of the exact measures needed and should tailor the strategies to its specific contexts, a bundle of measures at all three levels – macro, meso, micro – is likely to yield the best results.

References

Charles L, Triscott J, Dobbs B et al. (2016). Effectiveness of a core-competency-based program on residents' learning and experience. Can Geriatrics J, 19:50–57.

De Geest S, Moons P, Callens B et al. (2008). Introducing advanced practice nurses/nurse practitioners in health care systems: a framework for reflection and analysis. Swiss Med Weekly, 138:621–628.

Friedrichs A, Schaub H-A (2011). Academisation of the health professions – achievements and future prospects. GMS Z Med Ausbild, 28(4):Doc50.

Gravina EW. (2017). Competency-based education and its effect on nursing education: a literature review. Teaching and Learning in Nursing, 12:117–121.

Hale C (2003). Interprofessional education: the way to a successful workforce? Br J Ther Rehab, 10:122–127.

Kovner CT, Brewer C, Katigbak C et al. (2012). Charting the course for nurses' achievement of higher education levels. J Prof Nursing, 28:333–343.

Kroezen M, Dussault G, Craveiro I et al. (2015). Recruitment and retention of health professionals across Europe: a literature review and multiple case study research. Health Policy, 119:1517–1528.

Lahtinen P, Leino-Kilpi H, Salminen L (2014), Nursing education in the European higher education area – variations in implementation. Nurse Educ Today, 34:1040–1047.

Nousiainen M, McQueen SA, Hall J et al. (2016). Resident education in orthopaedic trauma. *Bone Joint J*, 98-B:1320–1325.

Reeves S, Perrier L, Goldman J et al. (2013). Interprofessional education: effects on professional practice and healthcare outcomes (update). Cochrane Database Syst Rev, 3:CD002213.

Salyers VL (2005). Web-enhanced and face-to-face classroom instructional methods: Effects on course outcomes and student satisfaction. Int J Nursing Educ Scholarship 2:Article 29. doi: 10.2202/1548-923x.1169.

Schoenstein M, Ono T, Lafortune G (2016). Skills use and skills mismatch in the health sector: what do we know and what can be done. In: Lafortune G, Moreira L, eds. Health workforce policies in OECD countries: right jobs, right kills, right places. OECD health policy studies. Paris. OECD Publishing. Paris, OECD Publishing, pp. 163–183.

4 Keeping people healthy: skill-mix innovations for improved disease prevention and health promotion

STEPHAN VAN DEN BROUCKE, KATARZYNA
CZABANOWSKA, HANNAH BUDDE, LAURA
PFIRTER, CLAUDIA B. MAIER

4.1 Introduction

Health services in most European countries were developed to meet the needs of demand-led health care. Although they still focus mostly on treatment, cure and care (Beaglehole & Dal Poz, 2003), the growing burden of noncommunicable diseases, along with newly emerging communicable diseases and increasing antimicrobial resistance, create strong and shifting demands on these services. At the same time, the growing prevalence of multimorbidity and the widening health inequalities pose additional threats to health systems that do not give enough attention to the factors that produce health. To address these challenges, it is necessary to reorient health services towards more preventive, people-centred and community-based approaches, with a more prominent role for disease prevention and health promotion, integrated within the wider health system.

Reorienting the health services is a key component of health promotion. The Ottawa Charter (World Health Organization, 1986) and the Astana declaration, which renewed the global policy commitment to public health and primary health care (World Health Organization/ UNICEF, 2018), explicitly mention it as an action area, next to building healthy public policies, developing personal skills, creating supportive environments and strengthening community action. But compared with the other action areas of health promotion, reorienting the health services has so far received relatively limited attention. This may be because there is limited understanding of the specific capacities that are needed for a health system to be more health-enabling.

In recent years, however, interest in integrating prevention and health promotion in health systems and strengthening their capacities for that purpose is growing. For instance, prevention and health promotion are included in the 10 Essential Public Health Operations listed in the WHO Regional Office for Europe's European Action Plan for Strengthening Public Health Capacities and Services (World Health Organization, 2016). In 2012, the European Commission commissioned a mapping of the public health capacities in EU Member States, focusing on enabling factors such as knowledge development, workforce, resources, organizational structure, partnerships, leadership and governance (Aluttis et al., 2013). More recently, the WHO Regional Office for Europe brought together a Coalition of Partners of experts from the public health community to accelerate the process of strengthening public health capacities and services by focusing on the enablers of these services (Van den Broucke, 2017).

A competent health workforce is one of these enablers. Whereas a well-trained health workforce has always been considered a key condition for the delivery of effective health services, the nature of the necessary competencies is being redefined in light of the current reorientation of these services. Primary care providers can play an important role in engaging individuals and communities in health promotion and disease prevention activities, yet this role is often underdeveloped or lacking due to high workloads, and lack of expertise and skills, or funding. The growing recognition of disease prevention and health promotion provides new opportunities to tackle these barriers. Within the diversifying primary care and public health workforce, new skills and tasks are being added to existing professional roles, new professional profiles emerge, and collaborations between professions become more important.

In the next section, we will provide an overview of skill-mix strategies that exist in primary and secondary prevention and health promotion, and consider the evidence of their effects while also pointing out the existing gaps in evidence and research. Next, we will summarize common trends and patterns of the major skill-mix developments and reforms that occurred across Europe, and present country examples in different contexts.

4.2 Research evidence on outcomes of skill-mix changes addressing prevention and health promotion

To document the skill-mix strategies that exist in primary and secondary prevention and health promotion, an overview of reviews was performed, resulting in a total of 35 systematic reviews on skill-mix changes (see Box 4.1). Ten reviews analysed the outcomes of skill-mix changes focusing on health promotion and prevention in healthy populations or population groups. Nineteen reviews analysed skill-mix interventions aimed at the prevention of diseases in specific groups through lifestyle-related risk factors (for example, people at risk of cardiovascular diseases, nutrition-related conditions and various other risk factors). Seven reviews specifically looked at skill-mix changes related to screening of various population groups. The reviews covered in this chapter are concerned with health promotion and prevention for the population at large and for subgroups, whereas Chapter 8 focuses particularly on vulnerable groups and their needs (see Chapter 8).

Skill-mix interventions in health promotion and prevention across the life cycle

Ten reviews analysed changes to the roles and skills of teams or individual professions to expand health promotion activities across the lifespan (Table 4.1). The settings and teams varied considerably, but most of the interventions took place in ambulatory health care settings. Some reviews also analysed skill-mix changes in non-health sectors, such as schools or the homes of at-risk groups. Selected reviews focused on health promotion activities and/or prevention for children, such as healthy eating and weight reduction programmes at schools run by nurses (Schroeder, Travers & Smaldone, 2016). The skill-mix interventions outside the

---

Box 4.1 Overview of the evidence on skill-mix innovations for health promotion and prevention

- Number of reviews: A total of 35 systematic reviews analysed the outcomes of skill-mix changes in health promotion and/or prevention, covering over 848 individual studies.
- Country coverage: The studies were conducted in over 40 countries.
- Methods: Thirteen reviews performed meta-analyses.

Table 4.1 *Skill-mix interventions for health promotion and primary prevention across the life cycle*

Skill-mix interventions					Outcomes°	
Description of intervention [Sources]	Content of interventions and skill-mix changes	Profession(s) in intervention and in comparator group	Population	Country	Population-/Patient-related outcomes	Health-system-related outcomes
Primary care provider-delivered diet-related health advice [1,2]	Interventions to promote healthy diet, including dietary counselling, advice and referrals, nutrition assessment, education on physical activity, motivational interviews	Intervention: Primary care professionals, including GPs, (school-) nurses, dieticians, health counsellors, physicians, exercise professionals Comparison: n/r	Schoolchildren attending primary, middle or high school [1] or healthy adults attending primary care [2]	UK, USA, IT, DK, JP, AU, NZ, NL, FI, Asia	• Significant reduction in weight and BMI (BMI (adults); –0.48, 95% CI –0.84 to –0.12; BMI z-score (children): –0.10, 95% CI –0.15 to –0.05) [1] • Statistically significant increase in fruit, vegetable and dietary fibre consumption [2] • Decrease in total fat intake [2] • Mean decrease in serum cholesterol of 0.10 mmol/L (95% CI –0.19 to 0.00) [2]	

Intervention	Description	Provider / Comparison	Population	Countries	Findings
Primary care provider-provided physical activity promotion for adults [3]	Interventions to increase physical activity, including advice or counselling given face to face or by phone, vouchers for or referrals to leisure centres, motivational interviews and written material	Intervention: Physicians, nurses, physical activity specialists, physiotherapists, health promotion specialists, working alone or in a team. Comparison: n/r	Sedentary adults, aged >16 years	UK, NZ, USA, CH, NL, AU, CA	• Significantly improved self-reported physical activity at 12 months (OR 1.42, 95% CI 1.17–1.73; SMD 0.25, 95% CI 0.11–0.38) • Positive effects on cardiorespiratory fitness at 12 months • 1/6 studies reporting on adverse events found a significant increase of 11% in falls and 6% in injuries during 12 months of follow up
Various skill-mix changes to enhance maternity and child health by various professions and lay health workers [4,5]	Various interventions to improve maternal or child health including care collaboration, education programmes, social service referrals, multilingual and culturally sensitive approaches	Intervention: Nurses, coordinators, case-managers, mental health professionals, dieticians, social workers, obstetricians, gynaecologists [4] or lay health workers (paid or voluntary) [5]. Comparison: n/r or usual care	Pregnant women, mothers or/ and their children in primary and community health care, with low socioeconomic status, from various ethnic groups	USA, AU, CA, NZ, UK, IE, BR, CN, IN, MX, PH, TH, ZA, TR, BD, BF, ET, GH, IQ, JM, PK, TZ, VN, Nepal	• Significantly improved gestational age and birth weight [4] • Significantly improved outcomes on breastfeeding [5] • Significantly improved immunization childhood uptake (RR 1.22, 95% CI 1.10–1.37; $P = 0.0004$) [4,5] • Significantly reduced child morbidity (RR 0.86, 95% CI 0.75–0.99; $P = 0.03$), child mortality (RR 0.75, 95% CI 0.55–1.03; $P = 0.07$) and neonatal mortality (RR 0.76, 95% CI 0.57–1.02; $P = 0.07$) [5] • Significantly improved care coordination [4] • Cost savings [4] • Insignificant increase in the likelihood of seeking care for childhood illness (RR 1.33, 95% CI, 0.86 to 2.05; $P = 0.20$) (3) [5]

Table 4.1 *(cont.)*

Skill-mix interventions					Outcomes°		
Description of intervention [Sources]	Content of interventions and skill-mix changes	Profession(s) in intervention and in comparator group	Population	Country	Population-/Patient-related outcomes		Health-system-related outcomes
Home visits for pregnant women or mothers [6,7] or prevention of child maltreatment [8]	Home visits to eliminate health disparities through action on social determinants of health [6] or to improve prenatal care utilization and birth weight [7] or to prevent child maltreatment [8]. Interventions included counselling, referrals, sometimes combined with phone calls, clinic visits and transport	Intervention: Home visitor or case managers, CHWs, nurses, social workers psychologists, or paraprofessionals, physicians, teams, firefighter Comparison: n/r	Pregnant women or mothers and/or their children who are underserved, ethnic minorities or who are at high medical or social risk	AU, USA (not consistently reported)	• Significantly improved parenting knowledge and self-efficacy skills [6] • Significantly reduced depressive symptoms among pregnant women after stressor reduction intervention [6] • 7/17 studies found a significant increase in birth weight [7] • 5/24 studies reported significantly improved gestational age[7]		• Significantly fewer overnight hospital stays ($P < 0.01$) [6] • 5/11 studies with statistically significant rise in prenatal care utilization. Significant decrease among African American women in one study [7] • Cost savings ranged from €9206.64 to €182 912.59 (based on lifetime maltreatment cost value of €195 735.02)[a] [8]
Pharmacist-delivered smoking cessation [9]	Smoking cessation interventions through counselling, either one-to-one or within group session	Intervention: Community pharmacists Comparison: Community pharmacists	Adults who smoke, attending community pharmacies	SE, UK, USA	• Improved smoking abstinence rates (RR 2.21, 95% CI 1.49–3.29) • Nicotine replacement therapy plus counselling showed better abstinence rates		

| Expanded professional roles in health literacy education [10] | Lifestyle interventions to improve health literacy including information, self-management support, goal setting, group education, group empowerment, motivational interviews and coaching, exercise logs, physical activity prescriptions, face to face and/or by phone | Intervention: Multidisciplinary teams, physicians, lay worker, nurse, others. Comparison: n/r | Adults with at least one SNAPW (smoking, nutrition, alcohol, physical activity, weight) risk factor and low health literacy | AU, CA, CH, JP, NL, NZ, SE, UK, USA | • Improved health literacy in 71% of the included studies (37 out of 52), in particular among moderate to high-intensity interventions
• By profession: physician-delivered interventions showed improved health literacy in 33% (3 out of 9) of the studies, dietician/educator/nurse-delivered in 92% of the studies (11/12) and in 91% if provided in multiprofessional teams (10/11) |

Abbreviations: BMI: body mass index; CHW: community health worker; CI: confidence interval; GP: general practitioner; mmol/L: millimoles per litre; n/r, not reported; OR, odds ratio; RR, relative risk; SMD: standard mean deviation; TB: tuberculosis.

Country abbreviations: AU: Australia; BD: Bangladesh; BF: Burkina Faso; BR: Brazil; CA: Canada; CH: Switzerland; CN: China; DK: Denmark; ET: Ethiopia; FI: Finland; GH: Ghana; IE: Ireland; IN: India; IQ: Iraq; IT:Italy; JM: Jamaica; JP: Japan; MX: Mexico; NL: the Netherlands; NZ: New Zealand; PH: Philippines; PK: Pakistan; SE: Sweden; TH: Thailand; TR: Turkey; TZ: Tanzania; UK: the United Kingdom; USA: the United States of America; VN: Vietnam; ZA: South Africa.

Notes: [a] no profession-specific outcomes were found. [b] Cost savings ranged from 15 000 Australian dollars to 298 000 Australian dollars, based on lifetime maltreatment cost value of 318 760 Australian dollars (converted on 12 September 2018, rate: 1 Australian dollar = 0.61 euros),

Sources: [1] Schroeder, Travers & Smaldone (2016); [2] Bhattarai et al. (2013); [3] Orrow et al. (2012); [4] Kroll-Desrosiers et al. (2016); [5] Lewin et al. (2010); [6] Abbott & Elliott (2017); [7] Issel et. al. (2011); [8] Dalziel & Segal (2012); [9] Saba et al. (2014); [10] Dennis et al. (2012).

traditional boundaries of the primary care settings involved home visit programmes by nurses or other professionals to prevent child maltreatment (Dalziel & Segal, 2012), and home visits for pregnant women at risk (Abbott & Elliott, 2017). In the other reviews, the interventions took place (mainly) in primary or ambulatory care settings.

The reviews evaluated the outcomes of skill-mix innovations with a large number of different interventions as well as outcome measures used.

- Two systematic reviews analysed the impact of interventions to reduce overweight and obesity among children or adults attending primary care providers, run by school nurses (Schroeder, Travers & Smaldone, 2016) or various primary care professions (Bhattarai et al., 2013). The interventions included a mix of education, changes to nutrition and physical activity programmes as well as counselling to school children and parents (Bhattarai et al., 2013; Schroeder et al., Travers & Smaldone, 2016). Meta-analysis revealed a significant reduction in children's weight (Schroeder, Travers & Smaldone, 2016) and a significant increase of the intake of fruits, vegetables and dietary fibre among individuals attending primary care providers, whereas fat intake decreased (Bhattarai et al., 2013).
- Physical activity promotion for sedentary adults was delivered by various primary care providers who applied different strategies, such as counselling, advice and motivational interviewing. Self-reported physical activity significantly improved and positive effects were reported for cardiorespiratory fitness. However, one of six studies also reported adverse events, notably a significant increase of 11% in falls and 6% in injuries within 12 months follow up (Orrow et al., 2012).
- Skill-mix interventions that focused on enhanced maternity and child health through improved education, counselling and collaboration among professions revealed an improvement on several outcome measures (Kroll-Desrosiers et al., 2016; Lewin et al., 2010), including improved birth weight, particularly among ethnic minorities (Kroll-Desrosiers et al., 2016) and significantly improved outcomes on breastfeeding and childhood immunization uptake (Lewin et al., 2010). Interventions that showed enhanced care coordination were also associated with cost savings (Kroll-Desrosiers et al., 2016).
- Two home visit programmes on health promotion and prevention for disadvantaged (pregnant) women or mothers resulted in fewer inpatient hospital stays, improved health, self-efficacy and fewer

depressive symptoms (Abbott & Elliott, 2017). Moreover, significant increases in prenatal care utilization and birth weight were also found (Issel et al., 2011). One home visit programme for children at risk of maltreatment resulted in cost savings (Dalziel & Segal, 2012). The most cost-effective programmes reported by Dalziel & Segal (2012) used professional home visitors (for example, nurses, midwives, social workers) in a multidisciplinary team, who targeted high-risk populations and included interventions beyond home visiting.

- Saba et al. (2014) analysed a smoking cessation programme through counselling by community pharmacists, targeted at patients with tobacco consumption and provided at an individual or group level. Overall, these smoking cessation sessions in community pharmacies were associated with improved abstinence rates.
- One review assessed the contribution of various primary care providers to enhance health literacy among various population groups, including healthy adults and people at risk for developing chronic conditions (Dennis et al., 2012). The skill-mix interventions varied considerably, ranging from expanded roles to include health literacy counselling, to intense, bundled packages of counselling, goal setting, group empowerment sessions to develop health literacy skills and lifestyle changes. Interventions delivered by physicians were generally brief, but those provided by nurses and other health professions tended to be more comprehensive and resulted in a higher number of studies with improved health literacy outcomes.

Skill-mix interventions in prevention targeting at-risk groups

A second group of reviews concerned interventions that were directed at specific risk groups. The groups again varied considerably: some interventions were targeted at groups that were at risk of cardiovascular diseases (Table 4.2), that were overweight or obese (Table 4.3), or that had multiple risk factors (Table 4.4). Several systematic reviews also included patients who had already been diagnosed with a disease, whereby the focus was to delay the progression of the disease and prevent the onset of multimorbidity, hence the inclusion of these reviews in this chapter. Interventions took place in the primary or community care setting in various countries around the world. The majority of interventions introduced new roles for different professionals or shifted tasks from physicians to other professions.

Table 4.2 *Skill-mix interventions for prevention targeting at-risk groups with cardiovascular risk factors*

Skill-mix interventions					Outcomes[a]	
Description of Intervention	Interventions and skill-mix changes	Profession(s)	Population	Countries	Patient-related outcomes	Health-system-related outcomes
Prevention and management of cardiovascular diseases (CVD) risk factors by pharmacist or nurses [1–5]	Interventions such as written or verbal patient educational interventions, intensified patient care, patient-reminder systems and medication management	Intervention: Expanded roles by pharmacists and/ or nurses, working alone [2,5] or in collaboration with physicians [1,3,4] Comparison: GPs, pharmacists, physicians, nurses, cardiologists [1–3,5], n/r [4]	Patients with risk factors or diagnosis for CVD or prescribed lipid-lowering medication	AE, AU, BR, CA, CH, CL, CN, ES, HK, IN, PT, TH, TW, USA, [1–3,5]; n/r [4]	• Significant reduced systolic/ diastolic blood pressure (−8.1 mmHg, 95% CI −10.2 to −5.9/−3.8 mmHg, 95% CI −5.3 to −2.3) [1] or similar findings [3,5] • Significant reduced total cholesterol (−17.4 mg/L, 95% CI −25.5 to −9.2) [1]; (MD 17.57 mg/L, 95% CI 14.95–20.19) [4] or similar findings [5] • Significant benefits for BMI [5] • Significant reduced risk of smoking [1] • Significant improved medication adherence on lipid-lowering intake [4] • Nurse-led education improved QoL [2]	• Nurse-led education reduced readmission and hospitalization [2] • Nurse-led interventions were more cost-effective than usual care [2]

	Interventions	Intervention:/Comparison:	Population	Countries	Outcomes
Pharmacist-delivered CVD interventions [6]	Interventions included education, follow up, identification of drug-related problems, recommendations to patient's physician	Intervention: Community pharmacists Comparison: n/r	Patients at risk for CVD	AU, BE, BR, CA, CL, MX, NE, NL, SP, TR, UK, USA	• Significantly improved outcomes in most of the studies • Reduced HbA1c and systolic blood pressure
Physiotherapist-delivered physical activity-interventions[b] [7]	Physiotherapist interventions aimed at increasing physical activity levels	Intervention: Physiotherapists Comparison: Physiotherapists	Adults with risk factors for NCD or suffering from NCDs	AU, DE, NL, NO	• Significantly more patients achieved the minimum recommended physical activity levels (OR 2.15, 95% CI 1.35–3.43, $P = 0.001$) • Significant effect on total physical activity level (SMD 0.15, 95% CI 0.03–0.27, $P = 0.02$) • Efficacy of interventions did not differ based on their length

Abbreviations: CI: confidence interval; CVD: cardiovascular disease; GP: general practitioner; HbA1c: glycated haemoglobin; MD: mean difference; n/r: not reported; NCD: noncommunicable disease; OR: odds ratio, QoL: quality of life; SMD: standardized mean difference.

Country abbreviations: AE: United Arab Emirates; AU: Australia; BE: Belgium; BR: Brazil; CA: Canada; CH: Switzerland; CL: Chile; CN: China; ES: Spain; DE: Germany; HK: Hong Kong; IN: India; MX: Mexico; NE: Nigeria; NL: the Netherlands; NO: Norway; PT: Portugal; SP: Spain; TR: Turkey; TH: Thailand; TW: Taiwan; UK: the United Kingdom, USA: the United States of America.

Notes: [a] No profession-specific outcomes were found. [b] Intervention group includes both at-risk populations and patients with the disease(s).

Sources: [1] Santschi et al. (2011); [2] Rice et al. (2018); [3] Santschi et al. (2014); [4] Deichmann et al. (2016); [5] Santschi et al. (2012); [6] Ifeanyi-Chiazor et al. (2015); [7] Kunstler et al. (2018).

The outcomes of these skill-mix innovations covered a range of different interventions as well as patient- and health-system-related outcome measures:

- Out of the seven reviews identified, five addressed the prevention and management of cardiovascular risk factors by various professions, including pharmacists and/or nurses, alone or in collaboration with other professions such as GPs. Nurse- and pharmacist-led interventions comprised educational programmes, medication management and reminder systems. Patient-related outcomes improved for both nurse and pharmacist-led interventions. Overall, total cholesterol (Deichmann et al., 2016; Santschi et al., 2011, 2012), risk of smoking (Santschi et al., 2011), body mass index (Santschi et al., 2012) and blood pressure (Santschi et al., 2011, 2012, 2014) were reduced significantly in the intervention groups and quality of life improved (Rice, Say & Betihavas, 2018). Deichmann et al. (2016) reported significantly improved medication adherence on lipid lowering intake. Cost-effectiveness was reported for nurse-led interventions. Moreover, nurse-led education to at-risk groups led to reduced readmission and hospitalization rates (Rice et al., 2018).
- Interventions provided by community pharmacists covered patient education and follow up as well as identification of drug-related problems and providing therapeutic recommendations to physicians. Most studies reported positive effects on patient-related outcomes. Interventions for patients with diabetes and hypertension showed clinically reduced blood pressure and glycated haemoglobin (Ifeanyi Chiazor et al., 2015).
- Clinic-based interventions by physiotherapists aimed at increasing physical activity generally involved face-to-face contact on a one-to-one basis, and often included additional telephone contact. The interventions showed significant positive effects on the total physical activity and significantly helped patients to achieve the minimum recommended level of physical activity (Kunstler et al., 2018).

Six systematic reviews reported on interventions directed at populations with a high body mass index, including adults and children with overweight or obesity and patients with special nutritional needs (Table 4.3).

- The effects of nurse-led weight management and lifestyle counselling were evaluated in three systematic reviews. The programmes

Table 4.3 *Skill-mix interventions for prevention targeting at-risk groups with body mass/nutrition-related risk factors*

Skill-mix interventions

Description of intervention	Interventions and skill-mix changes	Profession(s)	Population	Countries	Outcomes[a] Patient-related outcomes	Health-system-related outcomes
Nurse-delivered weight management interventions and lifestyle counselling[b] [1–3]	Lifestyle interventions, including behavioural counselling, goal setting, motivational interviewing, lifestyle education [1–3] and the use of theoretically based behaviour change techniques [1]	Intervention: Nurses, alone or with multidisciplinary teams (e.g. dieticians, CHWs, physiotherapists) Comparison: GPs, cardiologists, paediatric or public health nurses, nutritionists [2,3], n/r [1]	Children and adults, in most studies with socioeconomic, lifestyle or health-related risk factors, few with a diagnosis or chronic disease	UK, USA, FI, NL, NZ, AU, NO, SE, RU, TR, TW	• Statistically significant weight reduction [1–3] • Significant improvements in systolic and diastolic blood pressure, cholesterol, favourable dietary intake, fitness status, physical activity and health status [1] • Patient satisfaction increased statistically significant [3] or insignificant [1] • Practice nurses achieved equally good health outcomes compared to GPs [3]	• Practice nurses took longer in their consultations than GPs [3] • Nurses' more comprehensive approach: more likely to address weight, diet and physical activity than that of GPs[3]

Table 4.3 (cont.)

Skill-mix interventions					Outcomes[a]	
Description of intervention	Interventions and skill-mix changes	Profession(s)	Population	Countries	Patient-related outcomes	Health-system-related outcomes
Diet-related intervention by various professions [4,5]	Interventions to promote healthy diet, including dietary counselling, advice, information and referrals, assessment, motivational interviews, diagnosis and monitoring	Intervention: Health care professionals (e.g. dieticians, GPs, nurses, physicians, exercise professionals), working alone or in a multidisciplinary team Comparison: n/r	Adults, attending primary care, in most studies with lifestyle-related risk factors and few with chronic diseases	UK, USA, AU, BR, CA, DK, HK, IT, JP, KR, PT, TR, TW, NZ, NL, FI	• Significant improvements in dietary behaviours [4,5] • Significant increase in daily vegetable and fruit intake, fish intake and consumption of high-fibre bread [4] • Significantly improved glycaemic control, anthropometry and cholesterol, triglycerides [5]	
Skill-mix and organizational changes on weight reduction[b] [6]	Interventions to change the behaviour of health professionals or the organization of care to promote weight reduction	Intervention: Physicians, dieticians, nurses, NPs Comparison: Professionals delivering standard care	Children and adults with overweight or obesity, some with comorbidities	AU, UK, USA	• Reduced weight with care provided by a dietician (−5.60 kg, 95% CI −4.83 kg to −6.37 kg) and by a doctor-dietician team (−6.70 kg, 95% CI −7.52 kg to −5.88 kg) • Reduced BMI z-score with shared care (adjusted MD −0.05, 95% CI −0.14 to 0.03)	• Weight loss was achieved at a modest cost

Abbreviations: BMI: body mass index; CHW: community health worker; CI: confidence interval; GP: general practitioner; MD: mean difference; n/r: not reported; NP: nurse practitioner; OR: odds ratio; SMD: standardized mean difference.

Country abbreviations: AU: Australia; BR: Brazil; CA: Canada; DK: Denmark; FI: Finland; HK: Hong Kong; IT: Italy; JP: Japan; KR: South Korea; NL: the Netherlands; NO: Norway; NZ: New Zealand; PT: Portugal; SE: Sweden; TR: Turkey; TW: Taiwan; UK: the United Kingdom; USA: the United States of America.

Notes: [a] No profession-specific outcomes were found. [b] Intervention group includes both at-risk populations and patients with disease(s)

Sources: [1] Sargent, Forrest & Parker (2012); [2] Petit Francis et al. (2017); [3] Van Dillen & Hiddink (2014); [4] Ball et al. (2015); [5] Mitchell et al. (2017); [6] Flodgren et al. (2017).

encompassed consultation, motivational interviewing and education. Body mass index and overweight were significantly reduced in the intervention groups (Petit Francis et al., 2017; Sargent, Forrest & Parker, 2012; van Dillen & Hiddink, 2014). Significant improvements were also reported for weight control, blood pressure, cholesterol and physical activity (Sargent et al., 2012). Successful programmes involved nurses engaged in health promotion activities, operating within multidisciplinary teams and/or providing consultations, physical activity education and coaching over the phone (van Dillen & Hiddink, 2014).

- Individualized nutrition care for patients with special dietary needs delivered by health care professionals including dieticians and nurses working alone or in teams ranged from assessment and diagnosis to intervention and monitoring. These interventions led to a significant increase of the daily intake of vegetables, fruits, fish and high-fibre bread (Ball et al., 2015), and significantly improved glycemic control, dietary change, anthropometry, cholesterol, triglycerides (Mitchell et al., 2017).

- One Cochrane review analysed two types of interventions on weight reduction. Interventions by health professionals covered different strategies including educational programmes, whereas interventions addressing the care organization involved multidisciplinary teams and shared care models. Significantly reduced weight and body mass index scores were reported for the dietician-led and shared care (dietician–physician) interventions. Interventions directed at professionals, such as education, tailoring and clinical decision tools, showed only a small positive effect on weight loss. Weight loss was achieved at modest costs in the interventions provided by physicians only or in collaboration with dieticians (Flodgren et al., 2017).

Six systematic reviews were concerned with multiple risk groups (Table 4.4). The interventions focused on task shifting and the uptake of new roles by nurses, pharmacists or lay health workers. The results in terms of patient and health system outcomes were mixed.

- One review evaluated task shifting with regard to secondary prevention from physicians to nurses. Nurse practitioners and other specialized nurses with additional training took over tasks from physicians in the secondary prevention and performed them independently or under supervision of a physician. Prevention measures

Table 4.4 *Skill-mix interventions for prevention targeting at-risk groups with multiple risk factors*

Skill-mix interventions				Outcomes	
Description of intervention	Interventions and skill-mix changes	Profession(s)	Population	Countries	Patient-related outcomes	Health-system-related outcomes
Nurse task shifting interventions under autonomous or delegated responsibility[b] [1]	Physician–nurse task shifting for secondary/tertiary prevention. Tasks included assessments, history taking, diagnostics, monitoring, prescriptions, referrals, follow ups	Intervention: NPs, licensed nurses Comparison: Family physicians, paediatricians, geriatricians	Patients in primary care with wide range of diagnoses (e.g. type 2 diabetes, hypertension)	NL, RU, UK, ZA	• Most studies (84%) showed no significant differences between nurse-led care and physician-led care • Nurse-led care showed better outcomes in secondary prevention of heart diseases • Positive effect in managing dyspepsia and lowering CVD risk in diabetic patients • Significantly reduced differences for stroke risk and CHD risk	

Health-related lifestyle advice by professionals or lay health workers [2–4]	Lifestyle advice, including physical activity or nutrition counselling, goal setting, education, identifying barriers, introducing self-management. Delivered in person, by phone, post or online	Intervention: Various health care professionals [3,4] or trained, but unqualified health-related lifestyle advisors [2] Comparison: n/r	Patients with lifestyle-related risk factors (for CVD, diabetes, overweight, fatty liver disease, hypertension)	AU, FI, NL, SE, US [4]; n/r [2, 3]	• Significant reduction in weight (5/6) [3] • Increased physical activity [3] • Little evidence for the effectiveness of interventions for promotion of exercise or improved diets [2], significant decrease in blood pressure (6/7) [3], improved blood lipids [2] and blood glucose control (7/10) [3] • Improved cardiovascular risk factors [4] • Cost-effectiveness varied, but was predominantly positive [2]
Pharmacist-delivered interventions [5]	Interventions included education, follow up, recommendations for preventing or managing diabetes or CVD and/or their major risk factors	Intervention: Pharmacists Comparison: Pharmacists	Patients at risk or suffering from diabetes or CVD	n/r	• Some interventions (patient education, patient follow up, identification of drug-related problems and subsequent physician recommendations) were effective in the majority of studies

Table 4.4 *(cont.)*

Skill-mix interventions				Outcomes		
Description of intervention	**Interventions and skill-mix changes**	**Profession(s)**	**Population**	**Countries**	**Patient-related outcomes**	**Health-system-related outcomes**
Nurse-led prevention of falling [6]	Structured home-based health promotion to prevent falls	Intervention: Public health nurses, community nurses, specialist nurses Comparison: GPs and other health professionals	Older patients >75 years with long-term medical needs such as chronic heart failure, Parkinson's disease, stroke	UK	• Significantly reduced risk of death (OR 0.80, 95% CI 0.68–0.95) • Reduction in falls, but not significant	• No significant effect on hospital admission and number of individuals moving into residential care • Three studies on costs found potential cost savings, but face several limitations

Abbreviations: CHD: coronary heart disease; CVD: cardiovascular disease; n/r: not reported; NP: nurse practitioner.

Country abbreviations: AU: Australia; FI: Finland; NL: the Netherlands; RU: Russian Federation; SE: Sweden; UK: the United Kingdom; USA: the United States of America; ZA: South Africa.

Notes: ᵃ No profession-specific outcomes were found. ᵇ Intervention group includes both at-risk populations and patients with disease(s).

Sources: [1] Martínez-González et al. (2015); [2] Pennington et al. (2013); [3] Tapsell & Neale (2016); [4] Frerichs et al. (2012); [5] Evans et al. (2011); [6] Tappenden et al. (2012).

were delivered during the course of disease to patients with various diagnoses. Most studies included in this review did not show a difference in patient-related outcomes between nurse-led and physician-led care. Some studies showed better outcomes for nurse-led secondary prevention of heart diseases, for managing dyspepsia and for lowering cardiovascular risk in individuals with diabetes and for significantly lowering differences in mean fall from baseline for stroke risk (Martínez-González et al., 2015).

- Several reviews evaluated health-related lifestyle advice performed by either trained lay health workers (Pennington et al., 2013) or by various health care professionals (Frerichs et al., 2012; Tapsell & Neale, 2016). The interventions were directed at adults with different health conditions and encompassed education, counselling and support delivered in person, via telephone or electronically. Improved cardiovascular risk factors (Frerichs et al., 2012) and physical activity and significantly improved blood pressure, blood glucose control, weight (Tapsell & Neale, 2016) and blood lipids (Pennington et al., 2013) were reported. However, little evidence of effectiveness, measured via resource use, was reported for interventions promoting exercise or healthy diets. Where interventions were effective, their cost-effectiveness varied greatly. Incremental cost-effectiveness ratios were estimated at £6000 for smoking cessation, £14 000 for a telephone-based type 2 diabetes management and £250 000 or greater for promotion of mammography attendance and for HIV prevention among drug users (Pennington et al., 2013).

- One review focused on pharmacist interventions to prevent diabetes or cardiovascular diseases in patients at risk or to improve self-management in already diagnosed patients. The interventions combined patient education, follow up, identifying drug-related problems and providing recommendations for the prevention and management of the diseases. Patient education, patient follow up, identification of drug-related problems and subsequent physician recommendations were effective in the majority of studies (Evans et al., 2011).

- One review focused on nurse-led prevention of falling in older patients with multiple risk factors at risk of admission to hospital, residential or nursing care. The review showed a significantly reduced risk of death associated with the intervention, but could not show a significant effect on the number of falls and admissions to hospital and residential care. The identified economic evaluations tended to show cost savings, but faced several methodological shortcomings (Tappenden et al., 2012).

Table 4.5 *Skill-mix interventions with a focus on screening*

Skill-mix interventions					Outcomes[a]	
Description of intervention	Interventions and skill-mix changes	Profession(s)	Population	Countries	Patient-related outcomes	Health-system-related outcomes
Patient navigation [1-3]	Patient navigator such as face-to-face, mail, phone interventions including education or support in identifying barriers, setting up appointments and by making reminder calls	Intervention: Trained lay-persons or health professionals (e.g. bilingual), working in a team; Comparison: n/r [1,2]; Control group without PN or intervention group before intervention [3]	Patients in primary care, medically underserved (often vulnerable) [1-3] as well as non-proficient Anglophone populations [3]	USA, BD, CA	• Increased access to screenings (OR 2.48, 95 % CI 1.93-3.18, $P < 0.00001$) [1], improved breast, cervical or colorectal cancer screening [2], significant increased screenings rates for breast, cervical, or colorectal cancer (14/15 studies) [3] • Improved completion of diagnostics [2]	• Increased probability to attend recommended care events (OR 2.48, 95% CI 1.27-5.10, $P = 0.008$) [1] • Improved referral and follow up [2]
Transdisciplinary interventions with focus on social determinants of health [4]	Home visits conducted alone or as part of a transdisciplinary community secondary prevention to eliminate health disparities through action on social determinants of health	Intervention: CHWs, paraprofessionals, nurses, social workers, physicians, firefighter, research staff, case managers Comparison: n/r	Disadvantaged populations, including ethnic minorities	USA	• Significantly improved mammography attendance ($P < 0.01$), Papanicolaou screening ($P < 0.01$) and Hepatitis B screening ($P < 0.01$) • No significant difference in prostate cancer screening rates in low-income African-American men	

Interventions to improve cervical cancer screening [5]	Interventions to improve screening, diagnosis or treatment, through patient navigation or education with written or multimedia materials	Intervention: Nurses, NPs, lay health workers, community health aides, physicians, care managers Comparison: n/r	Racial and ethnic minority, as well as low-income women	USA	• Increase in cervical cancer screening rates when education was delivered by lay health workers in combination with other interventions, as well as through navigation and phone support • Significant increase in screening rates through multiple interventions and unique combinations in multiple interventions
Nurse-delivered colorectal cancer screening [6]	Nurse-led endoscopy in colorectal cancer screening	Intervention: Endoscopy nurses, NPs Comparison: Gastroenterologists, general surgeons, physician endoscopists	Asymptomatic males and females aged 45 years and older	USA, CA	• Nurses detected significantly higher adenomas compared with physicians and polyps at similar rates to endoscopists • Absence of complications during endoscopy • Greater patient satisfaction for nurse-led care • Nurse-led endoscopy produced lower costs compared with physician-led by approximately $100 (Nurse: $183, Physician: $283)

Table 4.5 *(cont.)*

Skill-mix interventions					Outcomes[a]	
Description of intervention	Interventions and skill-mix changes	Profession(s)	Population	Countries	Patient-related outcomes	Health-system-related outcomes
Nurse-delivered skin cancer screening [7]	Nurse-led clinical skin cancer assessment/ examination	Intervention: APNs, NPs, specialized nurses Comparison: Physicians, general or expert dermatologists	Patients eligible for skin cancer (melanoma) screening	UK, USA (not consistently reported)	• High sensitivity to identify malignant lesions by NPs (100%) • Dermatology nurses showed less sensitivity compared with dermatologists with expertise in skin cancer and general dermatologists	

Abbreviations: APN: advanced practice nurse; CHW: community health worker; CI: confidence interval; n/r: not reported; NP: nurse practitioner; PN: patient navigator; OR: odds ratio.

Country abbreviations: BD: Bangladesh; CA: Canada; UK: the United Kingdom; USA: the United States of America.

Notes: [a] No profession-specific outcomes were found.

Sources: [1] Al-Faisal et al. (2017); [2] Roland et al. (2017); [3] Genoff et al. (2016); [4] Abbott & Elliott (2017); [5] Glick et al. (2012); [6] Joseph, Vaughn & Strand (2015); [7] Loescher, Harris & Curiel-Lewandrowski (2011).

Skill-mix interventions targeting screenings

Seven reviews focused on interventions by health professionals or lay health workers to facilitate the access to screenings. There were also non-health professionals involved, such as firefighters.

- The role of a patient navigator was introduced in three reviews for patients completing screenings, mostly targeting vulnerable individuals. Patient navigators, including health professionals, trained lay persons and community health workers and provided assistance in person, via mail or phone to increase screening and diagnostic rates. As a result, patients were significantly more likely to attend recommended care events and attend screenings (Ali-Faisal et al., 2017). Roland et al. (2017)) also reported increased screening and mammography uptake and improved completion of diagnostics, referral and follow up. Genoff et al. (2016) showed significantly improved screening rates for breast, cervical and colorectal cancer.
- Transdisciplinary secondary prevention interventions in the community targeting the social determinants of health were conducted through home visits in the review by Abbott and Elliott (2017). These were delivered by physicians, nurses, social workers, community health workers and firefighters. Disadvantaged population groups reported significantly improved mammography attendances, Papanicolaou cervical screenings and Hepatitis B screenings. However, no significant difference was found for prostate cancer screening rates among low-income African-American men.
- Interventions to improve screening of cervical cancer in women through patient navigation or education resulted in increased screening rates when interventions were delivered by lay health workers (Glick et al., 2012).
- Nurse-delivered colorectal cancer screenings in asymptomatic adults aged 45 years or more showed that nurses detected significantly higher rates of adenomas compared with physicians, and polyps at comparable rates to endoscopists. Higher patient satisfaction and absence of complications were also among the positive outcomes. Regarding resource use, nurse-led screenings resulted in lower costs compared with physician-led services (Joseph, Vaughan & Strand, 2015).
- One review focused on skin cancer screening, including the assessment and examination performed by nurse practitioners, other

advanced practice nurses or specialized nurses. The interventions were compared to screenings conducted by physicians or general and expert dermatologists. Overall, nurses showed a high sensitivity to identify malignant lesions, although there were differences in their level of specialization and sensitivity (Loescher, Harris & Lewandrowski, 2011).

Education and training of the professionals involved in the skill-mix interventions

The training of the professionals was not systematically reported across the systematic reviews reported in the previous sections. However, some reviews provided information on the educational background of the professionals who had been included in the skill-mix interventions. For instance, Loescher, Harris & Lewandrowski (2011) noted that nurse practitioners and advanced practice nurses underwent additional training programmes for skin cancer screening ranging from 10 minutes to 4 months, demonstrating the variability in the length of training.

Limitations and strength of evidence

The systematic reviews presented above did not systematically report comparison groups and interventions. Due to the great heterogeneity of the interventions covered in the reviews, some of which report complex interventions that also alter the organization of care, the attribution of causality between skill-mix interventions and outcomes must be done with caution. Health-system-related outcomes were less frequently evaluated than patient/population-specific outcomes, whereas profession-specific outcomes are missing. The quality of the reviews also varied considerably: there were 13 meta-analyses, four cost-effectiveness analyses and two Cochrane reviews.

Conclusions: summary of the evidence

As documented in the majority of the reviews summarized above, skill-mix innovations for health promotion and prevention show evidence of positive outcomes for patients and for the health systems. Health promotion and primary prevention across the life cycle have become increasingly the remit of primary care professionals. Several skill-mix innovations have emerged that explicitly focus on health promotion or prevention, ranging from the allocation of tasks to nurses and pharmacists to shared care models. Overall, these have shown a positive impact on individuals or risk groups in terms of lifestyle choices and outcomes. Moreover, innovative programmes such as home visits to prevent child maltreatment can save costs. Outcomes associated with cardiovascular, body mass and various other risk factors have given proof of improved patient- and health-system-related effects. The introduction of patient navigators as well as transdisciplinary home visits can be an effective strategy to expand screening rates, particularly for vulnerable population groups or individuals who would otherwise not participate in screenings.

4.3   Skill-mix innovations and reforms: trends

The skill-mix innovations for primary or secondary prevention and health promotion reviewed in the previous section can be considered against the backdrop of three major trends that can be observed in the health sector, and particularly in public health.

More informed decision-making

Shared decision-making, defined as "an approach where clinicians and patients share the best available evidence when faced with the task of making decisions" (Elwyn et al., 2012), as opposed to clinicians making decisions on behalf of patients, is gaining increasing prominence in health care. The trend is not restricted to decisions on medical treatment, but is also seen in preventive health and health promotion (for example, screening participation, vaccination, breastfeeding, diet advice). Policy-makers are often favourable towards the idea of shared decision-making, not only because they support the right of patients and citizens to be involved in decisions concerning their own health, but also because of its potential to reduce overuse of interventions that are not clearly associated with benefits for all, to reduce unwarranted health care practice variations, and to enhance the sustainability of the health care system (Légaré et al., 2018). The value of shared decision-making is supported by evidence from a growing number of studies showing knowledge gain by patients, more confidence in decisions, more active patient involvement, and generally a choice for more conservative treatment options (Elwyn et al., 2012). However, to allow for shared decisions, patients and citizens who decide on preventive measures must have the capacity to act independently and to make their own choices. Shared decision-making therefore depends on tasks that help confer agency on the patients by providing them with information about the likely benefits and risks of different options, and by supporting the decision-making process, taking into account their personal values and preferences. This process involves a continuing dialogue between health providers and decision-makers. Apart from a sufficient level of health literacy on the part of the patient, it requires adequate communication skills on the part of health workers. But more importantly, it also implies an important shift in the role of health workers, from that of an expert making decisions for the patient to that of an educator and coach in the decision-making process. To make this possible, new tasks must be added to their task description. The reviews summarized above make clear that new tasks and roles with a focus on health promotion or prevention are being introduced in primary care. Not only are tasks allocated to other actors such as nurses, nurse-practitioners, pharmacists, community health workers, patient navigators and lay persons, but more elaborate shared care models are also beginning to emerge. Overall, these skill-mix innovations have shown a positive impact on individuals or at-risk groups in terms of lifestyle choices and outcomes.

Internet as a health information source

With the availability of the internet and changes in media health coverage, the context in which patients consume medical and health information has changed dramatically. A Eurobarometer study on European citizens' digital health literacy (Eurobarometer, 2014) revealed that six out of ten European respondents use the internet to search for health-related information, and over half of these do so at least once per month. Information about health topics is abundantly available, but not always accurate and often contradictory. As such, being well-informed about health is not so much a matter of finding information, but rather a question of finding out which information sources that are accessed give adequate and useful information, and whether they are reliable.

As these changes influence the ways in which individuals obtain, interpret and evaluate health information, they also have an impact on the role of health care providers. Whereas traditionally physicians were gatekeepers of health care information and services to their patients, most physicians are now experiencing the effects of patients coming to their offices armed with printouts from the internet and requesting certain procedures, tests or medications (Hesse et al., 2005). Although patients still rely on health care providers as their most trusted information source on health, the role of physicians may no longer be seen as solitary caretakers but as trusted partners in helping patients sort through information derived from an expanding network of personal and mediated information channels. Again, this new role requires a series of new skills and a reorganization of the task division within the health system, with tasks being allocated to a range of actors within the health sector to ensure that patients' information needs and questions are being addressed.

A diverse and expanding primary care and public health workforce

Unlike the medical workforce, with its clearly established professions and curricula, the workforce for public health is very diverse. In addition to public health specialists (epidemiologists, health policy-makers, health educators, environmental health experts, health economists) and professionals in primary or ambulatory health care (physicians, nurses, dentists, pharmacists, midwives), there is also an important role for those who are not directly involved in health organizations, but whose activities can contribute to improving population health, such as social workers, teachers, police or urban planners (Aluttis et al., 2014). In this regard, Davies (2013) makes a distinction between specialist and mainstreamed public health and health promotion workers. The first are specialists at both academic and professional levels who have been trained in public health or health promotion as a scholarly discipline and who possess the knowledge, skills and practical experience to perform their tasks. The second are people inside and outside the health sector who work to promote health as defined by the Ottawa Charter, regardless of their professional designation. They represent the social movement aspect of public health and health promotion, more than the discipline.

Within the specialist public health and health promotion workforce, tasks are increasingly shared by or reallocated between professions. Prevention and health promotion tasks are taken up by specialists from a growing range of disciplines. For instance, public health nurses are added to primary care centres and general practice in a number of countries, including France, the Netherlands and Slovenia. In a similar vein, pharmacists increasingly take up a role as health promotion actors. This was seen in Belgium, for example, where a programme was introduced allowing pharmacists to be paid a fee to provide medico-pharmaceutical advice to clients using new medication (Box 4.2).

This trend also necessitates an enhanced collaboration between different disciplines involved in prevention and health promotion. When tasks shift, the collaboration between health workers from different disciplines needs to be re-calibrated. This is seen in a pilot project on

---

Box 4.2 Pharmacists' support of novice users of medicines

In 2013, a New Medicines Service (NMS) was introduced in community pharmacies in Belgium to support asthma patients who were novice users of inhaler devices with corticosteroids. The protocol-based intervention used the Asthma Control Test (ACT) and the Medication Adherence Report Scale (MARS) to assess asthma control and medication adherence. The NMS was the first initiative that put advanced pharmaceutical care into practice in Belgium. An evaluation study involving telephone interviews with pharmacists, semi-structured interviews with patients eligible for NMS, focus groups with GPs and lung specialists, and a work system analysis in community pharmacies revealed that the introduction of the NMS programme was not sufficiently embedded in the Belgian health care organization (Fraeyman et al., 2017). As a result, there was low uptake and resistance to its implementation by pharmacists, patients and other health care professionals. Apart from practical barriers, pharmacists found it difficult to identify new asthma patients when they were not informed about the diagnosis. A lack of commitment from physicians, patients and pharmacists was also noted, especially in the early start-up phase of the programme. Many pharmacists did not see how NMS differed from existing pharmaceutical care. Physicians considered this service as part of their own tasks and discouraged ACT for asthma follow up in the community pharmacy. To increase the uptake of this type of service and its possible extension to other patient groups, more collaboration among the different health care professionals during design and implementation would be required, as well as systematic data collection to monitor the quality of the service, better training of pharmacists, and more information for patients and physicians.

Box 4.3 Introducing diabetes screening in the pharmacy

Diabetes mellitus is the fourth largest cause of death in the EU. Of the approximately 32 million people in the EU who live with type 2 diabetes, many are unaware of their condition. The high prevalence of undiagnosed diabetes and the risk of complications create a strong imperative for diabetes screening. Although testing for and diagnosing diabetes is a task for medical professionals, pharmacists can also play a role in screening patients at high risk for diabetes, assessing their health status, referring them to other health care professionals as appropriate, and monitoring outcomes, thus empowering patients to take informed decisions about their health. On the other hand, diabetes screening by pharmacists can be a challenge for the relationship between health care professionals, as it involves a shift in their respective roles and requires an optimization of the communication between them with regard to patient follow up. A project currently taking place in Belgium explores how the introduction of diabetes screening in pharmacies influences the health care relationship of pharmacists and GPs with their patients and the professional relationship between them, identifies the factors that encourage or impede this partnership relationship, and develop guidelines and tools to enhance a collaborative approach to diabetes screening.

---

setting up a system of regular and structured consultation between GPs and pharmacists in Brussels who sell diagnostic self-tests (Box 4.3).

Involvement of non-health professionals and citizens is also seen in mental health. Examples from Canada, the United Kingdom and France show the role of volunteers delivering "safe and well visits", mobile crisis teams, or firefighters responding to people who have been confronted with traumatic experiences.

4.4 Conclusions and outlook

The skill-mix innovations presented in this chapter respond to challenges within the health services that require a more prominent role for prevention and health promotion. The current healthcare landscape is characterized by a need for more informed decision-making, a rapidly expanding digitalization making the internet an important information source regarding health, new roles for primary care providers and a diversifying primary care and public health workforce. There are three different types of skill-mix innovations tackling the challenge: tasks are shifted and re-allocated, existing roles are expanded, and in some cases teamwork/consultation is introduced. In terms of proxy indicators, most examples have been successful in delivering services to needs which otherwise would have remained unaddressed. Several countries have introduced reforms with expanded roles for nurses, pharmacists, dieticians, GPs or other (often non-health) specialists, yet these reforms have so far remained at a small scale. Fully integrating individual health promotion and prevention activities into routine care remains a challenge in most countries, despite emerging evidence on the effectiveness of the interventions involving skill-mix innovations.

References

Abbott LS, Elliott LT (2017). Eliminating health disparities through action on the social determinants of health: a systematic review of home visiting in the United States, 2005–2015. Public Health Nurs, 34(1):2–30.

Ali-Faisal SF, Colella TJF, Medina-Jaudes N et al. (2017). The effectiveness of patient navigation to improve healthcare utilization outcomes: a meta-analysis of randomized controlled trials. Patient Educ Couns, 100(3):436–448. (http://www.sciencedirect.com/science/article/pii/S0738399116304839).

Aluttis C, Brand H, Michelsen K et al. (2013). Review of Public Health Capacity in the EU. Luxembourg, European Commission, DG SANCO.

Aluttis C, Maier CB, Van den Broucke S et al. (2014). Developing the public health workforce. In: Rechel B, McKee M, eds. Facets of Public Health in Europe. Maidenhead, Open University Press: 255–266.

Ball L, Leveritt M, Cass S et al. (2015). Effect of nutrition care provided by primary health professionals on adults' dietary behaviours: a systematic review. Fam Pract, 32(6):605–617.

Beaglehole R, Dal Poz M (2003). Public health workforce: challenges and policy issues. Hum Resour Health, 1: 4.

Bhattarai N, Prevost AT, Wright AJ et al. (2013). Effectiveness of interventions to promote healthy diet in primary care: systematic review and meta-analysis of randomised controlled trials. BMC Public Health, 13:1203. (https://www.ncbi.nlm.nih.gov/pubmed/24355095).

Dalziel K, Segal L (2012). Home visiting programs for the prevention of child maltreatment: cost-effectiveness of 33 programs. Arch Dis Childhood, 97(9):787.

Davies JK (2013). Health promotion: a unique discipline? Auckland, Health Promotion Forum of New Zealand.

Deichmann RE, Morledge MD, Ulep R et al. (2016). A meta-analysis of interventions to improve adherence to lipid-lowering medication. Ochsner J, 16(3):230–237. (https://www.ncbi.nlm.nih.gov/pubmed/27660570).

Dennis S, Williams A, Taggart J et al. (2012). Which providers can bridge the health literacy gap in lifestyle risk factor modification education: a systematic review and narrative synthesis. BMC Fam Pract, 13(1):44. (https://doi.org/10.1186/1471-2296-13-44).

Elwyn G, Frosch D, Thomson R et al. (2012). Shared decision making: a model for clinical practice. J Gen Intern Med, 27(10):1361–1367.

Eurobarometer (2014). European citizens' digital health literacy. A report to the European Commission. (https://ec.europa.eu/commfrontoffice/publicopinion/flash/fl_404_en.pdf, accessed 23 June 2020).

Evans C, Watson E, Eurich D et al. (2011). Diabetes and cardiovascular disease interventions by community pharmacists: a systematic review. Ann Pharmacother, 45:615–628.

Flodgren G, Gonçalves-Bradley DC, Summerbell CD (2017). Interventions to change the behaviour of health professionals and the organisation of care to promote weight reduction in children and adults with overweight or obesity. Cochrane Database Syst Rev (11). (https://doi.org//10.1002/14651858.CD000984.pub3).

Fraeyman J, Foulon V, Mehuys E et al. (2017). Evaluating the implementation fidelity of New Medicines Service for asthma patients in community pharmacies in Belgium. Res Soc Admin Pharmacy, 13(1):98–108.

Frerichs W, Kaltenbacher E, van de Leur JP et al. (2012). Can physical therapists counsel patients with lifestyle-related health conditions effectively? A systematic review and implications. Physiother Theory Pract, 28(8):571–587.

Genoff MC, Zaballa A, Gany F et al. (2016). Navigating language barriers: a systematic review of patient navigators' impact on cancer screening for limited English proficient patients. J Gen Intern Med, 31(4):426–434. (https://doi.org/10.1007/s11606-015-3572-3).

Glick SB, Clarke AR, Blanchard A et al. (2012). Cervical cancer screening, diagnosis and treatment interventions for racial and ethnic minorities: a systematic review. J Gen Intern Med, 27(8):1016–1032. (https://www.ncbi.nlm.nih.gov/pubmed/22798213).

Hesse BW, Nelson DE, Kreps GL et al. (2005). Trust and sources of health information: the impact of the Internet and its implications for health care providers: findings from the first Health Information National Trends Survey. Arch Intern Med, 165(22):2618–2624.

Ifeanyi Chiazor E, Evans M, van Woerden H et al. (2015). A systematic review of community pharmacists' interventions in reducing major risk factors for cardiovascular disease. Value in Health Regional Issues, 7:9–21. (http://www.sciencedirect.com/science/article/pii/S2212109915000102).

Issel LM, Forrestal SG, Slaughter J et al. (2011). A review of prenatal home-visiting effectiveness for improving birth outcomes. J Obstet Gynecol Neonat Nurs, 40(2):157–165.

Joseph J, Vaughan R, Strand H (2015). Effectiveness of nurse-performed endoscopy in colorectal cancer screening: a systematic review. Gastroint Nurs, 13:26–33.

Kroll-Desrosiers AR, Crawford SL, Moore Simas TA et al. (2016). Improving pregnancy outcomes through maternity care coordination: a systematic review. Women's Health Issues, 26(1):87–99. (http://www.sciencedirect.com/science/article/pii/S1049386715001607).

Kunstler BE, Cook JL, Freene N et al. (2018). Physiotherapist-led physical activity interventions are efficacious at increasing physical activity levels: a systematic review and meta-analysis. Clin J Sport Med, 28:304–315.

Légaré F, Adekpedjou R, Stacey D et al. (2018). Interventions for increasing the use of shared decision making by healthcare professionals. Cochrane Database Syst Rev, 7:CD006732.

Lewin S, Munabi-Babigumira S, Glenton C et al. (2010). Lay health workers in primary and community health care for maternal and child health and the management of infectious diseases (Review). Cochrane Database Syst Rev, 3:CD004015.

Loescher LJ, Harris JM Jr, Curiel-Lewandrowski C. (2011). A systematic review of advanced practice nurses' skin cancer assessment barriers, skin lesion recognition skills, and skin cancer training activities. J Am Acad Nurse Pract, 23(12):667–673.

Martínez-González NA, Tandjung R, Djalali S et al. (2015). The impact of physician-nurse task shifting in primary care on the course of disease: a systematic review. Hum Resour Health, 13:55.

Mitchell LJ, Ball LE, Ross LJ et al. (2017). Effectiveness of dietetic consultations in primary health care: a systematic review of randomized controlled trials. J Acad Nutr Dietet, 117(12):1941–1962. (http://www.sciencedirect.com/science/article/pii/S2212267217731002X).

Orrow G, Kinmonth A-L, Sanderson S et al. (2012). Effectiveness of physical activity promotion based in primary care: systematic review and meta-analysis of randomised controlled trials. BMJ, 344:e1389.

Pennington M, Visram S, Donaldson C et al. (2013). Cost-effectiveness of health-related lifestyle advice delivered by peer or lay advisors: synthesis of evidence from a systematic review. Cost Effect Resource Alloc, 11(1):30. (https://doi.org/10.1186/1478-7547-11-30).

Petit Francis L, Spaulding E, Turkson-Ocran R-A et al. (2017). Randomized trials of nurse-delivered interventions in weight management research: a systematic review. West J Nurs Res, 39(8):1120–1150.

Rice H, Say R, Betihavas V (2018). The effect of nurse-led education on hospitalisation, readmission, quality of life and cost in adults with heart failure. A systematic review. Patient Educ Couns 101(3):363–374. (http://www.sciencedirect.com/science/article/pii/S0738399117305578).

Roland KB, Milliken EL, Rohan EA et al. (2017). Use of community health workers and patient navigators to improve cancer outcomes among patients served by federally qualified health centers: a systematic literature review. Health Equity, 1(1):61–76.

Saba M, Diep J, Saini B et al. (2014). Meta-analysis of the effectiveness of smoking cessation interventions in community pharmacy. J Clin Pharm Ther, 39(3):240–247.

Santschi V, Chiolero A, Burnand B et al. (2011). Impact of pharmacist care in the management of cardiovascular disease risk factors: a systematic review and meta-analysis of randomized trials. JAMA Intern Med, 171(16):1441–1453.

Santschi V, Chiolero A, Paradis G et al. (2012). Pharmacist interventions to improve cardiovascular disease risk factors in diabetes: a systematic review and meta-analysis of randomized controlled trials. Diabetes Care, 35(12):2706–2717. (https://www.ncbi.nlm.nih.gov/pubmed/23173140).

Santschi V, Chiolero A, Colosimo AL et al. (2014). Improving blood pressure control through pharmacist interventions: a meta-analysis of randomized controlled trials. J Am Heart Assoc, 3(2):e000718.

Sargent GM, Forrest LE, Parker RM (2012). Nurse delivered lifestyle interventions in primary health care to treat chronic disease risk factors associated with obesity: a systematic review. Obesity Rev, 13(12):1148–1171. (https://www.ncbi.nlm.nih.gov/pubmed/22973970).

Schroeder K, Travers J, Smaldone A (2016). Are school nurses an overlooked resource in reducing childhood obesity? a systematic review and meta-analysis. J School Health, 86(5):309–321.

Tappenden P, Campbell F, Rawdin A et al. (2012). The clinical effectiveness and cost-effectiveness of home-based, nurse-led health promotion for older people: a systematic review. Health Technol Assessment, 16(20):1–72. (https://www.ncbi.nlm.nih.gov/pubmed/22490205).

Tapsell L, Neale E (2016). The effect of interdisciplinary interventions on risk factors for lifestyle disease: a literature review. Health Educ Behav, 43:256–270.

Van den Broucke S (2017). Strengthening public health capacity through a health promotion lens. Health Promo Int, 32(5):763–767.

van Dillen SME, Hiddink GJ (2014). To what extent do primary care practice nurses act as case managers lifestyle counselling regarding weight management? A systematic review. BMC Fam Pract, 15:197. (https://www.ncbi.nlm.nih.gov/pubmed/25491594).

World Health Organization (1986). Ottawa charter for health promotion. Health Promo, 1, iii–v.

World Health Organization (2016). Midterm progress report on implementation of the European Action Plan for Strengthening Public Health Capacities and Services. Copenhagen, WHO Regional Office for Europe.

World Health Organization / UNICEF (2018). Declaration of Astana. Global Conference on Primary Health Care From Alma-Ata towards universal health coverage and the Sustainable Development Goals Astana, Kazakhstan, 25 and 26 October 2018. (https://www.who.int/docs/default-source/primary-health/declaration/gcphc-declaration.pdf, accessed 31 July 2019).

5 Caring for people with acute conditions: transitional care, relocation of care and new division of work

IVY BOURGEAULT, CHRISTINE BOND, ROMY MAHRER-IMHOF, HANNAH BUDDE, BERND RECHEL, CLAUDIA B. MAIER

5.1 Introduction

There is an overall trend towards decreasing length of stay in hospitals. Earlier discharges and transitions to home and community care are increasing, as well as the use of outpatient clinics for acute care across European countries. How this is implemented varies significantly not only between but also within countries (Corbella et al., 2018). Some of the key drivers of these trends are: improvements in medical and surgical techniques and pharmacotherapies; increased use of e-health, m-health and digital technologies; efforts to reduce the risk of hospital-acquired infections; and tightening health care budgets where care in the community and ambulatory care settings is seen to be more cost effective (Busby, Purdy & Hollingworth, 2015; Marschang & Bernardo, 2015).

Earlier discharge and shorter hospital stays result in more patients with more complex conditions being treated in the community by health professionals in primary care and in specialized ambulatory care settings. All patients are vulnerable during care transitions from acute care, but most particularly adults with complex medical conditions and older adults with comorbidities or on polypharmacy regimens. Ineffective care transitions resulting from poor cross-site communication and collaboration can lead to suboptimal patient outcomes. Key factors fostering more effective care transitions include interdisciplinary coordination and collaboration of patient care across care sectors, shared accountability by all clinicians involved, provision of appropriate support and follow up after discharge (Sheikh et al., 2018), mutual respect, shared goals and good communication. New models of care easing the shift in the location of care use existing health professionals in new ways (for example, extended roles) or introduce new professionals (for example, physician assistants or retinal screeners). These changes reflect an ongoing and dynamic process.

We focus this chapter on the changing skill-mix of health professionals providing care for patients with acute illnesses. Acute illnesses are defined for the purpose of this chapter as all short-term, acute conditions, ranging from acute episodes of chronic conditions, such as stroke or myocardial infarction, which require highly specialized, coordinated health care across sectors (for example hospital–ambulatory care transitions), to minor acute illnesses that are often prevalent in primary care practices (such as influenza, pharyngitis, urinary tract infections). We begin with a review of the literature on the increasingly earlier shift of patients from hospital to outpatient, ambulatory and community care, with a focus on home care settings, and the use of the wider health care team in the management of acute presentations of conditions – both major and minor. We then provide an overview of recent trends across Europe and internationally of skill-mix changes and innovations. We present three case studies of skill-mix innovations and innovative models of care that optimize the scope of practice of health professionals.

Our analysis of literature reviews and recently published studies shows that there are some promising innovations involving various skill-mix interventions. Caution is necessary, however, in comparing seemingly similar models across different country contexts and assuming transferability across different clinical conditions and unique professional practices.

5.2   Evidence on outcomes based on an overview of reviews

Twenty-eight reviews were identified that focused on skill-mix changes for acute health conditions including acute episodes of chronic conditions (see Box 5.1). The majority ($n = 20$) assessed new skill-mix models across care settings or providers (transitional care). Four reviews assessed skill-mix changes due to relocation of services (hospital-at-home) and four assessed expanded roles for specific health professionals for (minor) acute illnesses.

Box 5.1 Overview of the evidence on skill-mix innovations in acute care patients

- Number of reviews: A total of 28 systematic reviews covering 637 individual studies, often RCTs, were identified.
- Country coverage: The studies were conducted in a large number of different EU countries and other, primarily high-income, countries, notably the USA.
- Methods: Of all reviews, six performed meta-analyses. One review was a Cochrane review.

Most reviews covered skill-mix changes to reduce disruptions at the interface between care sectors, with a focus on the transitioning of care from hospital to ambulatory care (Table 5.1). The population groups targeted by the interventions ranged from patients with stroke, acute myocardial infarction or other acute cardiovascular conditions, or acute pneumonia to pregnant women at risk, and transitional care between paediatric and adult care for patients with juvenile onset of rheumatic and musculoskeletal diseases.

5.3 Skill-mix strategies addressing acute conditions

Skill-mix interventions with a focus on transitional care

Improving the transition from one setting to another is critical for patients with acute conditions, as there is a risk of disruption in service delivery. Transitional care is defined as the various points where a patient moves to, or returns from, a particular physical location or makes contact with a health care professional for the purposes of receiving health care. This includes transitions between home, hospital, residential care settings and consultations with different health care providers in outpatient facilities (World Health Organization, 2016).

Skill-mix interventions to improve transitional care were analysed in 20 systematic reviews emanating from the overview of reviews. All reviews evaluated interventions before, at, or immediately after discharge from hospitals to ambulatory care services. The skill-mix interventions were clustered into transitional care roles performed by various professions. These reviews did not differentiate between the professions that performed the role of coordination or case management. Four and five

Table 5.1 *Summary of reviews: skill-mix on transitional care and early discharge planning*

Description of intervention	Content of interventions and skill-mix changes	Profession(s)	Population	Countries	Patient-related outcomes[a]	Health-system-related outcomes	Profession-specific outcomes
Transitional care roles, various professions [1–9]	Various roles including case manager role, care coordinator, transition coordinator. Interventions included structured pre- and/or post-discharge planning, pre-discharge education, home visits, medication reconciliation scheduling follow up and linkage with other services and sectors, mostly provided by multiprofessional teams in a community setting	Intervention: Nurses (incl. APN), clinical pharmacists, GPs, care coordinators, physiotherapists, social workers, stroke support workers, case managers, caregivers, transitional care teams (team composition including transition coordinator) Comparison: Pharmacists, family physician, cardiologist not consistently reported	Stroke patients [1,2], patients with community-acquired pneumonia [3] or older people [4], juvenile onset rheumatic and musculoskeletal disease patients [5], patients with heart failure [6,9], adults hospitalized for diverse conditions [7,8]	UK, USA, AU, CA, DE, BE, BR, NL, IT, IL, IE, IR, ES, CH, NZ, AT, CN, HK, TW, DK, IN, NO PT, SE, TH, SW, not consistently reported	• Improvement in mortality (OR 1.04, 95% CI 0.77–1.40, $P = 0.81$) in stroke patients [2] • Home-visits reduced mortality 3–6 months (RR 0.77, 95% CI 0.60–0.997), outpatient clinic-based interventions reduced mortality in patients with heart failure (RR 0.56, 95% CI 0.34–0.92) [9] • Reductions in post-discharge clinical adverse event rates [8] • Improved knowledge about the disease [1], adherence to appointments; quality of life; psychosocial and disease-specific health status [5]	• Case management reduced emergency visits [1,6]; increased outpatient appointments [1]; significantly reduced hospital stay (MD 5.5 days, 95% CI 2.9–8.2, $P < 0.0001$) [2,4] • Significant reduction of hospital readmission (RR 0.92, 95% CI 0.87–0.98) in heart failure patients [6,9], mixed results for older people, pneumonia [3,4,7,8] • High (vs low) intensity interventions with significantly improved effect for readmissions in heart failure [6] • No significant improvements in ED visits, GP visits and specialist clinic/outpatient visits for older people [4] and no difference for health service utilization [1]	

Intervention	Interventions covered	Provider	Population / Countries	Outcomes	Resource use
Pharmacist-led transitional care [10–13]	Interventions covered medication review, reconciliation and patient counselling and education	Intervention: Pharmacists, pre-graduate pharmacists, pharmacist technicians, nurses/ physicians (collaborator), GPs, community health care professionals Comparison: Physicians, nurses, care coordinators, others n/r	Patients with various acute conditions (e.g. heart failure, COPD, diabetes, coronary syndrome [13], (not consistently reported)) AU, BE, CA, CN, DK, ES, IR, SE, UK, USA	• No significant effect in physical functioning, mood, quality of life for patients and caregivers [1] • Little or no difference for mood status and subjective health status and participants' ADL [2] • Medication error significantly improved (OR 0.44, 95% CI 0.31–0.63) [11] • Mixed results on adverse drug event [10] • Mixed results on mortality [10] • No significant difference for all-cause mortality [12] • Improved medication adherence [13]	Resource use: • Community-initiated case management reported lower costs [4] • Estimated costs ranged from 23% lower to 15% higher costs for the intervention group [2] • ED visits reduced [10–12]; 2 meta-analyses: OR 0.42, 95% CI 0.22–0.78 [11] and RR 0.72, 95% CI 0.58–0.92 [12] • Mixed results on hospital readmissions [10–12] • Reduction in hospital visits due to adverse drug events (RR 0.33, 95% CI 0.20–0.53) [12] • No significant improvements for readmissions, hospitalizations, emergency visits and mortality [13] • Cost savings associated with difference in readmissions [13]

Table 5.1 (*cont.*)

Description of intervention	Content of interventions and skill-mix changes	Profession(s)	Population	Countries	Patient-related outcomes[a]	Health-system-related outcomes	Profession-specific outcomes
Nurse-led transitional care [14–18]	Initiated in hospital, community or post-discharge. Interventions included discharge planning, care coordination and plans, patient education, assessment, home visits, improve medication adherence, technology-based integrated counselling, care coordination, advocacy for options and services, involvement with family members	Intervention: Case manager/ specialist nurses, clinical nurse specialists, registered nurses, registered nurses and other professions Comparison: GPs, nurses, physiotherapists, caregivers, discharge planning nurses (not consistently reported)	Patients with various acute conditions (e.g. after cancer surgery, heart failure, elderly, high-risk pregnant women) or chronic illness [17,18]	CA, CN, DE, DK, ES, HK, IL, IT, LB, NL, Taiwan, UK, USA	• Improved treatment adherence [15], and medication adherence [16] • Risk of death significantly reduced by 50% in cancer patients [15] • Increased satisfaction for postpartum mothers and for heart failure patients after discharge [15] • Depression symptoms for caregivers in elderly care reduced [15] • Improved patient satisfaction and quality of life [17] • Mixed results for psychological outcomes [18]	• Readmission rates reduced (RR 0.51, 95% CI 0.29–0.91, $P = 0.02$) [15], (OR 0.74, 95% CI 0.60–0.92) [14] • Hospital stay reduced [14,15,18], (MD 1.28 days [14]) • No difference for ED / outpatient visits [14] • Primary care visits reduced [15] • Hospital readmissions [17,18], ED visits [18], duration of readmission and mortality reduced [17] • No reduction in index admission stay [17] Resource use: • Cost saving (case management) [14] and lower maternal and infants care costs [15] • Discharge planning reduced total and readmission costs [17] • Mixed results for costs [18]	

| Patient navigator roles [19,20] | Transitional care intervention from hospital to home through patient navigation. Intervention components included coordination, discharge planning and follow up, education and multiprofessional collaboration | Intervention: Nurse, advanced practice nurse, social worker, pharmacist Comparison: Family physician, not consistently reported | Older patients with chronic conditions | • Significantly improved depression symptoms (P < 0.001) [19]
• Significant improvement for disease self-management (P < 0.05) [19]
• Mixed results on quality of life: improved (P < 0.001) [19], no significant effect [20]
• Improved activities of daily living, communication with patients, caregivers, education for caregivers, self-management, knowledge of patient medication [19]
• Mortality was significantly reduced (RD −0.02, 95% CI −0.05 to 0.00) [20] | • Significantly fewer ED visits at 3 months post-discharge (RD −0.08, 95% CI −0.15 to −0.01); no effect at 1, 6, 12 months [20]
• Significantly lower at 6 months (RD −0.05, 95% CI −0.09 to −0.00), 12 months (RD −0.11, 95% CI −0.17 to −0.05), and at 24 months (MD −1.03, 95% CI −1.81 to −0.24) (for patients with chronic conditions) [20]; lower readmissions for patients with chronic conditions [19]
• Shorter time to readmission and fewer hospital days [19]
• Improved community referrals [19]

Resource use:
• Inconclusive effect on emergency costs [19] |

Abbreviations: ADL: activities of daily living; CI: confidence interval; CNS: clinical nurse specialist; COPD: chronic obstructive pulmonary disease; ED: Emergency Department; GP: general practitioner; MD: mean difference; n/r: not reported; OR: odds ratio; RD: risk difference; RR: relative risk.

Country abbreviations: AU: Australia; AT: Austria; BE: Belgium; BR: Brazil; CH: Switzerland; CN: China; DE: Germany; DK: Denmark; ES: Spain; FI: Finland; GE: Georgia; IT: Italy; IR: Iran; JP: Japan; NL: the Netherlands; NZ: New Zealand; SE: Sweden; UK: the United Kingdom; USA: the United States of America.

Notes: [a] Including caregiver-related outcomes.

Sources: [1] Allison et al. (2011); [2] Langhorne & Baylan (2017); [3] Domingo et al. (2012); [4] Huntley et al. (2013); [5] Clemente et al. (2016); [6] Vedel & Khanassov (2015); [7] Hansen et al. (2011); [8] Rennke et al. (2013); [9] Feltner et al. (2014); [10] Ensing et al. (2015); [11] De Oliviera et al. (2017); [12] Mekonnen, McLachlan & Brien (2016); [13] El Hajj et al. (2017); [14] Huntley et al. (2016); [15] Bryant-Lukosius et al. (2015); [16] Verloo et al. (2017); [17] Zhu et al. (2015); [18] Joo & Liu (2017); [19] Manderson et al. (2011); [20] Le Berre et al. (2017).

reviews, respectively analysed the effects of transitional care roles led by pharmacists and nurses, whereas two reviews specifically analysed patient navigator roles for older people (Table 5.1). Although the skill-mix interventions varied across the reviews, they all had in common that the main tasks were to improve the coordination and transitioning of care between the inpatient and outpatient sectors.

The reviews evaluated the effects of several, often bundled, interventions. These included discharge planning, care coordination, home visits, shared care plans, multisectoral care collaboration across social and health sectors, as well as care coordination between hospital and ambulatory care providers.

- Nine systematic reviews focused on transitional care roles and pre- and post-structured discharge interventions. Case management was central to all reviews, but interventions in one review combined health and social care to collaboratively provide primary care-based follow up for stroke patients post-discharge from hospital. The interventions comprised medication reviews, assessment of disability and caregiver needs. It also included the provision of information and linkage with other services provided by social workers, stroke support workers, care coordinators, case managers, GPs and caregivers (Allison et al., 2011). Seven reviews covered a range of different interventions such as home visits or rehabilitation in addition to case management delivered by nurses, pharmacists, family physicians or case managers (Domingo et al., 2012; Feltner et al., 2014; Hansen et al., 2011; Huntley et al., 2013; Langhorne & Baylan, 2017; Rennke et al., 2013; Vedel & Khanassov, 2015). Multiprofessional teams were introduced in the transition from paediatric to adult care settings for patients with juvenile onset rheumatic and musculoskeletal diseases. Transitional care teams that focused on the care transitioning across the two different phases of life (paediatric to adulthood) encompassed at least a transition coordinator, paediatric and adult rheumatologist trained in adolescent rheumatology and a clinical nurse specialist as well as several other professionals (Clemente et al., 2016).
- Pharmacist-led transitional care focused primarily on medication reviews and reconciliation and patient counselling at the hospital–home interface (De Oliviera et al., 2017; El Hajj et al., 2014; Ensing et al., 2015; Mekonnen, McLachlan & Brien, 2016). Nurse-led

transitional care interventions often covered more interventions compared with pharmacists, including discharge planning and coordination, home visits and patient assessments, among others (Bryant-Lukosius et al., 2015; Huntley et al., 2016; Joo & Liu, 2017; Verloo et al., 2017; Zhu et al., 2015). However, pharmacists were unique in providing expert medication reviews and reconciliation services.

• Two reviews covered patient navigator roles performed by different professions. The reviews included a wide range of interventions, but most of them focused on the role of patient navigation providing discharge planning and follow up, education and multiprofessional collaboration (Le Berre et al., 2017; Manderson et al., 2011).

Skill-mix interventions focusing on the relocation of care

Four reviews summarized the evidence on skill-mix interventions resulting from re-location of care settings (Table 5.2). All analysed hospital-at-home services.

Three reviews, including two Cochrane reviews, analysed the effects of shifting care location from hospitals to home in which various professions were involved, a concept referred to as hospital-at-home, in which a specialized team provides active treatment in the patient's home for a disease that usually would require hospital inpatient stays. Randomized controlled trials covered different patient groups: stroke, mixed conditions, elective surgery (Gonçalves-Bradley et al., 2017), heart failure (Qaddoura et al., 2015) and acute episodes of chronic obstructive pulmonary disease (COPD) (Shepperd et al., 2017). The interventions comprised several new team and skill-mix models, including teams working in hospital outreach services, community-based teams, as well as teams enhancing coordination of care across the settings. The professions covered a range of both specialists and lay workers, including specialist physicians and social care workers, various therapists (speech, etc.), care assistants, home helps and volunteers (Gonçalves-Bradley et al., 2017; Qaddoura et al., 2015; Shepperd et al., 2017).

Another Cochrane review focused on hospital-at-home skill-mix interventions. This time delivered by a specialist respiratory nurse under guidance of a medical hospital team targeting patients with acute exacerbations of COPD (Jeppesen et al., 2012).

Table 5.2 *Summary of reviews: skill-mix interventions and relocation of care from hospital settings to patients' homes*

Description of intervention	Content of interventions and skill-mix changes	Profession(s)	Population	Countries	Patient-related outcomes	Health-system related outcomes	Profession-specific outcomes
Hospital-at-home, various professions [1–3]	Hospital treatment at home provided by specialized team	Intervention: Physicians and various specialties, nurses, GPs, cardiologists, care assistants, home helps, dieticians, physiotherapists, social workers, volunteers, occupational or speech therapists, social workers Comparison: Health care staff in inpatient settings, inconsistently reported	Patients with heart failure [2], stroke [1, 4], mixed condition [1, 3], elective surgery patients [1] or acute episodes of COPD [3]	AU, CA, NO, SE, UK, ES, IT, NZ, RO, USA	Lower risk of living in an institutional setting for patients with stroke (RR 0.63, 95% CI 0.40–0.98) and mixed medical conditions (RR 0.69, 95% CI 0.48–0.99) [1] • Little to no difference in mortality at 6 months follow up (RR 0.77, 95% CI 0.60–0.99; $P = 0.04$) [3] • No effect on functional status, patient-reported outcomes and caregiver outcomes for stroke patients [1] • No or little difference in mortality at 3–6 months for stroke patients (RR 0.92, 95% CI 0.57–1.48) and little or no difference in hospital readmission (RR 1.09, 95% CI 0.71–1.66) [1]	• Reduced days of hospital stay for all three patient groups [1] or mixed results [3] • No effect on hospital readmission [1] and little or no difference in the likelihood of being transferred (or readmitted) to hospital (RR 0.98, 95% CI 0.77–1.23; $P = 0.84$) [3] • Increased time to first readmission (MD 14.13 days 95% CI 10.36–17.91) and decreased readmissions [2] • Reduced likelihood of living in residential care at 6-month follow-up (RR 0.35, 95% CI 0.22–0.57, $P < 0.0001$) [3]	

| Nurse specialist-delivered hospital-at-home, under guidance of medical hospital team | Nurse specialist-delivered hospital-at-home [4] | Intervention: specialist respiratory nurse, medical hospital team

Comparison: medical hospital team | Patients with acute exacerbations of COPD | AU, DK, IT, ES, UK | • Slight improvement in patient satisfaction [1]
• No effect on all-cause mortality (RR 0.94, 95% CI 0.67–1.32) [2]
• Improved health-related quality of life [2]

• Lower mortality, but not significant (RR 0.65, 95% CI, 0.40–1.04, $P = 0.07$)
• Mixed results in patient satisfaction | Costs:
• Reduced total costs in the intervention group [2]
• Slightly decreased treatment costs, but this benefit is offset when the costs of informal care are considered [3]

• A small and significant reduction in readmission rates for acute exacerbations of COPD (RR 0.76, 95% CI, 0.59–0.99, $P = 0.04$) [3]

Costs:
• Significant reduction in direct costs [3] |

Abbreviations: CI: confidence interval; COPD: chronic obstructive pulmonary disease; ESP: extended scope-of-practice physiotherapists; GP: general practitioner; RR: relative risk.

Country abbreviations: AU: Australia; CA: Canada, DK: Denmark; ES: Spain; IT: Italy; NO: Norway; NZ: New Zealand; RO: Romania; SE: Sweden; UK: the United Kingdom; USA: the United States of America.

Sources: [1] Gonçalves-Bradley et al. (2017); [2] Qaddoura et al. (2015); [3] Shepperd et al. (2017); [4] Jeppesen et al. (2012)

Skill-mix interventions focusing on new division of work for (minor) acute illnesses

New division of work for acute, often minor, illnesses was the focus of four reviews (Table 5.3). The triage of patients with acute musculoskeletal conditions was shown to be as effectively performed by physiotherapists with extended scopes-of-practice as by physicians. The role of physiotherapists with extended scopes-of-practice in the triage involved assessments of patients, undertaking diagnostic procedures and onward referrals to other departments, surgery or community services such as rheumatology and orthopaedic services (Oakley & Shacklady, 2015).

A systematic review that covered studies in the United Kingdom found that pharmacy-based and pharmacy-led minor ailment schemes were effective in the management of minor acute illnesses. It resulted in generally high patient satisfaction and improved GP satisfaction, as well as reducing costs of prescribing by 25% (Paudyal et al., 2013).

Two reviews analysed the effects of extending the role of mid-level dental care workers by taking over tasks that have traditionally been performed by dentists. One review focused on caries treatment for patients with acute dental health care needs as a means to expand the dental care workforce in primary care and reduce dentists' workloads (Wright et al., 2013). The other review assessed interventions such as irreversible procedures or local anaesthesia performed by dental hygienists and assistants (Dasanayake et al., 2012).

5.4 Outcomes of skill-mix interventions

Transitional care

All 20 reviews (Table 5.1) on transitional care skill-mix interventions found them to be associated with improvements in at least one patient-related or health-system-related outcome measure. There was no evidence on profession-specific outcomes.

Positive effects were found with transitional care roles performed by various professions for patients with stroke and heart failure. Skill-mix changes focused on improving transitional care reduced mortality in stroke patients (Langhorne & Baylan, 2017). Moreover, home visits and clinic-based interventions focusing on easing transitions were associated

Table 5.3 *Summary of reviews: skill-mix interventions and new division of work for (minor) acute illnesses*

Skill-mix interventions					Outcomes		
Description of intervention	Content of interventions and skill-mix changes	Profession(s)	Population	Countries	Patient-related outcomes	Health-system related outcomes	Profession-specific outcomes
Triage of acute care [1]	Triage performed by Extended Scope-of-Practice Physiotherapists (ESP)	Intervention: Physiotherapists with expanded scope-of-practice Comparison: Physicians, orthopaedic surgeons, rheumatology consultants, GPs	Patients with musculo-skeletal conditions	AU, CA, IE, NL, UK, USA	• No significant differences between the percentage of correct diagnoses between ESP and physicians • All studies showed generally high patient satisfaction with ESP. Patient satisfaction with ESP ranged from 77% to 89%		• High general GP satisfaction with ESP's work
Pharmacy-based minor ailment schemes (PMAS) [2]	Community PMAS offering the management of two or more minor ailments (consultation by pharmacists)	Intervention: Pharmacists Comparison: GPs	Patients with various minor ailments	UK	• The resolution of minor ailments following pharmacy-based consultation ranged from 68% to 94.4% • >90% expressed general satisfaction with the PMAS consultation, pharmacy staff attitude and expertise of pharmacy staff	• Significantly fewer GP consultations for minor ailments • Decline in prescribing volume in general practices through PMAS • Reduction of prescribing cost by 25%	• GP satisfaction with PMAS was reported • Community pharmacists expressed positive attitudes towards the scheme

Table 5.3 *(cont.)*

Skill-mix interventions

Description of intervention	Content of interventions and skill-mix changes	Profession(s)	Population	Countries	Outcomes		
					Patient-related outcomes	Health-system related outcomes	Profession-specific outcomes
New roles for mid-level professions [3, 4]	Mid-level providers in dental teams in primary care	Intervention: Mid-level providers (e.g. dental hygienists, dental nurse, dental assistants) and dentists in supervision Comparison: No care, dentist or other professions	Population requiring dental care [3, 4]	AU, CN, HK, NZ, USA, UK, CA, SE	• Reductions in caries/severity over time [3] • Most studies comparing dental hygienists with other professions (e.g. dentists) or no usual care, found lower levels of untreated caries in the intervention group [3] • Mixed results for the differences in caries severity in the interventions vs comparison groups [3] • Effect on patient satisfaction [4] • Better restorations and fewer failures [4]	• Increased productivity and reduced waiting times with dental hygienists [4] • 3% required re-visits after irreversible procedures were performed by mid-level providers [4] • More than 90% success after first attempt to perform local anaesthesia by dental hygienists [4] • Equal quality provided by dental hygienists compared with dentists [4]	• 90% of students favoured the expansion of dental assistants' role [4]

Abbreviations: ESP: extended scope-of-practice physiotherapists; PMAS: pharmacy-based minor ailment schemes.

Country abbreviations: AU: Australia; CA: Canada; CN: China; IE: Ireland; HK: Hong Kong; NL: the Netherlands; NZ: New Zealand; SE: Sweden; UK: the United Kingdom; US: the United States of America.

Sources: [1] Oakley & Shacklady (2015); [2] Paudyal et al. (2013); [3] Wright et al. (2013); [4] Dasanayake et al. (2012)

with a decrease in mortality in patients with heart failure (Feltner et al., 2014). Other positive effects ranged from improved knowledge about the condition (Allison et al., 2011), improved self-management (Manderson et al., 2011), adherence to appointments (Clemente et al., 2016) and medication (El Hajj et al., 2017; Verloo et al., 2017) and increased patient satisfaction (Zhu et al., 2015). Several positive benefits were also identified for caregivers (Bryant-Lukosius et al., 2015; Manderson et al., 2012).

Pharmacist-led transitional care was found to significantly reduce medication errors in one review (De Oliviera et al., 2017), whereas a second review showed mixed results on adverse drug events (Ensing et al., 2015). Nurse-led transitional care was associated with improved treatment and medication adherence (Bryant-Lukosius et al., 2015).

Overall, there were mixed effects on mortality. In two studies, mortality was significantly reduced for patients receiving transitional care, based on meta-analyses (Bryant-Lukosius et al., 2015; Le Berre et al., 2017) and one showed improved mortality rates (Feltner et al., 2014). One review showed a non-significant reduction (Langhorne & Baylan, 2017), one review showed mixed results (Ensing et al., 2015) and one showed no significant difference for all-cause mortality (Mekonnen, McLachlan & Brien, 2016).

Regarding health-system-related outcomes, transitional care was shown to reduce emergency department visits in the pharmacist-led models (De Oliviera et al., 2017; Ensing et al., 2015; Mekonnen, McLachlan & Brien, 2016), and with mixed results emanating from the reviews analysing nurse-led and mixed-profession-led transitional care (Huntley et al., 2016; Le Berre et al., 2017) and case management and structured discharge (Allison et al., 2011). In the case of nurse-led transitional care, hospital readmissions and hospital length of stay were reduced (Bryant-Lukosius et al., 2015; Huntley et al., 2016; Joo & Liu, 2017; Zhu et al., 2015). Transitional care interventions delivered by various professions showed a significant reduction in readmission rates (Vedel & Khanassov, 2015) or mixed results (Rennke et al., 2013). Several reviews analysed the costs and efficiency of transitional care interventions, of which one found lower costs in nurse-led case management across care settings for patients (Huntley et al., 2016), one demonstrated reduced costs for nurse-led transitional care for at-risk pregnant women and low-birthweight newborns (Bryant-Lukosius et al., 2015), one reported cost savings associated with the difference in readmissions in the pharmacist-led intervention (El Hajj et al., 2017). Inconclusive (Manderson et al., 2011) or mixed (Joo & Liu, 2017) evidence on costs was also shown.

Skill-mix and relocation of care

Meta-analyses showed that hospital-at-home skill-mix models were associated with a reduced risk of living in an institutional setting for stroke patients at follow up (for example at 6 months) and for patients with multiple medical conditions, as well as slight improvements in patient satisfaction (Gonçalves-Bradley et al., 2017). Reduced like-lihood of living in residential care was also found in Shepperd et al. (2017). Hence, there is some evidence to suggest that hospital-at-home may delay admission to residential care and nursing homes. In all three patient groups reported in Gonçalves-Bradley et al. (2017), the length of inpatient hospital stay was significantly reduced, but mixed results were found in Shepperd et al. (2017). The two Cochrane reviews on hospitals-at-home showed no or little difference on mor-tality (Shepperd et al., 2017) at 3–6 months for stroke patients (Gonçalves-Bradley et al., 2017). Little or no difference on hospital readmission was reported in two reviews (Gonçalves-Bradley et al., 2017; Shepperd et al., 2017). Mixed results on costs were reported in one review (Shepperd et al., 2017). The third systematic review on hospital-at-home for patients with heart failure reported improved quality of life, decreased readmissions and a reduction in the total costs (Qaddoura et al., 2015).

The Cochrane review that focused on hospital at home interven-tions for patients with COPD delivered by a specialist respiratory nurse showed a small significant reduction in readmission rates and a non-significant effect for mortality rates. Mixed results on patient sat-isfaction and a significant reduction in direct costs were found in the review (Jeppesen et al., 2017).

New division of work for minor acute illnesses

Only one review highlighted profession-specific outcomes in terms of satisfaction of GPs with the skill-mix intervention (Oakley &

Shacklady, 2015). The review on triage performed by extended scope-of practice physiotherapists showed high patient and physician satisfaction with their overall performance in terms of diagnostic accuracy. The evidence was based on a total of 14 studies in six countries assessing the correctness of the diagnoses, after physiotherapists were trained in performing triage functions. This review states, however, that there may be a lack of robustness to the evidence making it difficult to generalize findings to all extended scopes-of practice in musculoskeletal triage, especially in terms of the different aspects of satisfaction. There is also insufficient evidence concerning the content and length of training for triage purposes. Extended scopes-of practice have a variety of clinical roles; these need to be clearly described and updated with current extended scope-of practice clinical practice/competencies to allow findings to be of relevant clinical value (Oakley & Shacklady, 2015).

In the review by Wright et al. (2013), all studies with mid-level dental hygienists performing expanded procedures for acute dental conditions (such as caries) were associated with reductions in caries over time, less untreated caries and mixed results in the treatment of caries severity, suggesting that mid-level providers can take care of minor, routine caries cases and expand access to services. Dasanayake et al. (2012) demonstrate that tasks performed by dental hygienists show equal quality compared with dentists, and they also find high success rates in giving local anaesthesia and in carrying out reversible and irreversible procedures. Increased productivity, reduced waiting times and patient satisfaction were also reported.

Results of pharmacy-based minor ailment consultations by pharmacists suggest that these are being managed well and are less costly than by a general practitioner. Moreover, the review's findings show significantly fewer GP consultations and an overall satisfaction or positive attitudes among patients, GPs and pharmacists (Paudyal et al., 2013).

Education and training of professions involved in the skill-mix changes

While the majority of reviews provided information on the professions involved in the skill-mix changes, few reported details on the education, competencies and skills they acquired. Also, when comparator groups were mentioned, their education was not reported.

5.5   Strengths and limitations of the reviewed evidence

The systematic reviews covered a large number of studies (>600) conducted in many countries in Europe and other high-income countries. Several meta-analyses of RCTs were performed, as well as reviews that narratively reported the findings from other research. Several RCTs had a small sample size, faced high attrition or other limitations and the comparison groups were not reported or not consistently reported. The education and training of the professions and individuals were insufficiently reported, as were the details of the skill-mix interventions. Often, bundled interventions of new skill-mixes and new organizations of care were evaluated, which limits the attribution of causality.

5.6   Conclusions on skill-mix intervention effectiveness in acute and transitional care

Several reviews evaluated new skill-mix models in the provision of acute care, where the boundaries between the care settings have shifted considerably from inpatient to outpatient care. Transitional care roles were shown to have several positive patient outcomes for stroke and heart failure patients and other conditions, although the evidence on multiple conditions was more limited. Pharmacist-led transitional care roles were associated with reduced medication errors and improved adherence whereas nurse-led transitional care roles showed improved therapy and treatment adherence. The re-allocation of tasks and roles from physicians and dentists to other professions, namely nurses, pharmacists and physiotherapists, was shown to be generally effective for a wide range of conditions and roles (including transitional roles, hospital-at-home and minor acute care) within the professions' enlarged scopes-of-practice. The reviews suggest that skill-mix models with the primary aim to improve transitions across sectors can improve patient-related outcome parameters, such as enhanced knowledge about the condition and self-management as well as improved medication adherence. The evidence on hospital readmissions and Emergency Department use is inconclusive, although there are some promising country experiences.

5.7 Acute and transitional care skill-mix innovations and reforms

Overview of recent trends across Europe and internationally

Recent trends in skill-mix innovations in acute and transitional care across Europe and internationally have focused on discharge and transition from hospital to ambulatory community care and home settings; relocating care to the lowest level (hospital-at-home) and new forms of division of work for minor acute illnesses in primary outpatient care. New models of care have emerged, involving the utilization of new skills of existing providers. The expanded roles of two key professions, nurses and pharmacists, are emphasized in the literature, but there are also expanded roles of physiotherapists (particularly in the triage function), radiographers and physician assistants, and of team-based interventions more generally. We highlight some of the key trends below.

Transitional care

Expanded roles of nurses and pharmacists are two of the more recent innovations to ensure smooth discharge and transition from acute care.

Expanded roles of nurses

In several countries, the role of nurses in care coordination from acute to community settings has been expanded. Having nurses and other clinical staff involved in transitioning care can help in both identifying patients at high risk and focusing interventions to reduce readmissions and improve quality of care.

In the Netherlands, recent transitional care interventions include the Transitional Care Bridge programme for acutely hospitalized older patients, combining a Comprehensive Geriatric Assessment, an integrated care plan and a transitional care programme, including visits during hospitalization and soon after discharge by a community nurse (Buurman et al., 2016). Another intervention in the Netherlands, coordinated by nurses and directed at outpatients with a recent coronary syndrome included guidance on lifestyle factors, biometric risk factors and therapy adherence (Jorstad et al., 2013). The nurse-coordinated Cardiac Care Bridge transitional care programme aimed to reduce unplanned hospital readmission and mortality in older hospitalized cardiac patients at high risk of readmission and mortality. In this programme, a cardiac research nurse develops an integrated care plan with the patient, is involved with a community nurse in handover and discharge, and a community nurse visits the patient four times after discharge. Participating nurses followed a 5-day training course on case and disease management (Verweij et al. 2018).

In Germany, secondary prevention after acute hospital episodes is provided by a number of actors, including GPs and nurses. However, no home-based early post-discharge programmes are available. Several intervention trials explored whether a post-discharge nurse-based case management could improve health outcomes and reduce readmissions. The KORINNA ("Coronary infarction follow-up in the elderly") study, for example, evaluated the effects of nurse-based case management for older patients discharged after an acute myocardial infarction from a tertiary care hospital. The intervention consisted of a nurse-based follow up for 1 year including home visits and telephone calls (Meisinger et al. 2013).

In the United States of America (USA), the Centers for Medicare & Medicaid Services are implementing a range of policies to reduce read-missions. This includes penalties for hospitals with 30-day readmissions above their expected rates and support for demonstration projects aimed to improve the transition from hospital to the community (Linden & Butterworth, 2014). Hospitals have responded with a range of tran-sitional care interventions, including in some cases an expanded role for nurses (Jones et al., 2017). A nurse-driven intervention in an acute care hospital in California, for example, aimed to reduce readmissions through a multifaceted approach during hospitalization with pre-discharge planning and post-discharge follow up (Dizon & Reinking, 2017). The intervention involved the hiring of a nurse outpatient care manager for those patients discharged home who performed home visits and follow-up phone calls, follow-up phone calls by a nurse practitioner for high-risk patients discharged to a skilled nursing facility, a review of discharge instructions for high-risk patients by a pharmacist, and medication reconciliation by pharmacist technicians.

Expanded roles of pharmacists

Roles of pharmacists in transitional care are expanding in several countries, partly driven by the attempt to reduce costly readmissions to hospital. Several studies have shown that pharmacist involvement in the discharge process can reduce the incidence of adverse drug events and have a positive impact on patient satisfaction (Phatak et al., 2016). A pharmacist-led discharge medication reconciliation service, conducted in collaboration with the hospital-based physician, can improve the completeness and accuracy of discharge prescriptions (Holland, 2015).

Pharmacist roles differ widely between and within countries. In a survey among experts from 30 European countries, only respondents from the United Kingdom stated that medication reconciliation is standard practice in the country. In most countries, medication reconciliation is implemented only in some hospitals, for some patients, or in some projects (Gillespie & Eriksson, 2016), although in Ireland, medication reconciliation services are mandated for all patients in all transitions of care (Holland, 2015). In the United Kingdom, a National Health Service (NHS) scheme encourages providers to plan and maintain provision of care support for the first 14 days after discharge (Yang 2017). These post-discharge interventions include an expanded role of pharmacists, with one example being telephone follow up to provide support for medicine management (Yang 2017).

In the USA, various interventions expanding the roles of pharmacists have been undertaken. In one study using a comprehensive approach in a tertiary care academic medical centre, pharmacists were involved in (i) face-to-face medication reconciliation on admission, (ii) development of a personalized medication plan discussed with the patient's physician, (iii) addressing any medication discrepancies with the discharge instructions being given to the patient, (iv) medication counselling performed at discharge, and (v) three post-discharge phone calls at 3, 14 and 30 days (Phatak et al., 2016). Earlier pharmacist-facilitated hospital discharge programmes had been undertaken elsewhere (Arnold, Buys & Fullas, 2015; Ni et al., 2018; Walker et al., 2009).

Multiprofessional team-based interventions

Team-based interventions seem to have become more common in a number of countries. In the above-mentioned, nurse-coordinated Cardiac Care Bridge transitional care programme in the Netherlands, which aimed to reduce unplanned hospital readmission and mortality in older hospitalized cardiac patients at high risk of readmission and mortality, multiprofessional collaboration across sectors was an important part of the intervention. This included the in-hospital cardiac team (including the cardiac research nurse and the cardiologist, the clinical nurse specialist in geriatrics and the pharmacist) as well as the community nurse and the physiotherapist in primary care. There were face-to-face handovers before discharge and a joint home visit of the community nurse and the physiotherapist, as well as support from a pharmacist (Verweij et al., 2018).

Skill-mix and relocation of care

Several countries have implemented or are evaluating new skill-mix models that are also linked to the re-organization of care. One frequently mentioned example is hospital-at-home. However, other models are specialized clinics (for example, heart failure clinic) or new roles and locations, such as intermediate care, all aiming at reducing hospital admissions and stays and providing care as close to patients' homes as possible.

While hospital-at-home service delivery has been adopted in the USA and Australia, the idea has also been taken up in some European countries such as the United Kingdom, Germany and Switzerland as an alternative to standard hospital care. Highly specialized and experienced health professionals are required to provide quality care. A hospital-at-home programme to avoid hospital readmissions involving advanced practice nurses is described in Box 5.2.

A United States-based study examined the effect of a multiprofessional team-based specialized Heart Failure clinic on 90-day readmission rates or all-cause mortality (Jackevicius et al., 2015). The team consisted of a physician assistant, clinical pharmacist specialist and case manager, with care overseen by a cardiologist. Prompt outpatient follow up was identified as specifically important in the case of heart failure because of a high risk of hospital readmission and mortality.

A Canadian study involved an advanced practice nurse (specifically a nurse practitioner) in an intermediate care role for patients discharged from an acute care hospital to home who were at high risk for acute care readmission (Neiterman, Wodchis & Bourgeault, 2015).

Box 5.2 Hospital-at-home to avoid readmission

Hospital-at-home schemes, although in existence since the early 1960s, are becoming an increasingly popular way of delivering health care (Corrado, 2001). Schemes differ in the type of patients they cater for and in the intensity and complexity of treatment they provide, depending on the health care team composition and their skills. Advanced practice nurses often play an important role within such teams.

For example in South London a project has started, bringing patient-centred care to the place of residence of older people (NHS England, 2018). The goal is to improve hospital discharge so that patients stay in hospital only as long as they clinically need to be there. A multiprofessional team, led by nurse practitioners and community nurses, improves care received at home. In London, the team is situated in the hospital and reaches out to patients in the community so as to avoid hospitalization or to help shorten length of stay through a single-point access with a 2-hour response to the request for urgent medical assessment. The teams operate 365 days a year, 24 hours a day. The home visits are provided by an advanced practice nurse or a GP when required. The visits can be provided daily up to four times a day for 3–7 days. There are intensive nursing, physical therapy and occupational therapy inputs during the intervention.

Patients can expect high-intensity clinical monitoring, with short-term interventions in an acute episode of ill-health in a safe and timely manner. For acutely unwell patients, urgent clinical assessment is provided, including where necessary electrocardiograms and urgent blood tests. Treatment and ongoing monitoring include the provision of intravenous therapy, subcutaneous hydration, ongoing blood therapy and nebulizers. Nurses further provide environmental checks and self-management support (Panagioti et al., 2014).

Several conditions have been identified that can effectively be treated at home, including cellulitis, falls, chronic obstructive pulmonary disease, unstable diabetes, gastroenteritis, deep vein thrombosis, urinary tract infections and viral illnesses.

This intervention, which involved the nurse practitioner completing a personal health record with patients outlining and reconciling their medication, laboratory tests and primary care visits, helped to effectively triage patients by attending to their medical as well as social needs during post-discharge recovery.

An expanded role for pharmacists to help avoid hospital admissions or readmissions has also emerged as a trend internationally. Countries in which the role of community pharmacists has been expanded in recent years include Australia, Canada, England, the Netherlands, Scotland, and the USA (Mossialos et al., 2015). There are notable divergences in scope of practice across the United Kingdom. England has defined different tiers of community pharmacist roles in terms of the effective, safe and efficient use of medicines and the prevention and management of chronic conditions. Not all pharmacies provide all services, and many are commissioned locally. In Scotland, provision of the majority of extended services is a core contractual requirement; that is, every pharmacist will provide them. In Canada, the scope of practice of pharmacists has also expanded in recent years, shifting from more traditional functions such as medication dispensing towards services such as minor ailment prescribing, medication reviews, immunizations and strategies to promote medication adherence (Kelly et al., 2014).

The roles of physiotherapists in triage at emergency departments to avoid acute care admissions have been expanded in recent years in several countries, including the United Kingdom, the Netherlands and Australia. In the above-mentioned, nurse-coordinated Cardiac Care Bridge transitional care programme in the Netherlands, for example, physiotherapists provided two home-based cardiac rehabilitation sessions per week during the first 6 weeks post-discharge in older hospitalized cardiac patients at high risk of readmission and mortality (Verweij et al., 2018).

In Australia, an expanded role of physiotherapists in emergency departments has been extensively funded since 2012. A study on the implementation of an expanded scope-of-practice physiotherapist role in a regional (that is, rural) hospital emergency department found that this role included increased autonomy in management and discharge of patients treated in the emergency department and independent ordering and interpreting of plain film X-rays (Goodman et al., 2018). For sustainability in rural areas, a larger advanced-level physiotherapy workforce with easier access to expanded scope training was recommended (Bird, Thompson & Williams, 2016).

Finally, physician assistants, a profession established in the USA in the 1960s, are now also being introduced in Europe, especially in the United Kingdom (since 2003), but also in Germany (since 2005).

Early studies of their implementation in the United Kingdom suggest that they are being deployed in primary care and out-of-hours centres as well as in hospital settings. A current limitation to their role is that they are not a regulated United Kingdom profession and therefore are not allowed to prescribe, but expectations are that this will ultimately be addressed. Observational studies suggest that patient satisfaction is high and outcomes are good (Farmer et al., 2011). One study in 12 English general practices for same-day consultations included 2086 patients and showed that processes and outcomes of physician assistants and GP consultations were similar, but physician assistants cost less per consultation (Drennan et al., 2015).

Treatment of minor, acute illnesses in primary and ambulatory care settings

Skill-mix innovations in the treatment of minor acute illnesses in primary, community and ambulatory care also involve the use of new and expanded roles. This is perhaps most extensive in the case of nursing and community pharmacy.

A number of countries have implemented programmes in which the unscheduled acute care of patients with minor illnesses is delivered by nurse practitioners. These programmes are based on extensive evidence that indicates that nurse practitioners can provide patients who have minor illnesses with a high standard of care similar to that provided by GPs. Some countries, such as the United Kingdom, Canada and the USA, have also allowed nurse prescribing in primary care (Bhanbro et al., 2011).

There have also been initiatives in a number of countries to expand the role of community pharmacists, for instance in Switzerland (see Box 5.3). Swiss pharmacists in community pharmacies are providing care and triage for patients with minor acute conditions. In the United Kingdom, far-reaching reforms have taken place. There, contractual frameworks recognize new roles of community pharmacies, including the provision of advice on and administration of vaccines, the provision of a minor ailment service, a chronic medicine management service including repeat dispensing, and many public health services, the most important of which is the provision of smoking cessation advice. Especially in Scotland, community pharmacy staff are responsible for the vast majority of successful quit attempts. These extended roles are

Box 5.3 *The netCare Project:* **Swiss community pharmacists providing triage to patients with minor acute conditions**

In Switzerland, a new form of skill-mix change initiated by the Swiss Pharmacists Association involved expanded roles of pharmacists in collaboration with physicians (Erni et al., 2016). Pharmacists working in community pharmacies were trained to perform structured triage for individuals with a range of common acute illnesses. The pharmacists used 24 evidence-based decision trees for the patients presenting at their pharmacy. The services ranged by severity and urgency of the patient's condition from

(i)   management by the pharmacist and (as required) dispensing of over-the-counter medicines for minor, routine cases;
(ii) services by the pharmacists, in collaboration with telemedicine services provided by a physician; to
(iii) direct referral to a GP or Emergency Room.

A total of 162 pharmacies participated in the programme, which was evaluated from 2012 to 2014. Overall, 4118 triages were performed. The most common medical conditions treated were urinary tract infection (>40%), followed by conjunctivitis (23%) and pharyngitis (6%). The majority (84%) of patients treated by pharmacists reported complete relief or symptom reduction, as assessed in follow-up calls. A collaborative approach with physicians was undertaken for 17% of cases. Triage was undertaken more often on Saturdays (20% of all cases) than on weekdays.

   Overall, this new form of service delivery with extended roles for pharmacists was positively evaluated. It showed that pharmacists can take care of a range of common minor illnesses in the pharmacy setting, directly with patients or in collaboration via telemedicine with GPs as a back-up. This skill-mix change whereby community pharmacies act as first entry point to the primary care system shows promise as a low-threshold service for patients and may attract individuals who may – for various reasons – delay care or not go to a physician in the first place (Erni et al., 2016). From a cost perspective, an economic analysis found the programme to be cost-saving, compared with standard care provided in GP offices or other alternative treatment options (Trottmann et al., 2016).

further enhanced by the granting of prescribing rights to pharmacists (and nurses) who undertake a short (25 days of study, plus 12 days supervised practice) post-qualification, university-based course. This has enhanced the ability of pharmacists to manage a wider range of minor ailments, such as a urinary tract infection, whereby antibiotics can now be prescribed by an independent prescribing pharmacist according to an agreed local protocol or through an alternative arrangement called a "patient group directive".

Research evidence underpinned these developments. Early work (Sinclair et al., 2006) showed that pharmacist-led care for rhinitis resulted in good outcomes, which were similar to those of a group of patients who had seen their GP. Most recently, the Minor Ailment Study (MINA) programme of work has looked at the real-world evidence for this service after national roll-out (see Box 5.4).

Box 5.4 The MINA Programme

The MINA programme of work in the United Kingdom studied the real-world experience of pharmacist provision of a minor ailment service compared with the provision of a similar service by emergency departments or GPs. Study sites were in both England and Scotland. In the first phase, a systematic review was conducted to explore the evidence for pharmacy provision of minor ailment services. This review included 26 studies (reported in 31 evaluations) and showed that for the majority (76–98%) of patients, symptoms were resolved completely, and the cost was between £1.44 and £15.90 per consultation.

In the second phase, data were collected from general practices and emergency departments to identify which ones had the highest impact on these services and might reasonably have been managed by a pharmacist. This showed that this ranged from 5.3% (95% CI 3.4%–7.1%) for emergency departments to 13.2% (95% CI 10.2%–16.1%) for general practices.

In the third phase, a prospective cohort study was undertaken in community pharmacies, general practices and emergency departments. For similar conditions, symptom resolution did not differ across the three settings, and as in the studies included in the review, health care costs were lowest in the pharmacy [£29.30 (standard deviation (SD) 37.81)] setting, compared with the general practice [£82.34 (SD 104.16)] and

---

Box 5.4 (cont.)

emergency departments [£147.09 (SD 74.96)]. The main reason for people choosing the provider they did was convenience.

In the final phase, a simulated patient study was conducted to assess the quality of pharmacy provision of minor ailment services. Quality was assessed based on patient satisfaction but also using an agreed checklist of essential consultation components specific to each condition. Although patients were satisfied and reported that the pharmacists were very professional, few pharmacists delivered a consultation that met all the criteria and the authors recommend further continued support for pharmacists and their staff in order to improve consultation performance. Nonetheless, overall the conclusion is that pharmacists are a valuable addition to the NHS workforce to manage minor ailments and reduce the pressure on other providers.

In the United Kingdom, pharmacists are also increasingly employed in settings other than the hospital or community, and there have been government initiatives to increase pharmacy capacity within both GP surgeries and care homes. Pharmacists regularly run patient clinics for patients with diabetes, coronary heart disease, diabetes, asthma, COPD and sexual health services, and provide advice to GPs on their medicine management. As in the management of minor ailments, research suggests that pharmacists with prescribing rights can manage patients effectively, with outcomes as good as or better than those from GPs, at least in certain defined conditions such as chronic pain (Bruhn et al., 2013). Studies in Canada have also confirmed the success of pharmacist prescribing interventions (Famiyeh & McCarthy, 2017).

5.8   Conclusions

In summary, some elements of acute care have shifted from inpatient to outpatient care, supported by a re-allocation of tasks and roles. Three key developments are observed: first, transitional care (for example, transitional care coordinator), second, re-location of care (for example, specialized teams providing services in hospitals-at-home) and third, new division of work in ambulatory care for minor acute illnesses. Cutting across the reviews and recent studies and trends across Europe and internationally, there are similar drivers and challenges of new roles in better navigating the transition of care from acute to community settings, the avoidance of acute care settings altogether and the delivery of acute care in more community-based settings including the home. The main factors motivating the implementation are a response to growing costs associated with hospital-based care, a changing demand for new more accessible locations of care, complemented by the desire for expanded roles for nurses, pharmacists and physiotherapists.

There are many differences in the nature and number of extended roles. Some extended roles are still provided on a delegated and supervised basis, whereas in other cases the practitioners are working independently and autonomously (de Bont et al., 2016). The most important facilitators to introducing a new extended role within a team are the willingness of medical practitioners to relinquish tasks, technological developments and service redesign.

In most reviews, these skill-mix interventions were shown to be effective, yielding at least one positive outcome for acute care patients or for health systems. There is however very limited evidence on profession-specific outcomes. There are also a number of challenges in the development and implementation of expanded roles, often only implicitly referenced, including opposition from the medical profession, organization and funding of care in the health systems, and legislative and regulatory changes. Moreover, there is a limited body of knowledge especially in the European context, as well as more broadly, regarding the scale of the expanded roles, level of implementation, and barriers and enablers experienced in different contexts. There is much variation across countries and care contexts within countries making it difficult to generalize conclusions of case studies.

In addition to the strengths and limitations of the systematic reviews, there are a number of other inherent challenges to note in research on this topic, including lack of clarity on definitions, labels of professions, qualifications, health service systems, research culture, clinician buy-in, clinician priorities and understanding of research and research ethics, among a number of others. These limitations are compounded by the inherent limitation of the significant differences in usual scope of practice and skill-mix across different country contexts where local education, funding and regulation affect practice at point of care.

References

Allison R, Shelling L, Dennett R et al. (2011). The effectiveness of various models of primary care-based follow-up after stroke: a systematic review. Primary Health Care Res Dev, 12(3):214–222.

Arnold ME, Buys L, Fullas F (2015). Impact of pharmacist intervention in conjunction with outpatient physician follow-up visits after hospital discharge on readmission rate. Am J Health-Syst Pharm, 72(11 Suppl 1):S36–42. (https://doi.org/10.2146/sp150011).

Bhanbhro S, Drennan VM, Grant R et al. (2011). Assessing the contribution of prescribing in primary care by nurses and professionals allied to medicine: a systematic review of literature. BMC Health Serv Res, 11:330.

Bird S, Thompson C, Williams KE (2016). Primary contact physiotherapy services reduce waiting and treatment times for patients presenting with musculoskeletal conditions in Australian emergency departments: an observational study. J Physiother, 62(4):209–214. (https://doi.org/10.1016/j.jphys.2016.08.005).

Bruhn H, Bond CM, Elliott AM et al. (2013). Pharmacist-led management of chronic pain in primary care: results from a randomised controlled exploratory trial. BMJ Open, 3:e002361. doi:10.1136/bmjopen-2012.

Bryant-Lukosius D, Carter N, Reid K et al. (2015). The clinical effectiveness and cost-effectiveness of clinical nurse specialist-led hospital to home transitional care: a systematic review. J Eval Clin Pract, 21(5):763–781.

Busby J, Purdy S, Hollingworth W (2015). A systematic review of the magnitude and cause of geographic variation in unplanned hospital admission rates and length of stay for ambulatory care sensitive conditions. BMC Health Serv Res 15(1):324.

Buurman BM, Parlevliet JL, Allore HG et al. (2016). Comprehensive geriatric assessment and transitional care in acutely hospitalized patients: the transitional care bridge randomized clinical trial. JAMA Intern Med, 176(3):302–309.

Clemente D, Leon L, Foster H et al. (2016). Systematic review and critical appraisal of transitional care programmes in rheumatology. Semin Arthr Rheum, 46(3):372–379.

Corbella X, Barreto V, Bassetti S et al. (2018). Hospital ambulatory medicine: A leading strategy for Internal Medicine in Europe. Eur J Intern Med, 54:17–20.

Corrado OJ (2001). Hospital-at-home. Age Ageing 30-S3:11–14.

Dasanayake AP, Brar BS, Matta S et al. (2012). Are procedures performed by dental auxiliaries safe and of comparable quality? A systematic review. J Calif Dent Assoc, 40:65–78.

de Barra M, Scott CL, Scott NW et al. (2018). Pharmacist services for non-hospitalised patients. Cochrane Database Syst Rev, 9:CD013102.

de Bont A, van Exel J, Coretti S et al.; MUNROS Team (2016). Reconfiguring health workforce: A case-based comparative study explaining the increasingly diverse professional roles in Europe BMC Health Serv Res, 16(1):637.

De Oliveira G, Castro-Alves L, Kendall M et al. (2017). Effectiveness of pharmacist intervention to reduce medication errors and health-care resources utilization after transitions of care: a meta-analysis of randomized controlled trials. J Patient Safety, Epub 20 June.

Dizon ML, Reinking C (2017). Reducing readmissions: nurse-driven interventions in the transition of care from the hospital. Worldviews on evidence-based nursing. 14(6):432–439. (https://doi.org/10.1111/wvn.12260).

Domingo G, Reyes F, Thompson F et al. (2012). Effectiveness of structured discharge process in reducing hospital readmission of adult patients with community acquired pneumonia: a systematic review. JBI Database Syst Rev Implement Rep, 10(18):1086–1121.

Drennan VM, Halter M, Joly L et al. (2015). Physician associates and GPs in primary care: a comparison. Br J Gen Pract 65:e344–e350.

El Hajj MS, Jaam MJ, Awaisu A (2018). Effect of pharmacist care on medication adherence and cardiovascular outcomes among patients post-acute coronary syndrome: a systematic review. Res Social Adm Pharm, 14:507–520.

Ensing H, Stuijt C, van den Bemt B et al. (2015). Identifying the optimal role for pharmacists in care transitions: a systematic review. J Manag Care Specialty Pharm, 21(8):614–636.

Erni P, von Overbeck J, Reich O et al. (2016). netCare, a new collaborative primary health care service based in Swiss community pharmacies. Res Social Admin Pharm, 12(4):622–626.

Famiyeh IM, McCarthy L (2017). Pharmacist prescribing: a scoping review about the views and experiences of patients and the public. Res Social Admin Pharm, 13(1):1–16.

Farmer J, Currie M, Hyman J et al. (2011). Evaluation of physician assistants in National Health Service Scotland. Scott Med J, 56(3):130–134.

Feltner C, Jones CD, Cené CW et al. (2014). Transitional care interventions to prevent readmissions for persons with heart failure: a systematic review and meta-analysis. Ann Intern Med, 160:774–784.

Gillespie U, Eriksson T (2016). Medication reconciliation activities among pharmacists in Europe. Eur J Hosp Pharm, 25(2).

Gonçalves-Bradley D, Iliffe S, Doll H et al. (2017). Early discharge hospital at home. Cochrane Database Syst Rev, 6(6):CD000356

Goodman D, Harvey D, Cavanagh T et al. (2018). Implementation of an expanded-scope-of-practice physiotherapist role in a regional hospital emergency department. Rural Remote Health, 18(2):4212–4212. (https://doi.org/10.22605/RRH4212).

Hansen LO, Young RS, Hinami K, et al. (2011). Interventions to reduce 30-day rehospitalization: a systematic review. Ann Intern Med, 155:520–528.

Holland DM (2015). Interdisciplinary collaboration in the provision of a pharmacist-led discharge medication reconciliation service at an Irish teaching hospital. Int J Clin Pharm, 37(2):310–319. (https://doi.org/10.1007/s11096-014-0059-y).

Huntley A, Johnson R, King A et al. (2016). Does case management for patients with heart failure based in the community reduce unplanned hospital admissions? A systematic review and meta-analysis. BMJ Open, 6(5):e010933.

Jackevicius CA, de Leon NK, Lu L et al. (2015). Impact of a multiprofessional heart failure post-hospitalization program on heart failure readmission rates. Ann Pharmacother, 49(11):1189–1196. (https://doi.org/10.1177/1060028015599637).

Jeppesen E, Brurberg KG, Vist GE et al. (2012) Hospital at home for acute exacerbations of chronic obstructive pulmonary disease. Cochrane Database Syst Rev. 2012 May 16;(5):CD003573. doi: 10.1002/14651858.CD003573.pub2.

Jones J, Lawrence E, Ladebue A et al. (2017). Nurses' Role in Managing "The Fit" of Older Adults in Skilled Nursing Facilities. J Gerontol Nurs, 43(12):11–20. (https://doi.org/10.3928/00989134-20171110-06).

Joo JY, Liu MF (2017). Case management effectiveness in reducing hospital use: a systematic review. Int Nurs Rev, 64:296–308.

Jorstad HT, von Birgelen C, Alings AM et al. (2013). Effect of a nurse-coordinated prevention programme on cardiovascular risk after an acute coronary syndrome: main results of the RESPONSE randomised trial. Heart, 99(19):1421–1430.

Kelly DV, Young S, Philips L et al. (2014). Patient attitudes regarding the role of the pharmacist and interest in expanded pharmacist services. Can Pharm J (Ott), 147(4):239–247.

Langhorne P, Baylan S (2017). Early Supported Discharge Trialists. Early supported discharge services for people with acute stroke. Cochrane Database Syst Rev, 7(7):CD000443.

Le Berre M, Maimon G, Sourial N et al. (2017). Impact of transitional care services for chronically ill older patients: a systematic evidence review. J Am Geriatrics Soc, 65(7):1597–1608.

Linden A, Butterworth SW (2014) A comprehensive hospital-based intervention to reduce readmissions for chronically ill patients: a randomized controlled trial. Am J Managed Care, 20(10):783–792.

Manderson B, Mcmurray J, Piraino E et al. (2011). Navigation roles support chronically ill older adults through healthcare transitions: a systematic review of the literature. Health Soc Care Commun, 20(2):113–127.

Marschang S, Bernardo G (2015). Prevention and control of healthcare-associated infection in Europe: a review of patients' perspectives and existing differences. J Hosp Infect, 89(4):357–362.

Meisinger C, Stollenwerk B, Kirchberger I et al. (2013). Effects of a nurse-based case management compared to usual care among aged patients with myocardial infarction: results from the randomized controlled KORINNA study. BMC Geriatrics, 13:115.

Mekonnen A, McLachlan A, Brien J (2016). Effectiveness of pharmacist-led medication reconciliation programmes on clinical outcomes at hospital transitions: a systematic review and meta-analysis. BMJ Open, 6(2):p. e010003.

Mossialos E, Courtin E, Naci H et al. (2015). From "retailers" to health care providers: Transforming the role of community pharmacists in chronic disease management. Health Policy, 119(5):628–639.

Neiterman E, Wodchis W, Bourgeault I (2015). Experiences of older adults in transition from hospital to community. Can J Aging / Rev can vieillissement, 34:90–99. doi:10.1017/ S0714980814000518.

NHS England (2018). Hospital at home. (https://www.england.nhs.uk/ urgent-emergency-care/improving-hospital-discharge/, accessed 20 May 2020).

Ni W, Colayco D, Hashimoto J et al. (2018). Reduction of healthcare costs through a transitions-of-care program. Am J Health-Syst Pharm, 75(10):613–621. (https://doi.org/10.2146/ajhp170255).

Oakley C, Shacklady C (2015). The clinical effectiveness of the extended-scope physiotherapist role in musculoskeletal triage: a systematic review. Musculoskeletal Care, 13(4):204–221. (https://doi.org/10.1002/msc.1100).

Panagioti M, Richardson G, Murray E et al. (2014). Reducing Care Utilisation through Self-management Interventions (RECURSIVE): a systematic review and meta-analysis. Health Serv Deliv Res, 2(54):1–200. (https:// doi.org/10.3310/hsdr02540).

Paudyal V, Watson MC, Sach T et al. (2013). Are pharmacy-based Minor Ailment Schemes a substitute for other service providers? A systematic review BJGP 63(612):e472–481. doi: 10.3399/bjgp13X669194.

Phatak A, Prusi R, Ward B et al. (2016). Impact of pharmacist involvement in the transitional care of high-risk patients through medication reconciliation, medication education, and postdischarge call-backs (IPITCH Study). J Hosp Med, 11:39–44.

Qaddoura A, Yazdan-Ashoori P, Kabali C et al. (2015). Efficacy of hospital at home in patients with heart failure: a systematic review and meta-analysis. PLoS One, 10(6):e0129282.

Rennke S, Nguyen OK, Shoeb MH, et al. (2013). Hospital-initiated transitional care interventions as a patient safety strategy: a systematic review. Ann Intern Med, 158:433–440.

Sheikh F, Gathecha E, Bellantoni M et al. (2018). A call to bridge across silos during care transitions. Joint Commission J Qual Patient Safety, 44(5):270–278. (https://doi.org/10.1016/j.jcjq.2017.10.006).

Shepperd S, Cradduck-Bamford A, Butler C et al. (2017). A multi-centre randomised trial to compare the effectiveness of geriatrician-led admission avoidance hospital at home versus inpatient admission. Trials, 18(1):491. (https://doi.org/10.1186/s13063-017-2214-y).

Sinclair H, Bond C, Largue G et al. (2006). Community pharmacy provision of allergic rhinitis treatments a longitudinal study of patient reported outcomes IJPP, 13:249–256.

Trottmann M, Frueh M, Telser H et al. (2016). Physician drug dispensing in Switzerland: association on health care expenditures and utilization. BMC Health Serv Res, 16(1):238.

Vedel I, Khanassov V (2015). Transitional care for patients with congestive heart failure: a systematic review and meta-analysis. Ann Fam Med, 13:562–571.

Verloo H, Chiolero A, Kiszio B et al. (2017). Nurse interventions to improve medication adherence among discharged older adults: a systematic review. Age Ageing, 46(5):747–754.

Verweij L, Jepma P, Buurman BM et al. (2018) The cardiac care bridge program: design of a randomized trial of nurse-coordinated transitional care in older hospitalized cardiac patients at high risk of readmission and mortality. BMC Health Serv Res, 18(1):508. doi: 10.1186/s12913-018-3301-9.

Walker PC, Bernstein SJ, Jones JN et al. (2009). Impact of a pharmacist-facilitated hospital discharge program: a quasi-experimental study. Arch Intern Med, 169(21):2003–2010. (https://doi.org/10.1001/archinternmed.2009.398).

World Health Organization (2016) Transitions of care: technical series on safer primary care. Geneva, World Health Organization; Licence: CC BY-NC-SA 3.0 IGO.

Wright J, Graham F, Hayes C et al. (2013). A systematic review of oral health outcomes produced by dental teams incorporating midlevel providers. J Am Dental Assoc, 144(1):75–91.

Yang S (2017). Impact of pharmacist-led medication management in care transitions. BMC Health Serv Res, 17:722.

Zhu QM, Liu J, Hu HY et al. (2015). Effectiveness of nurse-led early discharge planning programmes for hospital inpatients with chronic disease or rehabilitation needs: a systematic review and meta-analysis. J Clin Nurs, 24:2993–3005.

6 Chronic conditions and multimorbidity: skill-mix innovations for enhanced quality and coordination of care

JULIANE WINKELMANN, GEMMA A. WILLIAMS, MIEKE RIJKEN, KATHERINE POLIN, CLAUDIA B. MAIER

6.1 Introduction

The prevalence of chronic diseases and multimorbidity is rising across Europe, triggered by increasing life expectancy and changing lifestyles. Chronic conditions are now the leading causes of premature death and disability in high-income countries (IHME, 2018; Jakab et al., 2018). In European countries, the number of people with multimorbidity, defined as the co-existence of two or more chronic conditions, is growing and may be an even greater challenge (Rijken et al., 2017, 2018).

The resulting pressures on health systems to address chronic and multimorbid conditions have become a major concern for policy-makers and providers. Traditional care delivery models are insufficient to respond to the complexity of such health conditions, with some patients experiencing disrupted care pathways. Continuous, coordinated, person-centred care is essential. Yet, many health service delivery models remain fragmented and focused on a single disease. As a result, a variety of new care models responding to chronic conditions and multimorbidity have been developed over the last decades, including disease management programmes, integrated care and multiprofessional team collaboration (Nolte & Knai, 2015). However, implementation remains patchy, limited to stand-alone programmes or projects, certain regions or single health conditions. These new health care models require new professional skills from individual providers and new competencies. Skill gaps include coordination and communication among providers, digital health know-how, coordination and transition between care levels (home, community, ambulatory, hospital), and developing patients' self-management through self-care and independent decision-making.

The aim of this chapter is to investigate the impact of skill-mix interventions in the care of patients with chronic and multimorbid conditions on health outcomes and health-system-related outcomes. Findings are based on the overview of systematic reviews, of which the methods are described in Chapter 1. Next, it presents the main skill-mix innovations and reforms for care of chronic conditions and multimorbidity that have emerged across Europe. The identification of these trends and reforms is based on the overview of systematic reviews on outcomes; on country case studies; and on an analysis of policies and grey literature.

This chapter focuses on trends in skill-mix changes for people with chronic conditions and multimorbidity. Across Europe, extensive research points to general positive effects of several skill-mix changes such as multiprofessional teams and expanded roles of certain professions (for example, nurses, pharmacists) to strengthen the coordination of care and patient self-management. Simultaneously, numerous other reforms and smaller-scale programmes have been adopted across Europe. In countries with a tradition of multiprofessional teamwork within the health and social care sectors, such as England, Italy and the Netherlands, nurses are more involved in care delivery and coordination of chronic care, such as in nurse-led clinics and nurse-delivered case management, and use of multiprofessional teams is more widespread (Nolte & Knai, 2015). In other countries with a traditionally physician-centred service delivery model in primarily solo practice, skill-mix changes have been less extensive. Germany for example introduced community nurses and "care assistants in family practice" to strengthen the role of nurses in providing patient self-management support or the delivery of selected medical tasks in anticipation of future shortages of family physicians. However, most often these tasks have remained under the supervision of the GP.

The chapter is structured as follows: Section 6.2 summarizes the main results from the overview of systematic reviews on the impact of skill-mix innovation on individual health outcomes and health-system-related outcomes. Within health-system-related outcomes, a focus was given on resource use and other outcome measures, including outcomes on the health workforce itself (profession-specific outcomes), as available. Section 6.3 outlines skill-mix reforms and trends in skill-mix interventions taking a cross-country perspective, identified in the literature and grey material. It also presents four case studies informed by the literature, country experts' feedback and national policy documents. These were selected based on the extent of their integration with routine care, the innovation potential for other geographies and the representation of the variety of skill-mix innovation and areas of intervention. Section 6.4 concludes the chapter and discusses implications for practice, research and policy.

6.2   Evidence on outcomes of skill-mix interventions for chronic conditions and multimorbidity

Overview of the systematic reviews included

A total of 78 systematic reviews on skill-mix interventions for chronic conditions and multimorbidity were identified and synthesized for this chapter (Box 6.1).

Included reviews evaluated skill-mix innovations aiming to improve care for a variety of chronic diseases. Single chronic conditions were assessed in 69 reviews, covering the following conditions: diabetes and chronic kidney disease (25 reviews[1]), mental health (16 reviews), cardiovascular disease (10 reviews), cancer (six reviews), chronic respiratory diseases (five reviews), HIV infection (three reviews), musculoskeletal disorders (one review) and various chronic conditions (three reviews).

Box 6.1   Overview of the evidence

- A total of 78 reviews were identified and synthesized for this chapter:
  - o   69 reviews focused on single chronic conditions (diabetes mellitus and chronic kidney disease, cardiovascular disease, cancer, mental health, chronic respiratory diseases, HIV infection and musculoskeletal disorders)
  - o   nine reviews focused on multimorbidity, with one of them focusing on both single chronic conditions and multimorbidity.
- The majority of original studies were conducted in the USA, the United Kingdom, Australia and Canada. The Netherlands and Spain were the most represented European countries after the United Kingdom in terms of original studies, with a small number from Sweden, Belgium, Denmark, France, Ireland, Austria and Switzerland. There were no studies from Eastern European countries.
- The quality of reviews was moderate overall, there were 10 Cochrane reviews and 43 reviews including a meta-analysis.

---

[1] Some of these reviews also focus on cardiovascular disease and/or hypertension. However, reviews are only counted once, under one condition.

Nine reviews focused solely on multimorbidity with four of them evaluating some aspect of multiprofessional teamwork, three studies focused on nurse-led clinics, nurse prescribing and nurse-led collaborative care, and one study focused on collaborative goal setting between patients and primary health professionals. One review evaluated both single chronic conditions and multimorbidity, focusing on nurse-delivered education to improve self-management. Details on the main skill-mix innovations covered are described in Box 6.2 and in subsequent boxes (Boxes 6.3–6.6) in the respective subsections. Almost all reviews reported on health outcomes, but few studies assessed other outcome measures such as cost-effectiveness, health care utilization or patient and staff satisfaction. There was little consideration of the education or qualifications of health professionals involved in skill-mix innovations, so it was not possible to draw conclusions on different outcomes regarding the training.

In the following section we synthesize the evidence from the included systematic reviews according to the professional groups primarily involved in skill-mix innovations: pharmacists, nurses, other single professions (for example, community health workers) and multiprofessional teams.

Box 6.2 Major skill-mix innovations in the care for patients with chronic conditions and multimorbidity

The majority of skill-mix interventions for the management of single chronic conditions (mainly diabetes, cardiovascular disease and hypertension) involved a pharmacist or nurse taking on new tasks (for example, patient education) or being re-allocated tasks from another health profession (most frequently a physician). In contrast, the management of mental health diseases and multimorbidity often involved collaborative care and interprofessional teamwork between primary care physicians, specialists, nurses, pharmacists and other health and social care professionals. New skill-mix innovations involved care coordinating roles such as case managers (for example, nurse or social worker) or patient navigators for example, lay persons) overseeing the care process and providing social and psychological patient support or patient education. Many skill-mix innovations, however, were multifactorial interventions using a collaborative care approach that included a case manager (nurse or pharmacist) that may support primary care teams, set up care planning, collaborative goal setting, patient education and follow up.

Pharmacist-delivered interventions

Key messages

- Skill-mix interventions involving pharmacists are effective at improving blood glucose levels and blood pressure control and have comparable results on health-related quality of life.
- Pharmacist-delivered care can improve medication adherence for patients with a variety of chronic conditions.
- There is some, albeit limited, evidence showing that skill-mix interventions involving pharmacists may be cost-effective and reduce the risk of hospital admissions.

Chronic conditions

Evidence on health and profession-specific outcomes

With respect to diabetes, included reviews provide strong evidence that pharmacist-involved interventions (for example, more advanced roles in patient education, medication and disease management) compared with usual care can significantly improve glycated haemoglobin (HbA1c) levels, irrespective of whether pharmacists work as part of

---

Box 6.3 Skill-mix interventions involving pharmacists

- Pharmacist interventions were evaluated in 18 systematic reviews on single chronic conditions (Table 6.1)
- In the majority of reviews pharmacists were allocated tasks traditionally performed by physicians or nurses
- New tasks commonly undertaken included: health screenings, immunizations, monitoring of drug interactions and medication adherence, providing therapeutic recommendations to patient's physician and education and guidance to patients on healthy behaviours and disease management
- One review additionally assessed pharmacist-delivered education of physicians to improve adherence to prescribing guidelines for diabetes care
- One review evaluated pharmacists providing direct care to diabetes patients within a multiprofessional primary health care team
- Two reviews on COPD and multiple single chronic conditions evaluated pharmacist-collaborative care with primary health practitioners to improve medication adherence, prescribing and patient outcomes

Table 6.1 *Skill-mix interventions involving pharmacists for single chronic conditions*

Skill-mix interventions			Outcomes			
Content of interventions and skill-mix changes	Source(s)	Chronic condition [Sources]	Profession(s) in comparator group [Sources]	Patient-related outcomes [Sources]	Health system-related/resource use outcomes [Sources]	Profession-specific outcomes [Sources]
Pharmacist-involved care to improve patients' self-management including: health education, consultation, collaborative drug therapy management, initiation or titration of drug therapy, collaborative practice model, direct care under clinical guidelines, multidisciplinary diabetes management, home visitations, patient self-management training programmes	[1–9]	Diabetes [1–5]; Various chronic conditions (COPD, depression, diabetes, CVD) [6, 7]; CVD/hypertension [8, 9]	• Usual care, professions not defined [1, 3, 5, 6, 9] • Pharmacists, primary care physicians or nurses [2] • Usual care generally from physician [8], but also nurses and pharmacists [4] • Primary health care professionals or no comparable service [7]	• Reduced HbA1c levels* [2–4, 6, 7] • Reduced SBP and DBP* [6–9] • Reduced LDL-C* [4] • Improved medication adherence* [3, 8, 9] • Increased attainment of goals for HbA1c [6] • Improved quality of life* [3, 5] • Some evidence of improvements in quality of life for patients with asthma, heart failure and high risk of medications related problems (three of eight studies) [7] • Improved modifiable lifestyle risk factors and improvements in HbA1c levels [1] • No difference in all-cause mortality [6] • No significant improvements in COPD and depression outcomes [7] • Decrease in number of medications prescribed, an improvement in testing and statin prescribing for patients with hyperlipidaemia [7]	• Some evidence of reduced costs for collaborative care models and when pharmacists provide pro-active consultation for high-risk patients and new/changed prescriptions [1] • Intervention dominant (cost-effective) [5] • Improvements in eliminating therapeutic duplication [7] • Similar rates of office visits, emergency department visits and hospitalizations compared with usual care [6]	• Increased adherence to American Diabetes Association standards of care for most care types [1] • Improvements in guideline adherence for prescribing for physicians (compared with no intervention) [7]

Table 6.1 (cont.)

Skill-mix interventions				Outcomes		
Content of interventions and skill-mix changes	Source(s)	Chronic condition [Sources]	Profession(s) in comparator group [Sources]	Patient-related outcomes [Sources]	Health system-related/resource use outcomes [Sources]	Profession-specific outcomes [Sources]
Pharmacists providing direct patient care within an interprofessional team	[10]	Diabetes	• Usual care without pharmacist interventions and/or diabetes education provided by health care professionals other than pharmacists	• Reduced HbA1c levels, SPB and LDL-C*		• Improvements in prescribing guideline adherence by physicians
Pharmacist managed warfarin services including medication adherence, screening for side effects and monitoring drug interactions	[11, 12]	CVD/hypertension	• Physician or nurse [11, 12]	• Comparable effects (usual care) on anticoagulation control, major bleeding, thromboembolic events [11] • Lower or comparable (usual care) risk of major bleeding and thromboembolic events [12]	• Cost savings* [11, 12] • Reduced emergency department visits, hospitalization rates* [11, 12]	
Pharmacist provided education counselling,	[13]	Cancer	• Nurses	• Improved nausea and vomiting control • Improved medication adherence	• Improvement for anti-emesis drug costs	

Intervention	Reference	Condition	Comparator	Outcomes
health screening and monitoring medication adherence and side effects for adult outpatients with cancer using antineoplastic drugs				• Increased knowledge–attitude–practice for chemotherapy and blood pressure management • Increased patient satisfaction and quality of life
Pharmacist provided education and counselling to improve medication adherence and symptoms	[14]	Depression	Usual care, professions not defined	• No improvement in depression symptom severity • Improved medication adherence*
Pharmacist-delivered patient care services in the community pharmacy setting for disease or medication management, re-fill reminders, pharmacist-administration of influenza immunization [15, 16], and pharmacist-collaborative care with primary health practitioners [16]	[15, 16ᵃ]	Various including asthma, diabetes, hypertension, CVD, HIV, COPD and multimorbidity	Usual care, professions not defined [15, 16]	• Improved medication adherence, appropriate medication use and immunization rates [15] • Improved blood pressure control but limited evidence of other improved health outcomes [15] • No evidence of improved safety outcomes or quality of life [15] • Some limited evidence of improved patient satisfaction [15] • Improvements in diet and diabetes self-care but no change in exercise rates [15] • Reductions in SBP, DBP, LDL-cholesterol, HbA1c and 10-year Framingham risk score* [16] • Increased average number of inpatient and outpatient claims for patients with diabetes [15] • Higher percentage of asthma patients with breathing-related emergency department visits or hospitalization [15]

Table 6.1 *(cont.)*

Skill-mix interventions				Outcomes		
Content of interventions and skill-mix changes	Source(s)	Chronic condition [Sources]	Profession(s) in comparator group [Sources]	Patient-related outcomes [Sources]	Health system-related/ resource use outcomes [Sources]	Profession-specific outcomes [Sources]
Pharmacist-delivered care in the management of adults with pre-dialysis CKD in addition to usual care	[17][b]	CKD	• Usual care, GP	• No effect on quality of life, renal outcomes and blood pressure outcomes		• Higher rate of prescribing for vitamin D and bicarbonate*
Pharmacist-delivered care and pharmacist-collaborative care providing education, medication management, patient-reminder, smoking cessation	[18]	COPD	• Usual care, pharmacists, medical staff and nursing staff	• Improved medication compliance of patients* • No significant effect on lung function	• Cost savings* • Reduction in risk of hospital admission* • No significant effect on emergency department visits	

Abbreviations: BP: blood pressure; CKD: chronic kidney disease; COPD: chronic obstructive pulmonary disease; CVD: cardiovascular disease; DBP: diastolic blood pressure; GP: general practitioner; HbA1c: glycated haemoglobin; HIV: human immunodeficiency virus; LDL-C: low-density lipoprotein cholesterol; SBP: systolic blood pressure.

Notes: [a] Studies included in this review also covered patients with multiple chronic conditions (patients receiving polypharmacy, patients prescribed at least one medication, and any general practice patients and patients at risk of adverse health problems); [b] Review is also covered in Tables 6.2 and 6.4. * Statistically significant results.

Sources: [1] Armor et al. (2010); [2] Aguiar et al. (2016); [3] Deters et al. (2018); [4] van Eikenhorst et al. (2017); [5]Wang, Yeo & Ko (2016); [6] Greer et al. (2016); [7] Nkansah et al. (2010); [8] Morgado et al. (2011); [9] Cheema, Sutcliffe & Singer (2014); [10] Fazel et al. (2017); [11] Entezari-Maleki et al. (2016); [12] Manzoor et al. (2017); [13] Colombo et al. (2017); [14] Readdean, Heuer & Scott Parrott (2018); [15] Blalock et al. (2013); [16] Tan et al. (2014); [17] Nicoll et al. (2018); [18] Zhong et al. (2014).

a multiprofessional team or autonomously (Table 6.1) (Aguiar et al., 2016; Armor et al., 2010; Deters et al., 2018; Fazel et al., 2017; Greer et al., 2016; Nkansah et al., 2010; van Eikenhorst et al., 2017).

The evidence also suggests that pharmacist-delivered care improves cardiovascular disease outcomes, with studies reporting improvements in systolic and diastolic blood pressure measures versus usual care (Blalock et al., 2013; Cheema, Sutcliffe & Singer, 2014; Fazel et al., 2017; Greer et al., 2016; Morgado et al., 2011; Nkansah et al., 2010; van Eikenhorst et al., 2017). Pharmacist-delivered care had comparable effects on health-related quality of life and mortality risk for patients on warfarin compared with usual physician-delivered care (Entezari-Maleki et al., 2016). Some evidence suggested pharmacist interventions improved quality of life for patients with asthma, heart failure and those at high risk of medications related problems (Nkansah et al., 2010). Evidence also indicated a lower risk of major bleeding and thromboembolic events for participants engaged in pharmacist-delivered interventions, albeit with significance only found in non-RCT studies (Entezari-Maleki et al., 2016; Manzoor et al., 2017).

Pharmacist-delivered care for patients living with cancer led to improved control of nausea and vomiting, patient satisfaction, medication adherence and increased knowledge of blood pressure management. It was also shown to improve quality of life and patient satisfaction for adults on antineoplastic medication (Colombo et al., 2017). However, no significant effect of pharmacist-delivered care was reported in one study on patients with chronic kidney disease for quality of life, renal outcomes and blood pressure (Nicoll et al., 2018), nor in one study on COPD care for lung function (Zhong et al., 2014). In addition, one review concluded that pharmacist-delivered care did not improve depression symptoms (Readdean, Heuer & Scott Parrott, 2018).

Compared with usual care, pharmacist-delivered interventions were able to significantly improve medication adherence for patients with hypertension (Blalock et al., 2013; Cheema, Sutcliffe & Singer, 2014; Morgado et al., 2011), diabetes (Blalock et al., 2013; Fazel et al., 2017; van Eikenhorst et al., 2017; Wang, Yeo & Ko, 2016), depression (Readdean, Heuer & Scott Parrott, 2018) and COPD (Zhong et al., 2014). One review on pharmacist-delivered patient care services in the community for people with various chronic conditions or multimorbidity concluded that it improved patient satisfaction but did not reduce safety outcomes or quality of life (Blalock et al., 2013).

With respect to profession-specific outcomes, limited evidence also suggests that pharmacist interventions can improve adherence to pre-scribing guidelines for physicians, resulting in a reduction in therapeutic duplication and the number of medications prescribed (Nkansah et al., 2010). Two studies also reported that pharmacist-involved care increased adherence to American Diabetes Association standards of care for most care types (Armor et al., 2010) and led to a higher rate of prescribing of vitamin D and bicarbonate for patients with chronic kidney disease (Nicoll et al., 2018).

Evidence on health-system-related outcomes

Five studies reported economic outcomes on pharmacist-involved inter-ventions. According to one review (Wang, Yeo & Ko, 2016), pharmacist-managed care resulted in higher quality-adjusted life-years with lower costs than usual care (so the intervention was dominant). Pharmacist-managed warfarin services were shown to significantly lower emergency department visits and hospitalization rates and to be cost saving over usual physician-delivered care (Entezari-Maleki et al., 2016; Manzoor et al., 2017). Pharmacist-delivered care was also shown to lower anti-emetic drug costs for cancer care (Colombo et al., 2017), while lower costs were reported for collaborative care models involving pharmacists and pharmacist-provided consultations for high-risk diabetes patients (Armor et al., 2010) and for COPD patients (Zhong et al., 2014).

Pharmacist-directed care and pharmacist-collaborative care were also found to significantly reduce risk of hospital admissions for patients with COPD, but had no effect on emergency department visits (Zhong et al., 2014). One review also found similar rates of emergency department visits, office visits and hospitalizations compared with usual care for people with chronic conditions (Greer et al., 2016). There was, however, some evidence of pharmacist-delivered care leading to a higher percent-age of asthma patients with breathing-related emergency department visits or hospitalizations (Blalock et al., 2013).

Multimorbidity

The one review evaluating care for multimorbidity involving pharma-cists, focused on pharmacist-directed care and pharmacist-collaborative care with primary health practitioners. This review found evidence that multiprofessional teamwork significantly improved systolic and diastolic blood pressure, low-density lipoprotein cholesterol (but not high-density lipoprotein cholesterol), HbA1c levels and 10-year Framingham risk score versus usual care (Tan et al., 2014).

Nurse-delivered skill-mix interventions

Key messages

- Nurse-delivered care leads to equivalent or better health outcomes compared with the usual care, in particular titration of medication by nurses and nurse-led clinics.
- There is insufficient evidence on the impact of skill-mix interventions involving nurses in expanded roles on health system outcomes and cost effectiveness, but some studies show a positive impact on hospital (re)admissions, physician visits and costs.
- Evidence on the impact of skill-mix innovations involving nurses on health outcomes for people with multimorbidity is inconclusive.

Chronic conditions

Evidence on health and profession-specific outcomes

The included reviews focusing on diabetes found a comparable effect on HbA1c levels for independent nurse prescribing compared with physician-led prescribing (Health Quality Ontario, 2013;

Box 6.4 Skill-mix interventions involving nurses

- 20 systematic reviews assessed nurse-delivered skill-mix interventions for single chronic conditions (Table 6.2), with four reviews focused on multimorbidity (Table 6.5)
- In the majority of reviews nurses were allocated tasks traditionally undertaken by physicians
- New tasks undertaken by nurses range from prescribing, lifestyle education for improved self-management, management of medication adherence and prescribing, that are delivered either independently (as a physician substitute) or within a multiprofessional team
- Three reviews assessed nurse-led clinics in cardiac and asthma care
- Two reviews focused on care delivered either autonomously or within a multiprofessional team by nurse practitioners or specialist nurses for people with various chronic conditions
- One review evaluated titration of medicines by nurses for diabetes care

Table 6.2 *Nurse-delivered skill-mix interventions for single chronic conditions*

Skill-mix interventions				Outcomes		
Content of interventions and skill-mix changes	Source(s)	Chronic condition [Sources]	Profession(s) in comparator group [Sources]	Patient-related outcomes [Sources]	Health system-related/resource use outcomes [Sources]	Profession-specific outcomes [Sources]
Brief psychosocial intervention delivered by nurses, psychotherapists or social workers to support families living in the community affected by cancer	[19]	Cancer	• Usual care, professions not defined	• Improvements in depression and anxiety • Improved QoL • Improved patient–carer relationship • Reduced carer burden • Mixed evidence on physical symptoms, with some reviews reporting adverse consequences • Increased depression in those receiving CBT • Worse psychosocial status in carers taught to give direct care		
Nurse titration of medications following a protocol	[20]	Diabetes/CVD	• Usual care, professions not defined	• Reduced HbA1c levels, SBP and DBP* • Improved medication adherence*	• Lower inpatient costs* • No significant differences in outpatient costs	

Intervention	References	Condition	Comparator	Outcomes
Nurse-delivered education to improve patient self-management	[21]	Diabetes	Usual care, GP or nurse or other health care professional under GP supervision	• No significant difference in HbA1c levels • Reduced SBP and DBP*
Nurse practitioners and specialized nurses providing clinical care (e.g. prescribing) and lifestyle education, either independently or as part of a multiprofessional team	[22, 23]	Various chronic diseases (COPD, CVD, CAD, diabetes, chronic wounds) [22]; diabetes [23]	Usual care from physicians	• Comparable effect to physician-delivered care on HbA1c levels working autonomously [22, 23] • Reduction in HbA1c levels with nurse-led multiprofessional team* [22] • Improved BP and cholesterol control for teamwork [22] • Improved patient satisfaction for teamwork; no differences autonomous care [22] • Increase in the proportion of individuals appropriately receiving influenza or pneumovax vaccinations, patient education related to smoking, exercise, diet, and medication side-effects* [22] • Specialized nurses more likely to intensify glucose-lowering therapy, intensify blood pressure medications [22] • Reduced hospitalizations for the CAD population for teamwork*; no differences for nurses providing autonomous care [22] • Increase in number of referrals for echocardiographs among patients with presumed CHF, assessment of blood pressure, smoking status, and body mass index/weight among CAD patients (1 of 1 study) [22] • Specialized nurses more likely to refer to an internist for starting insulin therapy [22] • No significant difference in job satisfaction, or inappropriate demands for teamwork [22]

Table 6.2 (cont.)

Skill-mix interventions			Outcomes		
Content of interventions and skill-mix changes	Source(s)	Chronic condition [Sources]	Profession(s) in comparator group [Sources]	Patient-related outcomes [Sources]	Health system-related/ resource use outcomes [Sources]	Profession-specific outcomes [Sources]
Nurse-delivered autonomous care involving a variety of activities, ranging from nurse prescribing to nurse-delivered lifestyle education	[24]	Various chronic diseases (asthma, COPD, hypertension, diabetes, CVD, gastritis, Parkinson's)	• Physicians, including family physicians, paediatricians, geriatricians	• Comparable effect to physician-delivered care on HbA1c levels • Reduction in patients with feet-at-risk • Reduction in total mortality • No long-term differences in blood pressure, BMI, weight, smoking • Improved intake of aspirin, low-fat diets and moderate physical activity • No long-term differences in correct inhalation technique and well-controlled asthma • Improvements in best hand score for Parkinson's patients*		• No difference in adherence to practical guidelines • Nurses provided more information than physicians on the causes of health problems or illness (2 of 3 trials), relief of symptoms, duration of illness, how to reduce recurrences and what to do if problems persisted (1 of 2 trials)

Intervention	Ref	Condition	Comparator	Outcomes
Nurse-delivered education to improve self-monitoring and disease management	[25][a]	Various chronic diseases (COPD, hypertension, diabetes, CVD)	• Usual care, primary care physician	• Reduction in DBP, LDL-C and HbA1c* • No conclusive evidence on total mortality, quality of life, fasting serum glucose levels, triglycerides
Nurse-led cardiac clinics	[26, 27]	CVD	• Usual care, professions not defined [26, 27]	• No long-term differences in blood pressure, self-perceived physical or mental health compared with other clinics [26] • Decreased risk of myocardial infarction* [27] • No significantly lower risk of major adverse cardiac event [27] • Improved medication adherence* [27] • No significant differences in hospitalizations [26]
Nurse-delivered counselling, education and motivation to increase medication adherence delivered autonomously or within multiprofessional team	[28]	CVD/hypertension	• Usual care, professions not defined	• Improved medication adherence for motivation and follow-up interventions but not education and counselling*

Table 6.2 *(cont.)*

Skill-mix interventions				Outcomes		
Content of interventions and skill-mix changes	Source(s)	Chronic condition [Sources]	Profession(s) in comparator group [Sources]	Patient-related outcomes [Sources]	Health system-related/ resource use outcomes [Sources]	Profession-specific outcomes [Sources]
Nurses or pharmacists providing care in the home to improve disease self-management and lifestyle	[29]	CVD/ hyper-tension	• Usual care, professions not defined	• Reduced all-cause mortality* • Improved quality of life for nurse-delivered interventions but not for pharmacist-delivered interventions*	• Average savings of $10 665 per patient • Reduced hospitalizations*	
Use of nurses as managers of antidepressant medication adherence programmes, either as case managers or as part of collaborative team	[30]	Depression	• Usual care, professions not defined	• Improved depression symptom severity • No improvements in medication adherence		
Self-management skills education by nurses, peers or health assistant	[31]	Mental health	• Usual care or within person pre- and post-intervention, professions not defined	• Improved self-management skills and small improvements in physical health	• Small reduction in use of crisis and emergency services	

Intervention	Reference	Disease	Comparator	Outcomes
Transition manager (mostly nurse-delivered) providing education, follow up, needs assessment and inpatient/outpatient provider communication	[32]	Mental health	Not defined	• Reduction of readmission rates for pre- and post-discharge interventions: patient psycho-education, needs assessment, telephone follow up, home visits, use of transition manager and inpatient/outpatient provider communication* • No significant reduction for bridging interventions • Improvement of staff encouragement*
Nurse-delivered disease management programmes to improve quality of life for patients with pre-dialysis chronic kidney disease	[33]	CKD	Usual non-nurse led disease management care	• Improvement of symptoms and sleep* • No significant improvement of patient satisfaction
Nurse-delivered care (involving nurses, specialist nurses, NPs) in the management of adults with pre-dialysis CKD	[34][b]	CKD	Usual care, nephrologists, GPs	• No significant effect on mortality, renal outcomes, composite ischaemic heart disease end-point • Higher mean number of total visits (including nurse visits), and lower mean number of physician visits (per year)* • Increase in prescribing of relevant drugs*

Table 6.2 (cont.)

Skill-mix interventions				Outcomes		
Content of interventions and skill-mix changes	Source(s)	Chronic condition [Sources]	Profession(s) in comparator group [Sources]	Patient-related outcomes [Sources]	Health system-related/ resource use outcomes [Sources]	Profession-specific outcomes [Sources]
Nurse-delivered self-management intervention	[35]	COPD	• Usual care, GP, specialist, respiratory nursing service	• Reduction of anxiety symptoms* • No significant difference in exacerbation frequency and patient satisfaction		
Nurse-led asthma clinics with varying degree of doctor participation [36] and nurse-delivered asthma management (specialized asthma nurse, NP, physician assistant supervised by physician) [37]	[36, 37]	Asthma	• Usual care, GPs, [36]; physician-delivered asthma care, physician, paediatrician, respiratory specialist [37]	• Reduced nocturnal awakenings* [36] • No significant difference in use of preventer medication [36] • No significant improvement of quality of life [36, 37] • No significant improvement of asthma severity and symptoms [37] • No significant difference in number of exacerbations [37]	• No significant difference in accident and emergency department attendance [36] • No significant difference in hospital admission [36, 37] • Lower costs for nurse-delivered outpatient visits* [37]	

Nurse-delivered home care and education for patients with obstructive sleep apnoea	[38]	Obstructive sleep apnoea	Physician-delivered care	• No significant difference in continuous-positive airway pressure, Epworth Sleepiness Scale and physical functioning

Abbreviations: BMI: body mass index; BP: blood pressure; CVD: cardiovascular disease; CAD: coronary artery disease; CBT: cognitive behavioural therapy; CKD: chronic kidney disease; COPD: chronic obstructive pulmonary disease; CHF: coronary heart failure; DBP: diastolic blood pressure; HbA1c: glycated haemoglobin; HIV: human immunodeficiency virus; LDL-C: low-density lipoprotein cholesterol; NP: nurse practitioner; SBP: systolic blood pressure.

Notes: * Statistically significant results; [a] 16 of 23 studies in this review cover single chronic conditions, only their results are reported. Results on multimorbidity are reported in Table 6.5; [b] Review is also covered in Tables 6.1 and 6.4.

Sources: [19] Hopkinson et al. (2012); [20] Shaw et al. (2013); [21] Parker et al. (2016); [22] Health Quality Ontario (2013); [23] Tabesh et al. (2018); [24] Martínez–Gonzalez et al. (2015); [25] Massimi et al. (2017); [26] Schadewaldt & Schultz (2010); [27] Al-Mallah et al. (2016); [28] Al-Ganmi et al. (2016); [29] Fergenbaum et al. (2015); [30] Heise et al. (2014); [31] Kelly et al. (2014); [32] Vigod et al. (2013); [33] Chen et al. (2016); [34] Nicoll et al. (2018); [35] Baker & Fatoye (2017); [36] Baishnab & Karner (2012); [37] Kuethe et al. (2013); [38] Gong et al. (2018).

Martínez-González et al., 2015; Tabesh et al., 2018). Moreover, titration of medication by nurses significantly reduced HbA1c levels and improved health behaviours and medication adherence (Shaw et al., 2013). Self-management education by nurses was nevertheless shown to have no significant impact on HbA1c levels (Parker et al., 2016), total mortality, quality of life or cholesterol levels (Massimi et al., 2017).

With respect to cardiovascular disease, nurse-titration of medication was reported to significantly reduce both systolic and diastolic blood pressure (Parker et al., 2016; Shaw et al., 2013). In addition, nurse-led cardiac clinics were found to provide equivalent or better care than clinics run by other health professionals or usual care of cardiovascular disease. Compared with usual care, studies reported significant reductions in total mortality and equivalent outcomes for self-reported mental or physical health compared with non-nurse led clinics (Schadewaldt and Schultz, 2010). Nurse-delivered motivational interviewing was shown to increase medication adherence for patients with cardiovascular disease (Al-Ganmi et al., 2016).

Moderate evidence also suggests that nurse-management of anti-depressant medication adherence programmes, with nurses working independently or as part of a multiprofessional team, helps to lower depression symptom severity and significantly improved patient satisfaction, but may not improve medication adherence (Heise & van Servellen, 2014). Limited evidence indicates that self-management education delivered by nurses, peers or health assistants can lead to small improvements in physical health and increased use of primary care services for people with a severe mental health condition (Kelly et al., 2014).

One review assessed psychosocial interventions for cancer patients and their families delivered predominantly by nurses (or psychotherapists and social worker) (Hopkinson et al., 2012). The review found some evidence of improved depression and anxiety symptoms and improved quality of life for cancer patients and improved patient–carer relationships. Nevertheless, there was also some evidence of worse psychosocial status in carers taught to give direct care and adverse consequences for the health status of cancer patients, including increased depression in those receiving cognitive behavioural therapy (Hopkinson et al., 2012).

Nurse-delivered care was found to lead to equivalent or better outcomes than usual care for patients with chronic kidney disease. Reviews reported significant improvement of symptoms and sleep, equivalent outcomes for patient satisfaction, mortality and renal outcomes (Chen et al., 2016; Nicoll et al., 2018).

Four reviews assessed nurse-delivered interventions for patients with respiratory diseases. Nurse-delivered self-management for patients with COPD was shown to significantly reduce anxiety symptoms (Baishnab et al., 2012) and nurse-led asthma clinics had a significant effect on nocturnal awakenings (Baker et al., 2017). For asthma patients, there was comparable effect on number of exacerbations (Baker et al., 2017; Kuethe et al., 2013), quality of life, disease severity and symptoms as well as use of preventer medication (Baishnab et al., 2012; Kuethe et al., 2013) and levels of correct inhalation technique and well-controlled asthma (Martínez-González et al., 2015). Nurse-delivered home care and education for patients with obstructive sleep apnoea was shown to have no significant effect on continuous positive airway pressure and physical functioning compared with physician-delivered care (Gong et al., 2018).

For patients with Parkinson's disease, nurse-delivered autonomous care was shown to significantly improve best hand score compared with usual care (Martínez-González et al., 2015), while nurse practitioner- and specialist nurse-delivered care within a team significantly increased the proportion of individuals with a chronic disease appropriately receiving influenza or pneumovax vaccinations as well as patient education related to smoking, exercise, diet, and medication side effects (Health Quality Ontario, 2013).

Four studies reported on professional-specific outcomes. For patients with various chronic conditions, nurse practitioner- or specialist nurse-delivered clinical care within a multiprofessional team was shown to lead to no significant difference in job satisfaction, or inappropriate demands for teamwork (Health Quality Ontario, 2013), while no difference in adherence to practical guidelines was found for nurse-delivered autonomous care (Martínez-González et al., 2015). However, nurse-led care for patients with chronic kidney disease was shown to lead to improvements in staff encouragement and an increase in prescribing of relevant drugs (Chen et al., 2016; Nicoll et al., 2018). Limited evidence also suggests that nurse practitioner- or specialist nurse-delivered clinical care increased the number of referrals for echocardiographs among patients with presumed coronary heart failure and the assessment of blood pressure, smoking status and body mass index/weight among coronary artery disease patients (Health Quality Ontario, 2013). Nurse practitioners and specialist nurses were also more likely to intensify glucose-lowering therapy, intensify blood pressure medications or refer patients with diabetes to an internist for the start of insulin therapy (Health Quality Ontario, 2013).

Evidence on health-system-related outcomes

Ten reviews reported on health-system-related outcomes of which most outcome measures covered the use of health resources. There is some evidence that nurse-led collaborative care can reduce hospitalizations for patients with coronary artery disease (Health Quality Ontario, 2013). Nurses providing interventions to improve the transition from inpatient to outpatient care were found to reduce readmission among adults with mental illness (Vigod et al., 2013). Nurse-delivered care in general was reported to improve secondary prevention of heart disease by appropriately increasing aspirin intake and adoption of low-fat diets and physically activity (Martínez-González et al., 2015). Furthermore, nurse-delivered care for patients with chronic kidney disease significantly reduced the number of physician visits, associated with an increased number of nurse visits (Nicoll et al., 2018). However, no significant difference was reported on accident and emergency department attendance and hospital admissions for patients attending nurse-led asthma and cardiac clinics (Baishnab et al., 2012; Kuethe et al., 2013; Schadewaldt and Schultz, 2010).

In terms of economic outcomes, nurse or pharmacist-delivered care in the home was shown to improve self-management of cardiovascular disease, reduce all-cause mortality and hospitalizations, resulting in average cost savings over usual care of $10 665 per patient (Fergenbaum et al., 2015). Nurse-delivered asthma management also led to significantly lower costs for outpatient visits (Kuethe et al., 2013), and nurse titration of medicines following a protocol led to lower inpatient costs but not significant differences in outpatient costs for patients at risk of cardiovascular disease (Shaw et al., 2013). Limited evidence suggests that titration of medication by nurses lowers inpatient costs as well as salary costs compared with usual care (Shaw et al., 2013).

Multimorbidity

Of the nine reviews on multimorbidity, four reviews analysed the expansion of roles for nurses and found improved or equivalent patient outcomes compared with usual care or physician-delivered care models (Table 6.5). Nurse-prescribing and community monitoring moderately reduced systolic but not diastolic blood pressure compared with physician-delivered care, while nurse-led clinics provided equivalent care to other clinics (Clark et al., 2011). All care models had a comparable effect on medication adherence compared with physician-delivered care (Clark et al., 2011). Nurse-delivered education to improve self-monitoring and disease management was shown to significantly reduce systolic and diastolic blood pressure and HbA1c levels, with a weak trend towards lower mortality (Massimi et al., 2017). Nurse-led collaborative care of patients significantly reduced depression severity for patients with depression and a physical health condition (Ekers et al., 2013), with limited evidence for improvements on patient, caregiver and health care staff satisfaction. No impact was observed on emergency admissions and bed days (Lupari et al., 2011).

Skill-mix interventions delivered by professions other than pharmacists and nurses for single chronic conditions

Key messages

- Peer educators and community health workers – if involving regular contact with patients – were shown to improve several health outcomes and peer-related outcomes and/or to have comparable effects.
- The evidence is mixed as to whether transition coordinators (by various health professions or multiprofessional teams) can improve certain health outcomes.
- Disease management delivered by different professions or multiprofessional teams was shown to improve HbA1c levels, self-reported health status and patient satisfaction.
- Skill-mix interventions involving patient navigators, transition coordinators or peers reported a positive impact on resource use for cancer and diabetes patients and patients with mental illness. However, evidence on impact of skill-mix interventions on resource use overall is mixed and remains insufficient.

Box 6.5 Skill mix interventions involving professions other than pharmacists and nurses

- Thirteen reviews evaluated skill-mix interventions involving professions other than pharmacists or nurses for single chronic conditions (Table 6.3)
- Five reviews assessed care delivered by non-health professionals (peers, parents) involved in patient navigation for breast cancer or case management, including for diabetes and mental health
- Two reviews evaluated interventions by community health workers providing education and chronic care management for diabetes and hypertension care
- Four reviews assessed interventions involving various professionals (GPs, dieticians, transition coordinators, specialists, social workers) in chronic disease management
- One review evaluated training for primary care physicians to provide depression care; one review assessed management of musculoskeletal disorders by physiotherapists acting as substitute for physicians and specialists

---

Evidence on health and profession-specific outcomes

Diabetes disease management delivered by different professions or multiprofessional teams significantly reduced HbA1c levels but had no impact on mortality risk (Pimouguet et al., 2011). The transition coordinator model did not lead to overall improvements in HbA1c levels (Chu et al., 2015).

Peer support (generally lay persons with experience of the same disease(s) or community health workers) was found to significantly reduce HbA1c levels compared with usual care, provided that there was a moderate to high frequency of contact with patients (Qi et al., 2015). Peer support was also shown to significantly improve blood pressure control, cholesterol, body mass index, physical activity levels, self-efficacy, depression and perceived social support (Dale, Williams & Bowyer, 2012). However, peers involved in case management for adults with severe mental illness had no significant effect on symptoms, patient satisfaction and quality of life (Wright-Berryman, McGuire & Salyers, 2011).

With respect to depression, training for primary care practitioners failed to improve clinical symptoms unless implemented alongside provision of specific care guidelines (Sikorski et al., 2012). Training for parents to better manage children with autism spectrum disorder had no impact on comprehension, child initiation, expression and joint

Table 6.3 *Skill-mix interventions delivered by professions other than pharmacists and nurses for single chronic conditions*

Skill-mix interventions

Content of interventions and skill-mix changes	Source(s)	Chronic condition	Profession(s) in comparator group	Outcomes		
				Patient-related outcomes	Health system-related/resource use outcomes	Profession-specific outcomes
Patient navigation in breast cancer care involving non-health professionals (breast cancer survivors, lay community health workers, nurse navigator in cooperation with lay navigator and social worker, laypersons)	[39]	Breast cancer	• Usual care, professions not defined	• Improved adherence to breast screening and diagnostic follow up due to navigation (follow up after abnormal radiographic screening, attending genetic counselling)	• Reduced waiting time for biopsy/diagnostic intervals • Decreased time to appointment with genetic counsellor	
GP-led follow-up care for child cancer survivors. Model 1: "GP only" model: GP solely responsible for follow up; Model 2: shared care follow up	[40]	Cancer	• Non-GP-led follow up (professions not described)	• Both models: Less patient travel, geographically convenient and "portable"	Both models: • Less attrition to follow-up appointments • Some evidence that more cost effective than follow-up in LTFU clinic • Reduced access to complex diagnostic testing	

Table 6.3 *(cont.)*

Skill-mix interventions				Outcomes		
Content of interventions and skill-mix changes	Source(s)	Chronic condition	Profession(s) in comparator group	Patient-related outcomes	Health system-related/resource use outcomes	Profession-specific outcomes
with close collaboration between the GP and paediatric cancer centre, primary cancer treatment team, or late effects clinic					GP only model: • Greater potential for discontinuity of care • May lose contact with original diagnosis centre	
Transition of coordination from paediatric to adult diabetes care by specialist physician, paediatric nurse, trained transition coordinator	[41]	Diabetes or sickle cell anaemia	• Usual care or no intervention, professions not defined	• No improvement in HbA1c levels (three of four studies)	• Higher rates of successful transfer and higher rates of attendance in adult clinics (three of five studies)	
Structured education sessions delivered by community health workers or peers with diabetes	[42]	Diabetes	• Usual care, professions not defined	• Reduction in HbA1c levels*		

Intervention	Ref	Condition	Comparator/Provider	Outcomes
Peer support models for adults living with diabetes including: face-to-face management programmes, peer coaching, telephone-based peer support and web- and email-based support	[43]	Diabetes	• Usual care and nurse care management	• Improvements* in glycaemic control, blood pressure, cholesterol, BMI, physical activity, self-efficacy, depression and perceived social support
Disease management defined as ongoing and proactive patient follow-up by various professionals or peer counsellors including at least two of the five activities: (i) patient education (dietary, exercise, self-monitoring, knowledge of disease and medication), (ii) coaching, (iii) treatment adjustment, (iv) monitoring, (v) care coordination	[44]	Diabetes	• Nurses, dieticians, primary care physicians	• Reduction in HbA1c levels* • No significant difference in mortality risk

Table 6.3 (cont.)

Skill-mix interventions				Outcomes		
Content of interventions and skill-mix changes	Source(s)	Chronic condition	Profession(s) in comparator group	Patient-related outcomes	Health system-related/resource use outcomes	Profession-specific outcomes
Community health workers providing chronic care management including: health coaching, health education, home visiting, environmental modification, advocacy, care coordination, connecting with health/social services	[45]	Various chronic conditions (Type 2 diabetes, asthma, HIV, hypertension, CVD)	• Professions not defined		• Significant decrease in preventable medication use • Evidence of cost savings and reduced per-patient annual costs • Significant decrease in emergency room visits, urgent care visits, and hospitalizations in 42% of RCTs	
Training for primary care physicians to provide depression care	[46]	Depression	• Usual care, professions not defined	• No improvement to symptom severity, unless implemented alongside care guidelines		
Substitution of doctors with physiotherapists	[47]	Musculoskeletal disorders	• Usual care, physicians and specialists	• No significant difference in health outcomes • Improved patient satisfaction*	• No difference in diagnostic and management decisions • Inconsistent results on resource utilization	

Intervention	Ref	Condition	Comparator	Outcomes	
Parent education in improving management, communication and interaction of/with children's autism spectrum disorder problems	[48]	Mental health/ autism spectrum disorder	• Usual care/ no treatment, student therapist, teacher, parents, professionals	• Improvement of autism characteristics' severity, shared attention in parent–child interaction* • No significant effect on comprehension, child initiation, expression, joint language	• Improved parent's satisfaction and confidence with therapy • Significant improvement of parents' synchrony
Consumer providers (peers) as practitioners on case management or assertive community treatment teams	[49]	Mental health	• Usual care	• No significant effect on symptoms, patient satisfaction and quality of life	• Better engagement in treatment and social relationships (i.e. staff, services) • Limited evidence on reduced use of services (emergency rooms, hospitalization, mental health services)
Self-management education provided in home to children, adolescents and/or caregivers by various health professionals	[50]	Asthma	• Usual care, less intensive education programme, professions not defined	• No significant effect on asthma symptoms, quality of life scores, number of school days missed	• No significant effect on emergency department visits • Mixed results on hospital admissions

Table 6.3 *(cont.)*

Skill-mix interventions			Outcomes			
Content of interventions and skill-mix changes	Source(s)	Chronic condition	Profession(s) in comparator group	Patient-related outcomes	Health system-related/resource use outcomes	Profession-specific outcomes
Case management carried out by single case manager (various professions: e.g. social worker, geriatrician, occupational therapists, psychologist) or multidisciplinary team	[51][a]	Various chronic conditions, frail elderly, frequent users of health services	• Usual care or no-case management	• Significant effect on self-reported health status in the short-term, patient satisfaction in the long-term* • No significant effect for mortality	• No significant effect for total cost of services, utilization of primary and non-specialist care or secondary care	

Abbreviations: ASD: autism spectrum disorder; BMI: body mass index; CVD: cardiovascular disease; GP: general practitioner; HbA1c: glycated haemoglobin; HIV: human immunodeficiency virus; LTFU: loss to follow up; RCT: randomized controlled trial.

Notes: * Statistically significant results; [a] Review also includes studies covering patients with multiple chronic conditions (but not explicitly indicated).

Sources: [39] Robinson-White et al. (2010); [40] Singer et al. (2013); [41] Chu et al. (2015); [42] Qi et al. (2015); [43] Dale, Williams & Bowyer (2012); [44] Pimouguet et al. (2011); [45] Jack et al. (2016); [46] Sikorski et al. (2012); [47] Marks et al. (2017); [48] Oono, Honey & McConachie (2013); [49] Wright-Berryman, McGuire & Salyers (2011); [50] Welsh, Hasan & Li (2011); [51] Stokes et al. (2015).

language but showed significant improvement of severity of autism characteristics, shared attention in parent–child interaction as well as parent satisfaction (Oono, Honey & McConachie, 2013).

Physiotherapists providing management of musculoskeletal disorders were shown to improve patient satisfaction compared with physician care, and had comparable effects on general health outcomes (Marks et al., 2017). Self-management education provided by various health professionals for asthma patients was shown to have comparable effects on asthma symptoms, quality of life scores and number of school days missed (Welsh, Hasan & Li, 2011). One review looked at case management carried out by various professionals either independently or within multiprofessional teams for patients with various chronic conditions (mostly frail elderly); the review found significant improvements of self-reported health status in the short-term and patient satisfaction in the long-term and comparable effects on mortality (Stokes et al., 2015).

Evidence on health-system-related outcomes

For cancer care, GP-led follow-up care for child cancer survivors delivered autonomously or collaboratively with paediatric cancer specialists was reported to reduce patient travel and attrition for follow-up appointments, with some evidence of improved cost-effectiveness compared with follow up in long-term follow-up clinics (Singer et al., 2013). Nevertheless, there was also evidence of reduced access to complex diagnostic testing compared with follow up in specialist care settings (Singer et al., 2013). Patient navigation for breast cancer care involving lay workers and peers was reported to improve adherence to screening and diagnostic follow up after abnormal radiographic screening and to reduce waiting times for appointments with genetic counsellors and for biopsy/diagnostic intervals (Robinson-White et al., 2010).

With respect to diabetes care, the transition coordinator and community health worker model produced higher rates of successful transfer and attendance in adult clinics compared with usual care (Chu et al., 2015) and a decrease of medication use and patient costs (Jack et al., 2016).

For musculoskeletal disorders, physiotherapists made similar diagnostic and management decisions to specialists. However, results on resource utilization are inconsistent and evidence on costs is lacking (Marks et al., 2017). Consumer–provider models in which mental health services are provided by peers improved patient engagement in treatment and social relationships but studies showed limited support for reduced hospitalizations (Wright-Berryman, McGuire & Salyers, 2011). For self-management education provided by various health professionals for asthma patients mixed evidence was found on hospital admissions and no effect on emergency department visits (Welsh, Hasan & Li, 2011).

Skill-mix interventions delivered by multiprofessional teams

Key messages

- Collaborative care and interdisciplinary care were shown to have a moderate impact on physical health (HbA1c levels, blood pressure, progression of chronic kidney disease, physical functioning), medication adherence and patient satisfaction, and may improve mental health symptoms and quality of life.
- Other multiprofessional care models (for example, primary care networks, multiprofessional clinics) led to few improvements in physical or mental health (of which included reduction in all-cause mortality) but reduced utilization of inpatient care and other health care services.
- Specialty-based shared multiprofessional care for HIV patients saw positive effects on health outcomes and treatment adherence, though it is limited around whether it is cost-effective.

Collaborative care models for people with comorbidities improved adherence to medication and some health outcomes (depression, Quality-Adjusted Life-Years), but showed limited evidence on cost savings.

Box 6.6 Skill-mix interventions involving multiprofessional teams

- 21 reviews evaluated skill-mix interventions involving multiprofessional teams for single chronic conditions (Table 6.4), with four reviews assessing multimorbidity (Table 6.5)
- The majority of reviews assessed chronic care interventions provided within a multiprofessional approach instead of usual care generally provided by primary care practitioners and physicians
- Most reviews evaluated consultation liaison, care coordination, shared care or case management involving various professionals (primary care physicians, specialists, nurse care coordinators, social workers, pharmacists, psychologists)
- One review assessed multiprofessional cardiac clinics; another evaluated the introduction of family medicine groups and primary care networks

Table 6.4 *Multiprofessional team skill-mix interventions for single chronic conditions*

Skill-mix interventions				Outcomes		
Content of interventions and skill-mix changes	Source(s)	Chronic condition [Sources]	Profession(s) in comparator group [Sources]	Patient-related outcomes [Sources]	Health system-related/ resource use outcomes [Sources]	Profession-specific outcomes [Sources]
Collaborative care involving primary care physicians and secondary care specialists	[52–54]	Various chronic diseases (cancer, CKD, diabetes, COPD, heart failure, dermatology, complex conditions, mental health) [52, 54]; diabetes, psychiatric conditions or cancer [53]	• Usual care, generally by primary care physician [52] • Usual care, professions not defined [53, 54]	• Limited impact on blood pressure control [52] • Reduction in HbA1c levels and depression symptoms* [53] • Increased patient satisfaction [52] • Improvements in physical functioning for people with heart failure [52] • No significant differences in clinical outcomes for physical health conditions [54] • Improvements in mental health outcomes and depression* [54]	• Moderately increased costs for intervention compared with usual care [52] • Increased clinical attendance rates [52] • No significant differences in health care utilization [52]	

Table 6.4 (*cont.*)

Skill-mix interventions				Outcomes		
Content of interventions and skill-mix changes	Source(s)	Chronic condition [Sources]	Profession(s) in comparator group [Sources]	Patient-related outcomes [Sources]	Health system-related/resource use outcomes [Sources]	Profession-specific outcomes [Sources]
Multiprofessional family medicine groups and primary care networks	[55]	Diabetes	• Usual care, professions not defined	• No significant differences in self-reported physical and mental health	• Reduced emergency department and hospital visits	
Multiprofessional cardiac clinics	[56]	CVD and/or hypertension	• Nurses, physicians	• Reduction in all-cause mortality *	• Reduction in hospitalization for those with non-stable heart failure*	
(i) Case management, (ii) shared care and (iii) interdisciplinary teams	[57]	Cancer	• Usual care, professions not defined	• No significant improvements in functional status, physical or mental health or quality of life	• No evidence of increased continuity of care	
Cancer care coordination from primary prevention, screening, detection, diagnosis, treatment, and survivorship to end-of-life care	[58]	Cancer	• Usual care, professions not defined	• No significant improvements in mental health or quality of life • Improved patient experience with care, and quality of end-of-life care	• Improved appropriate health care utilization in primary, acute and hospice care settings, emergency departments and ICU	
Collaborative care between mental health specialist and at least one other primary care provider (usually physician)	[59–62]	Depression	• Usual care, professions not defined [59, 61] • Primary care physicians [60, 62]	• Improved depression symptoms* [59–62] • Improved quality of life* [59, 61] • Improved patient satisfaction* [59, 61] • Improved medication adherence* [59, 61, 62]		

Intervention	Category	Comparator	Outcomes
[63] Consultation liaison between primary care provider (mostly GP) and mental health specialist for the delivery of mental health care	Mental health	• Mental health specialist and primary care practitioners working alone	• Improved mental health up to 3 months following the start of treatment, but not from 3 to 12 months • Improved adherence to treatment guidelines • Improved consumer satisfaction • Improved adequate treatment from primary care practitioners • Mean costs higher for intervention • More likely to be prescribing pharmacological treatment up to 12 months • No difference in number of health care visits up to 12 months
[64] Intensive case management (Assertive Community Treatment and Case Management) for adults with severe mental illness	Mental health	• Usual care (non-intensive case management), community psychiatric nurse, clinician	• No improvements in mental health, mortality risk, social functioning or quality of life • Reduced length of hospital stay
[65] Multiprofessional community mental health teams for older people	Mental health	• Usual care, psychiatrist	• Improved quality of life, social contact, reduction in distress behaviour and caregiver burden for dementia patients
[66] Consumer-provider roles as managers, facilitators, advocates or mentors	Mental health	• Usual care, professions not defined	• No differences in psychosocial, mental health and client satisfaction • Increased use of primary care services

Table 6.4 (cont.)

Skill-mix interventions

Content of interventions and skill-mix changes	Source(s)	Chronic condition [Sources]	Profession(s) in comparator group [Sources]	Outcomes		
				Patient-related outcomes [Sources]	Health system-related/ resource use outcomes [Sources]	Profession-specific outcomes [Sources]
Collaborative care intervention requiring a designated psychiatrist (0.25 FTE) and nurse care coordinator (0.5 FTE)	[67]	Mental health	• Usual care, psychiatrist	• Improvement of MHC of quality of life* • No significant effect on physical health component of the quality of life	• Lower proportion of participants psychiatrically hospitalized for year two of the 3-year follow up* • No significant difference of direct intervention costs	
Multidisciplinary care for patients with pre-dialysis CKD	[68]	CKD	• Usual care	• Delayed progression of CKD* • Improved cholesterol and anaemia control		
Multidisciplinary specialist care involving diabetologist, endocrine trainees, diabetic nurses, dietician, nephrologist, renal nurse, social worker	[69][a]	CKD	• Usual care, diabetologist, GP	• No effect on renal outcomes • No difference between groups for their composite cardiovascular end-point • Increase of proportion of patients without hypertension*	• Higher mean total number of outpatient clinic visits* • No difference in the number of hospitalizations or emergency department visits	

Care model	Ref.	Disease	Comparator	Outcomes	Other
Shared care models with primary care clinicians working with specialist	[70, 71]	HIV	• Specialty care, HIV specialists/experts, university clinic fellows [70] • Usual care, GPs [71]	• No significant adverse clinical outcomes [70, 71] • Reduction of perinatal infection and transmission rate [70] • Positive effect on treatment adherence [70]	• Higher cost-effectiveness for HIV screening [70]
Specialty-based care provided by physician, advanced practitioner-based care, team-based care and shared care co-management by multidisciplinary team in different locations	[72]	HIV	• Physicians (with less experience working with HIV); general medical practice	• Specialty-based care shows better clinical outcomes and reduced mortality • Increased antiretroviral use with more experienced or specialist HIV clinicians, but no significant effect among more experienced practices	• No significant differences in referral for or use of mental health services and hepatitis C screening

Abbreviations: CKD: chronic kidney disease; COPD: chronic obstructive pulmonary disease; FTE: full-time equivalent; GP: general practitioner; HbA1c: glycated haemoglobin; HIV: human immunodeficiency virus; ICU: intensive care unit; LDL-C: low-density lipoprotein cholesterol; MHC: Mental Health Component; SBP: systolic blood pressure.

Notes: * Statistically significant results; ª Review is also covered in Tables 6.1 and 6.2.

Sources: [52] Mitchell et al. (2015); [53] Foy et al. (2010); [54] Smith et al. (2017); [55] Carter et al. (2016); [56] Gandhi et al. (2017); [57] Aubin et al. (2012); [58] Gorin et al. (2017); [59] Archer et al. (2012); [60] Sighinolfi et al. (2014); [61] Thota et al. (2012); [62] Coventry et al. (2014); [63] Gillies et al. (2015); [64] Dieterich et al. (2010); [65] Abendstern et al. (2012); [66] Pitt et al. (2013); [67] Reilly et al. (2013); [68] Strand & Parker (2012); [69] Nicoll et al. (2018); [70] Wong, Luk & Kidd (2012); [71] Mapp, Hutchinson & Estcourt (2015); [72] Kimmel et al. (2017).

Table 6.5 *Skill-mix interventions for patients with multimorbidity*

Skill-mix interventions				Outcomes		
Profession involved in skill-mix	Content of interventions and skill-mix changes	Source(s)	Profession(s) in comparator group [Sources]	Patient-related outcomes [Sources]	Health-system-related/ resource use outcomes [Sources]	Profession-specific outcomes [Sources]
Nurses	Nurse prescribing, nurse-led clinics and community monitoring for people with comorbid diabetes and hypertension	[73]	Physicians	• Reduction in SBP but not DBP for community monitoring and nurse prescribing; no differences for nurse-led clinics* • No significant improvement in medication adherence • Reduction in SBP* but not DBP • Community monitoring comparable effects to physician-delivered care on achievement of blood pressure targets		
Nurses	Nurse-delivered education to improve self-monitoring and disease management	[74][a]	Physicians	• Reduction in HbA1c levels (one of two studies)* • No significant reduction in DBP and triglycerides • Mixed evidence for reduction of total cholesterol, LDL cholesterol and fasting serum glucose (one of three studies*)		

Nurses	Nurse-delivered case management for collaborative care	[75, 76]	Usual care, professions not reported	• Improvements in depression severity for patients with comorbid depression and a physical health condition* [75] • Improvements in patient and carer satisfaction* [76]	• No significant difference in costs [75] • No significant difference in emergency admissions or bed days [76] • Improvements in health care staff satisfaction* [76]
Primary health care practitioners	Collaborative goals setting between older patients with multimorbidity and primary health care practitioners	[77][b]	Usual care, professions generally not reported	• Interventions improved the application of goal setting, and the inclusion of goals in care plans	
Multiprofessional teams	Multiprofessional collaborative care models for comorbid diabetes or CVD and depression involving trained/specialist nurses, registered nurses, primary care physicians, non-physician mental health workers, psychologists	[78–80]	Usual care, professions not reported [78–80]	• Improvement in depression outcomes and HbA1c levels* [78] • Increased depression-free days and quality-adjusted life-years [79] • Improvement in depression remission at 6 months* but not 12 months [80] • No significant reduction in HbA1c levels [80]	• Higher rates of adherence to antidepressant medication and to oral hypoglycaemic agent* [80]

Table 6.5 (*cont.*)

Skill-mix interventions

Profession involved in skill-mix	Content of interventions and skill-mix changes	Source(s)	Profession(s) in comparator group [Sources]	Outcomes		
				Patient-related outcomes [Sources]	Health-system-related/ resource use outcomes [Sources]	Profession-specific outcomes [Sources]
Multiprofessional teams	Multiprofessional collaborative care models involving nurses, pharmacist and social workers for adults with multimorbidity	[81]	Usual care, professions not reported	• No evidence of improved health outcomes • Some evidence of improved medication adherence	• Evidence of improved prescribing	

Abbreviations: CVD: cardiovascular disease; DBP: diastolic blood pressure; HbA1c: glycated haemoglobin; SBP: systolic blood pressure.

Notes: * Statistically significant results; [a] Seven of 23 studies in this review cover multimorbidity, only their results are reported. Results on single chronic conditions are reported in Table 6.2; [b] Seven of eight studies included in this review cover multimorbidity (Bartels et al., 2014 does not cover multimorbidity, it covers mental illness).

Sources: [73] Clark et al. (2011); [74] Massimi et al. (2017); [75] Ekers et al. 2013; [76] Lupari et al. (2011); [77] Vermunt et al. (2017); [78] Atlantis, Fahey & Foster (2014); [79] Jeeva et al. (2013); [80] Huang et al. (2013); [81] Smith et al. (2012)

Chronic conditions

Collaborative care models and consultation liaison

Collaborative care between primary care physicians and specialists had a modest impact on reducing HbA1c levels, blood pressure outcomes and medication adherence compared with usual care in two studies (Foy et al., 2010a; Mitchell et al., 2015), although one study found no significant impact (Smith et al., 2017). Collaborative care did, however, significantly improve physical functioning, patient satisfaction and clinical attendance rates at a moderately increased cost compared with usual care for treatment of heart failure (Mitchell et al., 2015). Multiprofessional care models involving various health professionals were shown to have a significant effect in delaying progression of chronic kidney disease (Strand & Parker, 2012) and on the number of patients with hypertension, with no difference reported in renal outcomes and composite cardiovascular end-points (Nicoll et al., 2018).

Strong evidence suggests that collaborative care involving a mental health specialist and primary care physicians/providers significantly improved depressive symptoms (Archer et al., 2012; Coventry et al., 2014; Foy et al., 2010; Sighinolfi et al., 2014; Smith et al., 2017; Thota et al., 2012), patient satisfaction, quality of life and medication adherence versus usual care (Archer et al., 2012; Coventry et al., 2014; Thota et al., 2012). Similarly, consultation liaison between primary care providers (mostly GPs) and mental health specialists was shown to improve adherence to treatment guidelines, consumer satisfaction and delivery of adequate treatment from primary care practitioners (Gillies et al., 2015). Consultation liaison was also found to improve mental health in the short-term and to be similar to usual care at 12 months follow up, with no differences reported in the number of health care visits. There was, however, some limited evidence of higher costs over usual care (Gillies et al., 2015).

Multiprofessional care coordination and intensive case management

There is equivocal evidence on the impact of multiprofessional care coordination. Reviews on cancer care suggest that coordination of care failed to significantly improve functional status, physical or mental health or quality of life (Aubin et al., 2012; Gorin et al., 2017) or continuity of care (Aubin et al., 2012). It may nevertheless enhance patient satisfaction, quality of end-of-life care and the odds of appropriate health care utilization in primary, acute and hospice care settings (Gorin et al., 2017).

Findings from one review suggest that intensive case management does not lead to significant improvements for mental health conditions, mortality risk, social functioning or quality of life, although it did lead to a slight reduction in length of hospital stay for adults with severe mental illness (Dieterich et al., 2010). Another review reported that intensive case management did improve quality of life and social contact and reduce distress behaviour and caregiver burden in older adults with dementia (Abendstern et al., 2012).

Other multiprofessional care models

Primary care networks and family medicine groups for diabetes care did not improve self-reported physical and mental health, but were shown to reduce emergency department and hospital visits (Carter et al., 2016). Multiprofessional cardiac clinics led to fewer hospitalizations and a significant reduction in all-cause mortality (Gandhi et al., 2017).

Studies on mental health reported that consumer–provider models where mental health service users worked in partnership with mental health professionals did not improve mental health or client satisfaction outcomes, but led to small reductions in the use of crisis and emergency services (Pitt et al., 2013). Collaborative care interventions in which a designated psychiatrist and a nurse care coordinator worked together to address physical and mental health needs of people with severe mental illness demonstrated significantly lower hospitalization rates for patients, but only for the second year of the 3-year follow-up period. In comparison to the standard care group, the intervention significantly improved the Mental Health Component of quality of life but not the Physical Health Component of this measure (Reilly et al., 2013).

Shared care models and other specialty-based multiprofessional care for HIV-positive individuals showed positive effects on treatment adherence, infection and transmission rates and mortality (Wong, Luk & Kidd, 2012; Kimmel et al., 2017). Shared care models with primary care clinicians seem also to be more cost-effective for HIV screening compared with specialist care (Wong, Luk & Kidd, 2012). However, evidence is limited to determine whether HIV shared care is cost-effective (Mapp, Hutchinson & Estcourt, 2015).

Multimorbidity

Collaborative care models for people with comorbid depression and diabetes or cardiovascular disease were shown to improve depression outcomes (Atlantis, Fahey & Foster, 2014; Huang et al., 2013; Jeeva et al., 2013), reduce HbA1c levels (Atlantis, Fahey & Foster, 2014; Huang et al., 2013) and improve quality-adjusted life-years (Huang et al., 2013; Jeeva et al., 2013) and also to lead to higher rates of adherence to antidepressant medication and to oral hypoglycaemic agent (Huang et al., 2013). No statistically significant cost savings between intervention and usual care groups were identified (Jeeva et al., 2013).

Patient-focused education and collaborative care by nurses, pharmacists and social workers for people with multimorbidity improved prescribing and drug adherence, although there was little evidence of improved health outcomes, reduced health care utilization or cost savings (Smith et al., 2012).

Collaborative goal-setting between older patients with complex multimorbidity and a primary care physician within an integrated care strategy significantly improved goal-setting, the number of advance directives and the inclusion of goals in care plans for multifactorial, but not for single-factorial, interventions (Vermunt et al., 2017).

Strengths and limitations of the evidence

Evidence from the overview of reviews reveals that several skill-mix models (expanded roles for nurses and pharmacists and, based on weaker evidence, other professional roles and multiprofessional teams) have overall positive impacts on health outcomes for patients with chronic conditions, but uncertain effects on economic benefits and quality of care.

Allocating tasks such as patient education and health screenings to pharmacists was shown to effectively improve blood glucose levels, blood pressure control and medication adherence, with outcomes for chronic kidney disease, COPD and depression similar to those for usual care. There was also some evidence suggesting that pharmacist-involved care could improve professional-specific outcomes, most notably in terms of enhancing physician adherence to prescribing or other care guidelines. Included reviews also provided limited evidence that pharmacist-delivered care for diabetes, cardiovascular disease, hypertension and COPD could be cost saving compared with physician- and nurse-delivered care, with mixed evidence showing pharmacist interventions either improved the rate, or led to a similar rate, of health care utilization compared with usual care.

Nurse-delivered autonomous care including prescribing, titration of medication and nurse-led clinics also provided equivalent or better care compared with that provided by physicians or other health professionals, although nurse-led collaborative care in general did not improve health outcomes. There is insufficient evidence to make any assessments on the cost-effectiveness of skill-mix interventions involving nurses or their impact on health care utilization.

Evidence does not strongly indicate that multiprofessional care models lead to better physical health outcomes. However, it suggests that interdisciplinary care coordination, especially between primary and secondary care, can significantly improve mental health outcomes for patients with severe mental health issues or multimorbidity and may increase patient satisfaction.

Overall, the evidence base was considerable, as shown by a large number of reviews. Moreover, 43 reviews conducted a meta-analysis and sufficiently accounted for biases and heterogeneity in original studies when interpreting results. Nonetheless, there are a number of limitations in the evidence base. First, there was limited evidence on skill-mix interventions for the management of multimorbidity care. Second, the description of comparison groups was often sparse, and the education/training of professionals was generally not described. Third, although there was good evidence on health outcomes, few reported on other relevant outcomes such as health care utilization, economic benefits or professional-related outcomes. Third, systematic reviews were dominated by studies from the USA, the United Kingdom, Australia and Canada. As the impact of skill-mix interventions is likely to differ depending on specific geographical and cultural contexts and health system models, the generalizability and transferability of results may be limited. Similarly, and lastly, the contexts in which skill-mix initiatives were implemented and in which studies were undertaken differ across the included reviews and generalized conclusions must be made cautiously.

Overall, more research is needed to assess a wider spectrum of outcomes in more countries to determine whether skill-mix interventions can cost-effectively improve patient outcomes and quality of care for patients with single chronic conditions or multimorbidity.

6.3 Country developments and trends in skill-mix innovation for chronic care and multimorbidity across Europe

As reflected in the evidence synthesis, which evaluated a large variety of skill-mix models to improve the care of patients with chronic conditions and multimorbidity, a diversity of different skill-mix innovations and policies are being introduced across Europe. Yet, the extent to which they are integrated into routine care varies. Skill-mix changes have been implemented as either stand-alone tactics or embedded within broader strategies to improve quality of care and health outcomes. Three main types of skill-mix innovations implemented across Europe and other OECD countries can be identified in the management of chronic conditions and multimorbidity:

- The first is the expansion of existing roles of nonmedical primary care professionals (nurses, pharmacists, physiotherapists) through policies or programmes that facilitate the reallocation of tasks and responsibilities within primary care or by transferring care traditionally performed by medical specialists to primary care. As a result, health professionals, mostly specialized nurses, manage chronic conditions in primary care settings under varying levels of physician oversight.
- The second relates to collaboration and multiprofessional team-based care across primary and specialty/secondary care settings. These models introduced teamwork and collaborative care and have proliferated in integrated care networks and Disease Management Programmes (DMPs).
- Third is the introduction of new care coordinating roles for patients with chronic and multimorbid conditions. These roles, including care coordinators and patient navigators, having integration at their core, arrange care and develop single, shared care plans for patients' health and well-being. Depending on the country context and health conditions, these roles have been shown to be performed by health professionals or lay persons with training, for example, as peer educators (Gilburt, 2016).

These different approaches were often found in different combinations within new care models and strategies.

The following section provides an overview of skill-mix innovations involving nurses, pharmacists and other health professionals, followed by sections on collaboration and multiprofessional team-based care and new care coordinating roles. Descriptions are based on evidence from policies, projects and programmes in different country contexts.

The expansion of existing roles of nurses, pharmacists and other health professionals

The role expansion of nurses and other health professionals for the management of patients with chronic conditions

New forms of division of work and re-allocation of responsibilities have emerged across Europe, involving nurses in the management of patients with chronic conditions. The increases in patient volumes and complexity have led to changes in the division of work. In these models, physicians often take care of the more complex patients, whereas stable chronic patients are treated by nurses or other professions. Examples include task shifting and sharing between physicians and other professions, such as nurses, pharmacists, physician assistants or medical assistants, which is facilitated by expanding their scopes-of-practice. This follows a global trend to expand the role of nurses for specific, chronic conditions in primary care. For example, reforms have been introduced in Australia, Canada, Finland, Ireland, the Netherlands, New Zealand, the United Kingdom and the USA to widen the scope of practice of nurse practitioners and other advanced practice nurses[2] in the care of patients with chronic conditions (Maier, Aiken & Busse, 2017). Similarly, a new profession, physician assistants, has expanded globally, but they are numerically smaller and work less often in primary care than nurses or pharmacists (Hooker & Everett, 2012).

Nurses' roles are often broadened when medical shortages are anticipated. In France, skill-mix and professional cooperation initiatives were launched with support from key stakeholders in the face of such shortages between 2004 and 2008 (Mousquès et al., 2010). One was the ASALEE project (French acronym for Health Action by Teams of Self-employed Health Professionals) that was initiated in 2004 as a non-profit organization of several GP practices in a rural

---

[2] With usually a Master's degree in these countries

area of France to improve care, especially in the most remote or deprived areas, for patients with chronic conditions and multimorbidity. It employed nurses directly to collaborate closely with two to three independently practising GPs, after specific training. The nurses were delegated tasks in prevention and chronic disease management that were previously performed by GPs (such as therapeutic education consultations for diabetes and high blood pressure, cognition and cardiovascular risk factor screenings for individuals aged over 75 years and computerized management of patient data) (Supper et al., 2017; Bourgueil et al., forthcoming). The project has since expanded to all regions of France, involving about 2% of all practising GPs, 300 full-time equivalent nurses and 300 000 patients. Initially funded by innovation funds, ASALEE is now financed by national insurance, conditional upon economic evaluation since 2017 (Bourgueil et al., forthcoming). Evaluations of the management of type 2 diabetes showed improved glycaemic control and follow up of patients treated within ASALEE, without additional cost (Bourgeuil et al., 2008).

An important, related reform trend is the introduction of laws on nonmedical prescribing. Between 2010 and 2016 alone, seven countries (Cyprus, Estonia, Finland, France, the Netherlands, Poland and Spain) adopted laws that grant specialized nurses (nurse specialists, clinical nurse specialists or professional nurses with additional education) the authority to prescribe medication (Maier, Aiken & Busse, 2017). Ireland, the United Kingdom, Denmark and Sweden had authorized limited nurse prescribing before 2010. Since 2012, nurse specialists in the Netherlands with a 2-year Master's degree in Advanced Nursing Practice can prescribe licensed medicines for medical conditions within their specialty area. Since 2014, registered nurses with a Bachelor's degree and a completed pharmacotherapy module in diabetes, lung and oncology care may prescribe a limited number of prescription-only medications after diagnosis by a physician (Kroezen, 2014). In Finland, where nurses are authorized to prescribe a limited set of medicines since 2010, the shifting of prescribing rights to nurses is less extensive than in the Netherlands, but with considerable change in the division of responsibility, in particular for patients with chronic conditions, as they can receive prescriptions and follow-up care from nurse prescribers in health centres (see Box 6.7, below).

Box 6.7 Nurse prescribers in Finland take care of the routine management of patients with specific chronic conditions

Since the adoption of a new law in 2010 and its implementation in 2011, Finnish nurses can work in considerably expanded roles in primary care centres, in collaboration with physicians. Nurses who complete postgraduate education (as nurse prescribers) are authorized to issue prescriptions for common minor illnesses and continued prescribing for three chronic conditions (hypertension, diabetes, asthma). In 2018, a total of 376 nurse prescribers were registered in Finland. The majority were employed to treat patients with the above chronic conditions in municipal health centres, often in rural or underserved areas. Requirements for nurses to take care of patients are: employment with a municipal health centre, 3 years previous working experience and postgraduate education of 45 credit points following the European Credit Transfer System on prescribing. Further, they need to be authorized by a physician, registered as a prescriber and have an identification number from the National Supervisory Authority for Welfare and Health (Heikkilä, 2018; Maier, Aiken & Busse, 2017; Savolahti, 2016).

Finnish nurse prescribers take over certain medical tasks previously performed by physicians (physical examinations, arrangements of clinical tests, initial or continued prescribing depending on the medicine and issuing of sickness certificates of <5 days), but also exercise extended tasks for the care of chronic patients. Examples include designing treatment plans, including prescribing of medication (in cooperation with physicians), discussing personal health targets on health promotion and (secondary) prevention and performing counselling on self-management. Though physicians maintain overall responsibility for treatment plans and decide on new prescriptions, nurse prescribers are able to relieve physicians in routine case treatment, particularly in underserved regions, and so fill in coverage gaps, for example, by contributing to extended opening hours.

Since the Law's implementation, the role of nurse prescribers has fundamentally changed the division of work between nurses and physicians (Maier, Köppen & Busse, 2017). However, it also showed that successful collaboration requires development of thorough care plans and guidelines, clear task allocation and organization of consultations as well as mutual trust between nurse prescribers and GPs (Hopia, Karhunen & Heikkilä, 2017; Savolahti, 2017; Sulkakoski, 2016). To enable nurse prescribing beyond the opening hours of health centres, the Law on Health Care Professionals is to be amended by expanding nurse prescribing to all outpatient services (home care, nurse appointment in specialized care) and to the private sector.

Pharmacists are increasingly involved in the management of patients with chronic conditions

The role of pharmacists working in community pharmacies has substantially expanded over the last 10 years. As community-based accessible health care providers, pharmacists are well positioned to provide low threshold clinical and counselling services and drug therapy expertise to local populations. Their role is not only promising regarding medication management but also for disease management, including measurement and testing of clinical parameters, support in self-care/management-related interventions (Pharmaceutical Group of The European Union, 2017), structured patient education and adherence improvement counselling.

Services and activities provided by pharmacists are mostly provided at national level and are defined either in law or specific government policy. Pharmacies led the management of common chronic diseases such as asthma/COPD, diabetes and hypertension in more than one third of 30 European countries in 2016. Also, the share of pharmacies offering measurement and testing services for chronic conditions (blood pressure, weighing, hypertension, cholesterol) has significantly increased over the last 5 years across Europe. In 2012, about half of 30 European countries' pharmacies offered blood pressure measurement and weighing; in 2016 these services were offered in about 90% of the countries (Pharmaceutical Group of The European Union, 2013, 2017). Case study 2 describes how the scope of pharmacists' tasks in Portugal has grown substantially in the last decade.

Disease management as a single-disease integrated care model

Around 2000, many European countries began implementing DMPs as a way to effectively and efficiently improve the management of chronic disease care. DMPs are designed to create a continuum of care for single chronic diseases (mostly diabetes, cardiovascular disease and COPD), provided by a multiprofessional team of health care professionals, and to encourage patient self-management (Rijken and Bekkema, 2011). Although in several countries, GPs direct the care processes within a DMP, care managers (usually nurses or allied health care professionals) are increasingly appointed to assume the coordinating tasks. Called nurse-delivered or nurse-led DMPs, these have added to the types and implementation of collaborative care models and care coordination (see also next section).

Box 6.8 Expanding professional roles of pharmacists in Portugal

In the last 30 years, pharmaceutical care in Portugal has been characterized by pharmacist commitment to holistic care and new ways of service delivery impacting on their roles. Pharmacy services began point-of-care tests and disposal of unwanted medicines in the 1980s and in 1999, a strategy to implement pharmacy-based DMPs was adopted, steered by the National Association of Pharmacies (ANF). Pilot projects of community pharmacies providing consultation services and management of chronic patients started 2 years later with positive patient health outcomes (Costa, Santos & Silveira, 2006). In particular, a diabetes management pilot programme (2003–2010), where certified pharmacists followed up with patients through scheduled visits in the pharmacy using a standardized assessment system (SOAP) and a Drug-Related Problem Classification system, achieved significant decreases in blood glucose levels, HbA1c, cholesterol levels and blood pressure. These positive outcomes supported the agreement with the Ministry of Health to provide continuity in national health system co-payment of advanced pharmacy-based services (Costa, Santos & Silveira, 2017; International Pharmaceutical Federation, 2017; Martins et al., 2008).

Since 2007, the range of services provided by pharmacies has been expanded by law and includes immunization, specific counselling campaigns, home care support, screening activities and pharmaceutical care programmes. For patients with chronic conditions (asthma/COPD, diabetes and hypertension), the latter also comprises disease management and monitoring, counselling, disease or therapy education, adherence promotion and campaigns to identify non-controlled patients (Costa, 2017; Félix et al., 2017; International Pharmaceutical Federation, 2017).

A new law in 2018 has enabled community pharmacies to provide complementary interventions with other health care professionals, including nursing services, prevention and treatment of diabetic foot, adherence and therapeutic management, automated dose dispensing and rapid screening tests. In 2017, the ANF and the Portuguese National Nursing Association also agreed to establish a regulatory framework for the provision of nursing care in pharmacies to further improve the integration into pharmacy-based services. In the same year, the ANF signed a memorandum with the Association of Family Health Units to define a framework for joint primary care activities and multidisciplinary cooperation among pharmacists, family doctors and nurses. Simultaneously, the Ministries of Health and Finance signed an agreement with the ANF on the intervention of pharmacies in areas such as diabetes, rational use of medicines particularly in adherence, and management of therapies (International Pharmaceutical Federation, 2019).

Moreover, several skill-mix changes implemented as part of integrated chronic care models demonstrate the interrelatedness of skill-mix interventions and organizational re-design as was shown by the EU-funded INTEGRATE project. The skill-mix innovations that are frequently implemented in combination include nurse involvement in care delivery, multiprofessional teams and protocols/pathways, continuous training of health professionals, involvement of a case manager/care coordinator role, regular team meetings to discuss a patient's treatment, and the creation of a new position, role or function specifically to deliver integrated chronic care (Busetto et al., 2017).

Collaboration and multiprofessional team-based care

Many European countries have changed their chronic disease management strategies over the last decade as DMPs were increasingly criticized as inappropriate to meet the needs of the growing numbers of patients with multiple chronic conditions (Nolte, Knai & Saltman, 2014; Rijken et al., 2014; Starfield, 2008). Care for multimorbidity comprises specialized care, intersectoral coordination and collaboration between primary care and specialized care (Hujala, Taskinen & Rissanen, 2017; Rijken et al., 2018; Struckmann et al., 2017). To better respond to the needs of patients with multiple chronic conditions, countries are moving towards more comprehensive models of integrated care by looking beyond disease-specific interventions. Skill-mix innovation plays a major role in these care models. Three broad trends can be identified. They support the delivery of (i) integrated, multiprofessional care, (ii) improve collaboration of care outside integrated care paradigms and (iii) facilitate continuity and co-ordination of care across organizational boundaries through holistic care approaches.

First, the EU-funded ICARE4EU project identified 101 integrated multimorbidity care initiatives in 25 European countries. Of these, a quarter reported to be well-established care programmes and about 40% to be routine care. Skill-mix innovations were frequently reported among their main objectives, mostly improving multiprofessional collaboration (80%) and care coordination (71%). GPs were involved in most programmes (81%), followed by medical specialists (66%) and nurses (50%). Other occupations included physiotherapists (45%), social workers (40%), home help (37%) and psychologists (33%). Pharmacists and informal carers, who are considered important providers of multimorbidity care, were involved in only one third of the programmes (van der

Heide et al., 2015). In about half of the cases, integrated multimorbidity care initiatives were used to adapt or drive new multiprofessional care delivery structures. Case managers were introduced in about 40% of the initiatives; changes in job descriptions were introduced in a quarter of these initiatives (van der Heide et al., 2015).

New teamwork and collaborative care paradigms have also developed next to integrated care networks and disease management programmes with the goal of establishing closer working relationships between primary care (family doctors, GPs and practice nurses) and specialists. Primary care professionals increasingly work together in multiprofessional teams, in complex care hubs/networks and in new patient-centred care models. Most commonly, collaborative care models have been integrated into routine care for the treatment of mental health conditions. In ageing societies, mental illness is frequently comorbid with physical illness, requiring mental health specialists and primary care workers to collaborate closely. Several countries have explored such collaborative care models targeting the reduction in patient hospitalizations. For example, the United Kingdom, Ireland, Italy, the Netherlands, Denmark and Belgium have policies prioritizing community-based, multiprofessional care (Vitale, Mannix-McNamara & Cullinan, 2015). These care delivery approaches provide mental health and medical care in primary care settings at the community level, and coordinate with social care (see Case study 3). They have also been shown to be more effective than usual care for improving depression outcomes (see Section on Skill-mix interventions delivered by multiprofessional teams; Sighinolfi et al., 2014).

Multidisciplinary primary care teams have been set up in various countries (Belgium, Estonia, Finland, France, Italy, the Netherlands, Portugal, Spain and Sweden) to overcome the limitations of solo practices and benefit from interprofessional teamwork and multiprofessional competencies. The principal aim of multidisciplinary primary care teams is to offer a comprehensive set of services and to respond to the specific needs of patients with chronic and multimorbid conditions. There is large variation in team composition across countries; teams may include different social and health professionals besides family physicians and registered nurses (for example, psychologists, health promotors, nutritionists, clinical community pharmacists, physical activity counsellors, community health workers and front desk staff). In particular, the team-based model allows the provision of more complex services such as prevention and health promotion, patient education and self-management support, patient and family caregiver empowerment, psychological counselling, social services, referral and care coordination, which can usually not be offered by single-handed practices (De Maesseneer et al., 2018).

Box 6.9 Collaborative care models in mental health care in the United Kingdom, Ireland and Belgium

Community mental health teams (CMHTs) were established in the United Kingdom and Ireland in 1990 to provide continuity of care through a multiprofessional approach. Different types of mental health professionals from health and social care backgrounds (psychiatrists, community psychiatric nurses, psychologists, occupational therapists and social workers) provide and coordinate health and social care in the community for people with complex mental health problems. The multiprofessional perspectives and collaborative work through regular meetings and shared information enable joint mental health assessment, treatment and set-up of care plans that cover the needs and goals of an individual, and coordinate care. The CMHT may locally also include Assertive Outreach Teams, specialized community mental health teams focused on providing treatment and support to people who have complex needs and require more intensive support. However, experiences in both countries reveal difficulties in the implementation of this collaborative care model (Gilburt, 2016). In Ireland, the multiprofessional input from CMHTs was limited to psychiatrists, trainee doctors and nurses (Vitale, Mannix-McNamara & Cullinan, 2015). In the United Kingdom, blurred professional role boundaries, lack of training for role development, and models of decision-making and the adoption of generic working practices by staff within these teams became the main barriers to team continuity (Belling et al., 2011; Gilburt, 2016).

Conversely, more positive experiences with community-level mental health teams are found in Belgium, where they were introduced by a nationwide reform of mental health care delivery in 2008. Care networks established by psychiatric hospitals provide inpatient and outpatient mental health services, primary care, outreach, day care, vocational services, housing, and other social care services. Additionally, multiprofessional mobile outreach teams cooperate closely with primary health care workers, social workers and medical specialists in the treatment of chronic psychiatric patients (Lorant et al., 2016; Nicaise, Dubois & Laurant, 2014; World Health Organization, 2018). There were 22 active care networks in 2016 (Sermeus, 2019).

New care coordinating roles to improve the care trajectory of patients with chronic and multimorbid conditions

Reforms and programmes have introduced new professional roles working across organizational boundaries meant to provide coordinated, continuous and holistic care. These new roles range from case managers and social workers to care navigators, coordinators and community facilitators (Gilburt, 2016). Adapted to local health needs, they are especially useful to patients with long-term, multimorbid health conditions as well as people with low levels of literacy or cognitive deficits by helping navigate the fragmented sectors and services involved in covering their care needs (health, social care, housing, employment and education). Their main role is to support patients to plan, organize and access support by linking and coordinating resources and providers through a person-centred approach and provide social and psychological support. Case managers, for example, may also perform clinical needs assessment and clinical monitoring, provide patient and caregiver education and self-management support and establish care goals with the patients coupled with the development of their self-efficacy skills (De Maesseneer et al., 2018).

Box 6.10 New nursing roles in integrated case management of patients with complex needs in Valencia, Spain

An evaluation of home care in the Spanish region of Valencia in 2005–2006 showed that fragmentation of health care delivery and lack of care continuity were major obstacles for the quality of care of patients with advanced chronic diseases, multimorbidity or those in need of palliative care. As a result, a pilot initiative to increase cooperation between primary and hospital care was implemented between 2007 and 2010 and a Strategy for Chronic Care including an Integrated Care Model for Complex Cases was developed. The latter integrates hospital, primary and community-based health services under joint-case management to improve transitional care periods for highly complex home care patients, and to enable them to remain at home. This model introduced two new nursing roles: the community nurse case manager (CNCM) and the hospital nurse care manager (HNCM) to take care of the patient during critical stages in the care process. HNCMs are responsible for identifying highly complex chronic patients and for planning discharge to ensure continuity of care during and after hospital or hospital-at-home stay. CNCMs arrange care at home and mobilize the community-based collaborative care process.

> **Box 6.10 (cont.)**
>
> In this model, the care process starts with a comprehensive assessment of the patient, including living environment, family support and carers. An individualized care plan with medication reviews is then designed and implemented by multiprofessional primary care teams (GPs, nurses and social workers) with the support of the CNCM. Both the CNCM and HNCM remain jointly responsible for monitoring the patient, interacting with primary care teams and others and ensuring appropriateness and continuity of care. Innovative use of information and communication technologies supports the constant communication between and work of the CNCM and HNCM and the identification of high-risk patients. CNCMs and HNCMs are required to attend 100 hours of specific training and 1-month on-the-job training to start working as a case manager. Other professionals receive ongoing training related to care integration and care for complex cases.
>
> The dual-case manager model has gradually expanded. In 2015, there were 79 nurse case managers for approximately 1.4 million people (30% of the population). The case management model has shown positive impact for patients and family carers in terms of proactive care and administrative and emotional support. Moreover, health professionals increasingly value enhanced cooperation, though some reluctance remains, especially among hospital doctors (Barbabella et al., 2015; Gallud, Soler & Cuevas, 2012).

With this broader perspective, these new roles can also facilitate the implementation of effective, integrated care packages (Ivbijaro et al., 2014). The nurse-delivered case management programme in Valencia (Spain) describes an integrated care model that introduced case managers to support patients with multiple chronic conditions, including through arranging care transitions and settings (Case study 4). While these coordinating roles are an emerging trend in many countries, evidence and experiences are still limited.

6.4 Conclusions

The majority of skill-mix innovations and reforms in Europe have focused on single chronic conditions and to a smaller extent on multimorbidity. This uneven distribution is also reflected in the evidence. Systematic reviews assessing skill-mix innovations suggest that skill-mix innovations for the management of chronic diseases and multimorbidity reveal overall positive impacts on health outcomes. In particular, primary care teams with expanded roles for nurses or pharmacists are effective and show at least equivalent or better health outcomes. The effect of collaborative care and multiprofessional care models has shown some, albeit less strong, evidence of positive impacts on patient outcomes. As to the economic benefits and quality of care there was mixed and limited evidence.

The overview of systematic reviews revealed that there are gaps in the evidence base, which are critical to comprehensively capturing the efficacy and appropriateness of skill-mix reforms. On interventions targeting multimorbidity, in particular, the evidence base is weak, and more research is needed. Few reviews reported on non-health outcomes, including patient satisfaction, health care utilization or cost-effectiveness, which are important dimensions to understanding the potential impact of interventions. Moreover, many studies were undertaken in the USA, the United Kingdom, Australia and Canada and the findings may not be relevant to other health systems and countries. Finally, training of professionals in the skill-mix intervention and comparison groups was often not described. However, it is critical to ascertain the practical impact of skill-mix innovations and how this may differ across geographical contexts.

The overview of systematic reviews, review of country policies, and assessment of developments and trends of skill-mix innovations in Europe show that many new and promising skill-mix configurations targeting people with chronic conditions and multimorbidity exist in the region. The evidence and practice examples demonstrate that new and extended professional roles are promising solutions to fill gaps in primary care, improve the quality of care and alleviate provider shortages. In particular, pharmacists are well placed in the community to be involved in the care of patients with single chronic conditions and multimorbidity through, for example, providing medication management and education counselling, and also as part of multiprofessional teams. Also, nurses are well positioned to undertake titration, prescribing and management of medication and providing counselling around medical adherence as well as disease management, independently or as part of a multiprofessional team, and have a positive impact on patient health outcomes and cost. Evidence on the emerging care coordinating roles show a positive impact on health outcomes and resource use, although evidence and experiences are still very limited. Overall, multiprofessional teams involving various professionals are increasingly used in primary care with positive impact, in particular on mental health and utilization of inpatient care.

The developments in skill-mix innovations reveal that interventions have been implemented in different ways throughout Europe. Often, the interventions involve several skill-mix changes, including enhanced care coordination roles, teamwork interventions, sometimes combined with outreach activities. However, skill-mix innovations often remain patchy and not always fully integrated into routine care. In some countries, skill-mix changes are part of a broader reorganization of care that include multiprofessional teamwork, integrated care and new models of care, developed through existing staff working in new and different ways. Lack of regulation of scope of practice, education/training and reimbursement schemes as well as traditional role definitions and opposition from the medical profession are the most important barriers for successful implementation of skill-mix changes. Official authorization of expanded scopes-of-practice, incentives for increased cooperation, adapted training programmes coupled with decent working conditions (respecting work–life balance) are key prerequisites (Dussault & Buchan, 2018) to ensure that innovative skill-mix solutions reach patients with chronic conditions and multimorbidity.

To date, only a few countries in Europe have formalized new professional roles in chronic care within legal frameworks, and set up training schemes and requirements (for nurse prescribers, nurse practitioners and advanced practice nurses in the United Kingdom, Finland and the Netherlands), while the number of professionals working in new roles remains small in several other countries. However, the positive impact that these skill-mix innovations have on patient outcomes and the use of health resources shows that there is opportunity and scope to scale up programmes and introduce supportive policies. Such reforms can also reduce pressure on specialist services and GPs and deliver even better outcomes for patients and benefits to health systems.

References

Abendstern M, Harrington V, Brand C et al. (2010). Variations in structures, processes and outcomes of community mental health teams for older people: a systematic review of the literature. Aging Ment Health, 16(7):861–873. doi:10.1080/13607863.2011.651431

Aguiar PM, Brito G de C, Lima Tde M et al. (2016). Investigating sources of heterogeneity in randomized controlled trials of the effects of pharmacist interventions on glycemic control in type 2 diabetic patients: a systematic review and meta-analysis. PLoS One, 11(3):e0150999.. doi:10.1371/journal. pone.0150999

Al-Ganmi AH, Perry L, Gholizadeh L et al. (2016). Cardiovascular medication adherence among patients with cardiac disease: a systematic review. J Adv Nurs, 72(12):3001–3014. doi:10.1111/jan.13062

Archer J, Bower P, Gilbody S et al. (2012). Collaborative care for depression and anxiety problems. Cochrane Database Syst Rev, 10:CD006525. doi:10.1002/14651858.CD006525.pub2

Armor BL, Britton ML, Dennis VC et al. (2010). A review of pharmacist contributions to diabetes care in the United States. J Pharm Pract, 23(3):250–264. doi:10.1177/0897190009336668

Atlantis E, Fahey P, Foster J (2014).Collaborative care for comorbid depression and diabetes: a systematic review and meta-analysis. BMJ Open, 4(4):e004706. doi:10.1136/bmjopen-2013-004706

Aubin M, Giguère A, Martin M et al. (2012). Interventions to improve continuity of care in the follow-up of patients with cancer. Cochrane Database Syst Rev, 7:CD007672. doi:10.1002/14651858.CD007672.pub2

Baishnab E, Karner C (2012). Primary care based clinics for asthma (Review). Cochrane Database Syst Rev Prim, 4:CD003533. doi:10.1002/14651858. CD003533.pub2.www.cochranelibrary.com

Baker E, Fatoye F (2017). Clinical and cost effectiveness of nurse-led self-management interventions for patients with copd in primary care: a systematic review. Int J Nurs Stud, 71:125–138. doi:10.1016/j.ijnurstu.2017.03.010

Barbabella F, Hujala A, Quattrini S et al. (2015). The Strategy for Chronic Care in Valencia Region [Internet]. 2015. (http://www.icare4eu.org/pdf/Case_report_ Valencia__final.pdf, accessed 15 October 2018).

Bartels SJ, Pratt SI, Mueser KT et al. (2014). Longterm outcomes of a randomized trial of integrated skills training and preventive healthcare for older adults with serious mental illness. Am J Geriatric Psychiatry, 22:1251–1261.

Belling R, Whittock M, McLaren S et al. (2011). ECHO Group. Achieving continuity of care: facilitators and barriers in community mental health teams. Implement Sci, 6: 23.[3]

Blalock SJ, Roberts AW, Lauffenburger JC et al. (2013).The effect of community pharmacy-based interventions on patient health outcomes: a systematic review. Med Care Res Rev, 70(3):235–266. doi:10.1177/1077558712459215

---

[3] https://www.ncbi.nlm.nih.gov/pmc/articles/PMC3073925/ (accessed 15 April 2019)

Bourgueil Y (forthcoming). Skill-mix innovation in the workplace and classroom in France: moving from task transfer to the paradigm of cooperation? In: Wismar M, Glinos I, Sagan A eds. Skill-mix innovation in primary and chronic care: mobilizing patients, peers, professionals. European Observatory on Health Systems and Policies. Volume 1. Copenhagen, WHO Regional Office for Europe on behalf of the European Observatory on Health Systems and Policies.

Bourgueil Y, Le Fur P, Mousquès J et al. (2008). GPs teamed up with nurses: a skill mix experiment improves management of type 2 diabetes patients, main results of the ASALEE experiment. IRDES, Questions d'économie de la santé, 2008. (http://www.irdes.fr/EspaceAnglais/Publications/IrdesPublications/QES136.pdf, accessed 15 April 2019).

Busetto L, Luijkx K, Calciolari S et al. (2017). Exploration of workforce changes in integrated chronic care: Findings from an interactive and emergent research design. PLoS One 12(12):e0187468, (https://doi .org/10.1371/journal.pone.0187468)

Carter R, Riverin B, Levesque JF et al. (2016). The impact of primary care reform on health system performance in Canada: a systematic review. BMC Health Serv Res 16:324. doi:10.1186/s12913-016-1571-7

Cheema E, Sutcliffe P, Singer DR (2014). The impact of interventions by pharmacists in community pharmacies on control of hypertension: a systematic review and meta-analysis of randomized controlled trials. Br J Clin Pharmacol, 78(6):1238–1247. doi:10.1111/bcp.12452.

Chen C, Chen Y, Liu X et al. (2016). The efficacy of a nurse-led disease management program in improving the quality of life for patients with chronic kidney disease : a meta-analysis. PLoS One, 11(5):e0155890. doi:10.1371/journal.pone.0155890

Chu PY, Maslow GR, von Isenburg M et al. (2015). Systematic review of the impact of transition interventions for adolescents with chronic illness on transfer from pediatric to adult healthcare. J Pediatr Nurs, 30(5):e19–e27. doi:10.1016/j.pedn.2015.05.022

Clark CE, Smith LF, Taylor RS et al. (2011). Nurse-led interventions used to improve control of high blood pressure in people with diabetes: a systematic review and meta-analysis. Diabet Med, 28(3):250–261. doi:10.1111/j.1464-5491.2010.03204.x

Colombo LRP, Aguiar PM, Lima TM et al. (2017). The effects of pharmacist interventions on adult outpatients with cancer: A systematic review. J Clin Pharm Ther, 2017; 42:414–424.

Costa S. Economic evaluation of pharmacy services in Portugal. In: Zaheer-Ud-Din Babar, ed. Economic evaluation of pharmacy services. Amsterdam, Elsevier Science Publishing Co Inc.; 183–192.

Costa S, Santos C, Silveira J (2006). Community pharmacy services in Portugal. Ann Pharmacother, 40:2228–2234.

Coventry PA, Hudson JL, Kontopantelis E et al. (2014). Characteristics of effective collaborative care for treatment of depression: a systematic review and meta-regression of 74 randomised controlled trials. PLoS One, 9(9):e108114. doi:10.1371/journal.pone.0108114

Dale JR, Williams SM, Bowyer V (2012). What is the effect of peer support on diabetes outcomes in adults? A systematic review. Diabet Med, 29(11):1361–1377. doi:10.1111/j.1464-5491.2012.03749.x

De Maesseneer J, Borgermans L, Beran D et al. (2018). Transforming individual health services: towards integrated multidisciplinary primary health care. In: Jakab M, Farrington J, Borgermans L, Mantingh F, eds. Health systems respond to NCDs: time for ambition. Copenhagen, WHO Regional Office for Europe.

Deters MA, Laven A, Castejon A et al. (2018). Effective interventions for diabetes patients by community pharmacists: a meta-analysis of pharmaceutical care components. Ann Pharmacother, 52:198–211.

Dieterich M, Irving CB, Park B et al. (2010). Intensive case management for severe mental illness. Cochrane Database Syst Rev, 10:CD007906. doi:10.1002/14651858.CD007906.pub2

Dussault G, Buchan J (2018). Noncommunicable diseases and human resources for health: a workforce fit for purpose. In: Jakab et al. (eds) Health systems respond to NCDs: time for ambition. Copenhagen, WHO Regional Office for Europe; 182–199.

Ekers D, Murphy R, Archer J et al. (2013). Nurse-delivered collaborative care for depression and long-term physical conditions: a systematic review and meta-analysis. J Affect Disord 149(1–3):14–22. doi:10.1016/j.jad.2013.02.032

Entezari-Maleki T, Dousti S, Hamishehkar H et al. (2016). A systematic review on comparing 2 common models for management of warfarin therapy; pharmacist-led service versus usual medical care. J Clin Pharmacol, 56(1):24–38. doi:10.1002/jcph.576

Fazel MT, Bagalagel A, Lee JK et al. (2017). Impact of diabetes care by pharmacists as part of health care team in ambulatory settings: a systematic review and meta-analysis. Ann Pharmacother, 51(10):890–907. https://doi.org/10.1177/1060028017711454

Félix J, Ferreira D, Afonso-Silva M et al. (2017). Social and economic value of Portuguese community pharmacies in health care. BMC Health Serv Res, 17:606.

Fergenbaum J, Bermingham S, Krahn M et al. (2015). Care in the home for the management of chronic heart failure: systematic review and cost-effectiveness analysis. J Cardiovasc Nurs, 30(4 Suppl 1):S44–S51. doi:10.1097/JCN.0000000000000235

Foy R, Hempel S, Rubenstein L et al. (2010). Meta-analysis: effect of interactive communication between collaborating primary care physicians and specialists. Ann Intern Med, 152(4):247–258. doi:10.7326/0003-4819-152-4-201002160-00010

Gallud J, Soler P, Cuevas D (2012). New nursing roles for the integrated management of complex chronic and palliative care patients in the region of Valencia. Int J Integr Care, 12:1–6.

Gandhi S, Mosleh W, Sharma UC et al. (2017). Multidisciplinary heart failure clinics are associated with lower heart failure hospitalization and mortality: systematic review and meta-analysis. Can J Cardiol, 33(10):1237–1244. doi:10.1016/j.cjca.2017.05.011

Gilburt H (2016). Supporting integration through new roles and working across boundaries. The King's Fund, 2016. (www.kingsfund.org.uk/sites/default/files/field/field_publication_file/Supporting_integration_web.pdf, accessed 28 August 2018).

Gillies D, Buykx P, Parker AG et al. (2015). Consultation liaison in primary care for people with mental disorders. Cochrane Database System Rev, 9:CD007193. DOI: 10.1002/14651858.CD007193.pub2.

Gong F, Chen X, Wu Y et al. (2018). Nurse vs. physician-led care for obstructive sleep apnoea: A systematic review and meta-analysis of randomized trials. J Adv Nurs, 2018;74:501–506. doi:10.1111/jan.13346

Gorin SS, Haggstrom D, Han PKJ et al. (2017). Cancer care coordination: a systematic review and meta-analysis of over 30 years of empirical studies. Ann Behav Med, 51(4):532–546. doi:10.1007/s12160-017-9876-2

Greer N, Bolduc J, Geurkink E et al. (2017). Pharmacist-led chronic disease management: a systematic review of effectiveness and harms compared with usual care. Ann Intern Med, 165:30–40.

Health Quality Ontario (2013). Specialized nursing practice for chronic disease management in the primary-care setting: an evidence-based analysis. Ontario Health Technol Assessment Ser, 2013.

Heikkilä J. (2018). Development and status of nurse prescriber education in Finland. Presentation at the 10th ICN NP/APN Conference Rotterdam (26–29 August 2018), 2018. (http://www.npapn2018.com/wp-content/uploads/2018/09/518-Development-and-status-of-nurse-prescriber-education-in-Finland.pdf, accessed 9 May 2019).

Heise BA, van Servellen G (2014). The nurse's role in primary care antidepressant medication adherence. J Psychosoc Nurs Ment Health Serv, 52(4):48–57. doi:10.3928/02793695-20131126-08

Hooker RS, Everett CM (2012). The contributions of physician assistants in primary care systems. Health Care Soc Commun, 20(1):20–31.

Hopia H, Karhunen A, Heikkilä J (2017). Growth of nurse prescribing competence: facilitators and barriers during education. J Clin Nurs, 26:3164–3173. https://doi.org/10.1111/jocn.13665

Hopkinson JB, Brown JC, Okamoto I et al. (2012). The effectiveness of patient-family carer (couple) intervention for the management of symptoms and other health-related problems in people affected by cancer: a systematic literature search and narrative review. J Pain Symptom Manage, 43(1):111–142. doi:10.1016/j.jpainsymman.2011.03.013

Huang Y, Wei X, Wu T et al. (2013).Collaborative care for patients with depression and diabetes mellitus: a systematic review and meta-analysis. BMC Psychiat, 13:260. doi:10.1186/1471-244X-13-260

Hujala A, Taskinen H, Rissanen S, on behalf of the ICARE4EU consortium(2017). How to support integration to promote care for people with multimorbidity in Europe? Policy Brief 26, European Observatory on Health Systems and Policies. Copenhagen, WHO Regional Office for Europe.

Institute for Health Metrics and Evaluation (IHME) (2018). Findings from the Global Burden of Disease Study 2017. Seattle, WA: IHME.

International Pharmaceutical Federation (FIP). (2017). Pharmacy at a glance – 2015–2017. The Hague, the Netherlands, International Pharmaceutical Federation.

International Pharmaceutical Federation (FIP) (2019). Beating non-communicable diseases in the community. The contributions of pharmacists. 2019. (https://www.fip.org/files/fip/publications/NCDs/beating-ncds-in-the-community-the-contribution-of-pharmacists.pdf, accessed 06 May 2019).

Ivbijaro GO, Enum Y, Khan AA et al. (2014). Collaborative care: models for treatment of patients with complex medical-psychiatric conditions. Curr Psychiat Rep, 16(11):506.

Jack HE, Arabadjis SD, Sun L et al. (2016). Impact of community health workers on use of healthcare services in the United States : a systematic review. J Gen Intern Med, 32(3):325–344. doi:10.1007/s11606-016-3922-9

Jakab M, Farrington J, Borgermans L et al. (eds) (2018). Health systems respond to NCDs: time for ambition. Copenhagen, WHO Regional Office for Europe.

Jeeva F, Dickens C, Coventry P et al. (2013). Is treatment of depression cost-effective in people with diabetes? A systematic review of the economic evidence. Int J Technol Assess Health Care, 29(4):384–391. doi: 10.1017/S0266462313000445.

Kelly EL, Fenwick KM, Barr N et al. (2014). A systematic review of self-management health care models for individuals with serious mental illnesses. Psychiatr Serv, 65(11):1300–1310. doi: 10.1176/appi.ps.201300502.

Kimmel AD, Martin EG, Galadima H et al. (2017). Clinical outcomes of HIV care delivery models in the US: a systematic review. AIDS Care, 28(10):1215–1222. doi:10.1080/09540121.2016.1178702.

Kroezen M (2014). Nurse prescribing: a study on task substitution and professional jurisdictions. Utrecht, NIVEL, 2014. (https://www.nivel

.nl/sites/default/files/bestanden/Proefschrift-Marieke-Kroezen-2014.pdf, accessed 15 April 2019).

Kuethe M, Vaessen-Verberne A, Elbers E et al. (2013). Nurse versus physician-led care for the management of asthma (Review). Cochrane Database Syst Rev Nurse, 2:CD009296. doi:10.1002/14651858.CD009296.pub2.

Lorant V, Grard A, Van Audenhove C et al. (2016). Assessment of the priority target group of mental health service networks within a nation-wide reform of adult psychiatry in Belgium. BMC Health Serv Res, 16:187.

Lupari M, Coates V, Adamson G et al. (2011). 'We're just not getting it right' – how should we provide care to the older person with multi-morbid chronic conditions?. J Clin Nurs, 20(9–10):1225–1235. doi:10.1111/j.1365-2702.2010.03620.x

Maier C, Aiken L, Busse R (2017a). Nurses in advanced roles in primary care: Policy levers for implementation. OECD Health Working Papers, No. 98. Paris, OECD Publishing. (http://dx.doi.org/10.1787/a8756593-en).

Maier C, Köppen J, Busse R (2017b). Multiprofessionelle Behandlungsteams: neue Berufe (Nurse Practitioners und Physician Assistants) und neue Formen der Aufgabenteilung im internationalen Vergleich. Berlin, Berlin University of Technology.

Manzoor BS, Cheng W-H, Lee JC et al. (2017). Quality of pharmacist-managed anticoagulation therapy in long-term ambulatory settings: a systematic review. Ann Pharmacother, 51(12):1122–1137. (https://doi.org/10.1177/1060028017721241).

Mapp F, Hutchinson J, Estcourt C (2015). A systematic review of contemporary models of shared HIV care and HIV in primary care in high-income settings. Int J STD AIDS, 26(14):991–997. doi:10.1177/0956462415577496

Marks D, Comans T, Bisset L et al. (2017). Substitution of doctors with physiotherapists in the management of common musculoskeletal disorders: a systematic review. Physiotherapy, 103(4):341–351. doi:10.1016/j.physio.2016.11.006

Martínez-González NA, Rosemann T, Tandjung R, Djalali S (2015). The effect of physician-nurse substitution in primary care in chronic diseases: a systematic review. Swiss Med Wkly, 145:w14031. doi:10.4414/smw.2015.14031

Martins AP, Horta MR, Costa S et al. (2008). Evaluating the Portuguese pharmacy-based diabetes management program. where do we stand now? Poster session presented at: 68th International Congress of FIP, 2008. (https://www.fip.org/abstracts?page=abstracts&action=generatePdf&item=2551, accessed 20 September 2018).

Massimi A, De Vito C, Brufola I et al. (2017). Are community-based nurse-led self-management support interventions effective in chronic patients? Results of a systematic review and meta-analysis. PLoS One, 12(3):e0173617. doi:10.1371/journal.pone.0173617.

Mitchell GK, Burridge L, Zhang J et al. (2015). Systematic review of integrated models of health care delivered at the primary-secondary interface: how effective is it and what determines effectiveness? Aust J Prim Health, 21(4):391–408. doi:10.1071/PY14172

Morgado MP, Morgado SR, Mendes LC et al. (2011). Pharmacist interventions to enhance blood pressure control and adherence to antihypertensive therapy: review and meta-analysis. Am J Health Syst Pharm, 68(3):241–253. doi:10.2146/ajhp090656.

Mousquès J, Bourgueil Y, Le Fur P et al. (2010). Effect of a French experiment of team work between general practitioners and nurses on efficacy and cost of type 2 diabetes patients care. Health Policy, (https://doi.org/10.1016/j.healthpol.2010.06.001).

Nicaise P, Dubois V, Lorant V et al. (2014). Mental health care delivery system reform in Belgium: The challenge of achieving deinstitutionalisation whilst addressing fragmentation of care at the same time. Health Policy, 115(2–3):120–127.

Nicoll R, Robertson L, Marks A et al. (2018). Models of care for chronic kidney disease: a systematic review. Nephrology, 23:389–396. doi:10.1111/nep.13198

Nkansah N, Mostovetsky O, Yu C et al. (2010). Effect of outpatient pharmacists' non-dispensing roles on patient outcomes and prescribing patterns. Cochrane Database Syst Rev, 7:CD000336. doi:10.1002/14651858.CD000336.pub2

Nolte E, Knai C, Saltman RB, eds. (2014). Assessing chronic disease management in European health systems. Concepts and approaches. European Observatory on Health Systems and Policies. Copenhagen, WHO Regional Office for Europe.

Nolte E, Knai C (2015). Assessing chronic disease management in European health systems country reports. Observatory Studies Series 39. European Observatory on Health Systems and Policies. Copenhagen, WHO Regional Office for Europe.

Oono I, Honey E, Mc Conachie H (2013). Parent-mediated early intervention for young children with autism spectrum disorders (ASD) (Review). Cochrane Database Syst Rev, 4: CD009774. doi:10.1002/14651858.CD009774.pub2.www.cochranelibrary.com

Parker D, Maresco-Pennisi D, Clifton K et al. (2016). Practice nurse involvement in the management of adults with type 2 diabetes mellitus attending a general practice: results from a systematic review. Int J Evid Based Health, 14(2):41–52. doi:10.1097/XEB.0000000000000080

Pharmaceutical Group of The European Union (2013). Annual report 2013: measuring health outcomes in community pharmacy. Brussels 2013: PGEU. (https://www.pgeu.eu/en/library/224:annual-report-2013.html, accessed 28 August 2018).

Pharmaceutical Group of The European Union (2017). Annual report 2017: measuring health outcomes in community pharmacy. Brussels 2017: PGEU. (https://www.pgeu.eu/en/library/587:annual-report-2017.html, accessed 28 August 2018).

Pimouguet C, Le Goff M, Thiébaut R et al. (2011). Effectiveness of disease-management programs for improving diabetes care: a meta-analysis. CMAJ, 183(2):E115–E127. doi:10.1503/cmaj.091786

Pitt V, Lowe D, Hill S et al. (2013). Consumer-providers of care for adult clients of statutory mental health services. Cochrane Database Syst Rev, 3:CD004807. doi:10.1002/14651858.CD004807.pub2

Qi L, Liu Q, Qi X et al. (2015). Effectiveness of peer support for improving glycaemic control in patients with type 2 diabetes: a meta-analysis of randomized controlled trials. BMC Public Health, 15:471. (https://doi .org/10.1186/s12889-015-1798-y).

Readdean KC, Heuer AJ, Scott Parrott J (2018). Effect of pharmacist intervention on improving antidepressant medication adherence and depression symptomology: A systematic review and meta-analysis. Res Social Adm Pharm, 14(4):321–331. doi:10.1016/j.sapharm.2017.05.008

Reilly S, Planner C, Gask L et al. (2013). Collaborative care approaches for people with severe mental illness (Review). Cochrane Database Syst Rev Collab, 11:CD009531. DOI: doi:10.1002/14651858.CD009531.pub2. www.cochranelibrary.com

Rijken PM, Bekkema N. (2011). Chronic Disease Management Matrix 2010. Results of a survey in ten European countries. Utrecht: Nivel, 2011. (https://www.nivel.nl/sites/default/files/bestanden/Rapport-chronic-disease-management-matrix-2010.pdf, accessed 27 July 2018).

Rijken M, Bekkema N, Boeckxstaens P et al. (2014). Chronic disease management programmes: an adequate response to patients' needs? Health Expect, 17(5):608–621.

Rijken M, Struckmann V, van der Heide I et al., on behalf of the ICARE4EU consortium (2017). How to improve care for people with multimorbidity in Europe? Policy Brief 23. Health Systems and Policies Analysis. Nivel/TU Berlin, European Observatory on Health Systems and Policies.

Rijken M, Hujala A, van Ginneken E et al. (2018). Managing multimorbidity: profiles of integrated care approaches targeting people with multiple chronic conditions in Europe. Health Policy, 122(1):44–52. doi: 10.1016/j. healthpol.2017.10.002.

Robinson-White S, Conroy B, Slavish KH et al. (2010). Patient navigation in breast cancer. Cancer Nurs, 33:127–140. doi: 10.1097/ NCC.0b013e3181c40401

Savolahti MR (2016). Nurses with prescriptive authority in the Finnish healthcare. Best practices and management. JAMK University of Applied Sciences.

Master's Thesis. (http://www.theseus.fi/bitstream/handle/10024/125279/Savolahti%20Marja-Riitta.pdf?sequence=1&isAllowed=y)

Schadewaldt V, Schultz T (2010). A systematic review on the effectiveness of nurse-led cardiac clinics for adult patients with coronary heart disease. JBI Libr Syst Rev, 8(2):53–89. doi:10.11124/01938924-201008020-00001

Sermeus W (forthcoming). Interdisciplinary teams, new professions and new roles in Belgium: pilot projects in need of scaling up. In: Wismar M, Glinos I, Sagan A eds. Skill-mix innovation in primary and chronic care. Mobilizing patients, peers, professionals. European Observatory on Health Systems and Policies. Volume 1. Copenhagen, WHO Regional Office for Europe on behalf of the European Observatory on Health Systems and Policies.

Shaw RJ, McDuffie JR, Hendrix CC et al. (2013). Effects of nurse-managed protocols in the outpatient management of adults with chronic conditions. Washington DC, Department of Veterans Affairs (US).

Sighinolfi C, Nespeca C, Menchetti M et al. (2014). Collaborative care for depression in European countries: a systematic review and meta-analysis. J Psychosom Res, 77(4):247–263. doi:10.1016/j.jpsychores.2014.08.006

Sikorski C, Luppa M, König H et al. (2012). Does GP training in depression care affect patient outcome? - A systematic review and meta-analysis. BMC Health Serv Res, 12:10. https://doi.org/10.1186/1472-6963-12-10

Singer S, Gianinazzi ME, Hohn A et al. (2013). General practitioner involvement in follow-up of childhood cancer survivors: a systematic review. Pediatr Blood Cancer, 60(10):1565–1573. doi:10.1002/pbc.24586

Smith SM, Soubhi H, Fortin M et al. (2012). Managing patients with multimorbidity: systematic review of interventions in primary care and community settings. BMJ, 345:e5205.

Smith SM, Cousins G, Clyne B et al. (2017). Shared care across the interface between primary and specialty care in management of long term conditions. Cochrane Database Syst Rev, 2(2):CD004910. doi:10.1002/14651858.CD004910.pub3

Starfield B (2008). Foreword I: A health system perspective. In: Nolte E, McKee M, eds. Caring for people with chronic conditions. A health system perspective. European Observatory on Health Systems and Policies. Copenhagen, WHO Regional Office for Europe.

Stokes J, Panagioti M, Alam R et al. (2015). Effectiveness of case management for 'at risk' patients in primary care: a systematic review and meta-analysis. PLoS One, 10(7). doi:10.1371/journal.pone.0132340

Strand H, Parker D (2012). Effects of multidisciplinary models of care for adult pre-dialysis patients with chronic kidney disease: a systematic review. Int J Evid Based Healthcare, 10:53–59. doi:10.1111/j.1744-1609.2012.00253.x

Struckmann V, Quentin W, Busse R et al. (2017). How to strengthen financing mechanisms to promote care for people with multimorbidity in Europe? Policy Brief 24. European Observatory on Health Systems and Policies. Copenhagen, WHO Regional Office for Europe.

Sulkakoski M (2016). Collaboration between nurse prescribers and GPs at the Finnish health center receptions. Department of Health Sciences, University of Jyväskylä, Heath Education. Master's Thesis. (https://jyx.jyu.fi/bitstream/handle/123456789/50877/1/URN%3ANBN%3Afi%3Ajyu-201607213650.pdf, accessed 15 August 2018).

Supper I, Bourgueil Y, Ecochard R et al. (2017). Impact of multimorbidity on healthcare professional task shifting potential in patients with type 2 diabetes in primary care: a French cross-sectional study. BMJ Open, 7:e-016545. doi: 10.1136/bmjopen-2017-01654

Tabesh M, Magliano DJ, Koye DN et al. (2018). The effect of nurse prescribers on glycaemic control in type 2 diabetes: A systematic review and meta-analysis. Int J Nurs Stud, 78:37–43. doi:10.1016/j.ijnurstu.2017.08.018

Tan EC, Stewart K, Elliott RA et al. (2014). Pharmacist services provided in general practice clinics: a systematic review and meta-analysis. Res Social Adm Pharm, 10(4):608–622. doi:10.1016/j.sapharm.2013.08.006

Thota AB, Sipe TA, Byard GJ et al. (2012). Collaborative care to improve the management of depressive disorders: a community guide systematic review and meta-analysis. Am J Prev Med, 42(5):525–538. doi:10.1016/j.amepre.2012.01.019

van der Heide I, Snoeijs S, Melchiorre MG et al, on behalf of the ICARE4EU project team (2015). Innovating care for people with multiple chronic conditions in Europe. An overview. Utrecht, Nivel (http://www.icare4eu.org/pdf/State-of-the-Art_report_ICARE4EU.pdf).

van Eikenhorst L, Taxis K, van Dijk L et al. (2017). Pharmacist-led self-management interventions to improve diabetes outcomes. a systematic literature review and meta-analysis. Front Pharmacol, 8:891. doi:10.3389/fphar.2017.00891

Vermunt NPCA, Harmsen M, Westert GP et al. (2017). Collaborative goal setting with elderly patients with chronic disease or multimorbidity: a systematic review. BMC Geriatr, 17(1):167. doi:10.1186/s12877-017-0534-0

Vigod SN, Kurdyak PA, Dennis C et al. (2013). Transitional interventions to reduce early psychiatric readmissions in adults: systematic review. Br J Psychiat, 202:187–194. doi:10.1192/bjp.bp.112.115030

Vitale A, Mannix-McNamara P, Cullinan V (2015). Promoting mental health through multidisciplinary care: Experience of health professionals working in community mental health teams in Ireland. Int J Mental Health Promo, 17(4):188–200.

Wang Y, Yeo QQ, Ko Y (2016). Economic evaluations of pharmacist-managed services in people with diabetes mellitus: a systematic review. Diabet Med 33(4):421–427. doi:10.1111/dme.12976

Welsh E, Hasan M, Li P (2011). Home-based educational interventions for children with asthma (Review). Cochrane Database Syst Rev, 10: CD008469. doi:10.1002/14651858.CD008469.pub2

Wong WCW, Luk CW, Kidd MR (2012). Is there a role for primary care clinicians in providing shared care in HIV treatment ? A systematic literature review. Sex Transm Infect, 88:125–132. doi:10.1136/sextrans-2011-050170

World Health Organization (2018). Mental health – Belgium: switching to community mental health care. (https://www.who.int/mental_health/evidence/outreach_teams_belgium/en/, accessed 15 October 2018).

Wright-Berryman JL, McGuire AB, Salyers MP (2011). A review of consumer-provided services on Assertive Community Treatment and intensive case management teams: Implications for future research and practice. J Am Psychiatr Nurses Assoc, 17(1):37–44. doi:10.1177/1078390310393283.

Zhong H, Ni X-J, Cui M et al. (2014). Evaluation of pharmacist care for patients with chronic obstructive pulmonary disease : a systematic review and meta-analysis. Int J Clin Pharm, 36:1230–1240. doi:10.1007/s11096-014-0024-9

7 Long-term and palliative care at home: skill-mix innovations for enhanced responsiveness and satisfaction of patients and caregivers

ELKE BERGER, RAMONA BACKHAUS,
JAN HAMERS, PETER PYPE, PAULINE
BOECKXSTAENS, LAURA PFIRTER,
CLAUDIA B. MAIER

7.1 Introduction

Timely access to long-term care and palliative care that takes patients' individual choices into account has been an area of concern to policy-makers in many European countries. The majority of Europeans wish to receive long-term care in their homes for as long as possible (European Commission, 2007). They are often primarily cared for by their families and supported by health and social care professionals. Moving to a nursing home or a similar institution is the first preference of only approximately 10% of Europeans. As to palliative care, the majority of patients prefer to stay at home under the care of the regular health care providers with whom they often have longstanding relationships.

Hence, the policy focus in many countries is on strengthening its health and social care workforce as well as informal caregivers to ensure people can stay in their homes (OECD/EU, 2016). Similarly, the importance of the home care setting for persons with palliative care needs has increased as well. Therefore, this chapter focuses on skill-mix innovations in the ambulatory and in particular home care settings, and not on institutionalized care.

Although both long-term and palliative care are targeting people with functional limitations and the need for help with activities of daily living or with psychosocial needs, their underlying concepts are distinctly different. Long-term care at home aims to support people with limitations and their families' support (formal or informal) to live at home for as long as possible and as independently as possible. Typically, this refers to self-management support, preventive and rehabilitative care, help with activities of daily living, such as bathing, dressing and getting in and out of bed, performed by a team of health professionals, including nursing and other professions, but mostly by family caregivers (Colombo et al., 2011).

Following the WHO definition, the concept of palliative care aims to improve the quality of life of patients and their families facing incurable, often life-threatening, illness, through the prevention and relief of suffering by means of early identification, assessment and treatment of pain and other problems (physical, psychosocial and spiritual) (World Health Organization, 2018a). According to the WHO, long-term and palliative care should be designed to provide high-quality care, in a way that is people-centred and consistent with their rights, fundamental freedoms and human dignity (World Health Organization, 2017).

In light of an increased demand due to a rising burden of noncommunicable diseases, ageing populations and changing family constellations (World Health Organization, 2018b), there are existing skill gaps in both areas of care. Reasons include a lack of skilled providers, poor work environments, limited career options and insufficient financing and payment of services. Additional skill gaps in long-term care include a lack of (sufficient time for) communication, self-management, support, social care, patient-centred services and limited choices as to people's preferred place of living. In palliative care, skill gaps are also frequent, due to a shortage of palliative-care specialists with skills in pain management for severe pain and end-of-life palliation. Other skill gaps include support for spiritual needs as well as addressing patients' individual needs and wishes during the phase of transition from acute care to palliative care and at the end-of-life.

Across Europe, several skill-mix changes in policy and practice have emerged in long-term care over the past decade, ranging from small-scale programmes to larger scale reforms. Two major trends can be observed: current and expected future workforce shortages that generate a need to attract more health professionals into providing long-term care of high quality; and interventions that specifically focus on skills enhancements to empower and support the people and their caregivers. As to palliative care, there are only a few skill-mix developments like in pilot programmes for palliative care teams with specialized skills in Belgium, Germany, the Netherlands and the United Kingdom.

This chapter aims to describe and analyse main skill-mix changes for patients receiving long-term and palliative care at home and their caregivers. In order to do so, a summary of the evidence on existing skill-mix innovations is given in the first section based on the overview of reviews (for the methodology, see Chapter 1), including evidence on their effectiveness in terms of health outcomes, resource use and professional outcomes. The second section shows trends in skill-mix innovations for both areas of care from a cross-country perspective.

7.2 Evidence on outcomes

The overview of reviews identified 17 systematic reviews (Box 1). Overall and especially in palliative care, the number of systematic reviews was relatively low when compared to those identified for the other Chapters.

Long-term care

Skill-mix interventions in long-term care

Interventions in long-term care comprised a broad range of skill-mix innovations (Table 7.1) of which the introduction of case management was the most prominent. Ten systematic reviews summarized the effects of case management for people requiring long-term care at home and

---

Box 7.1 Overview of the evidence on long-term and palliative care

Number of reviews: 17 systematic reviews covering a total of 286 studies were identified, with six systematic reviews related to palliative care and 11 related to long-term care.

Country coverage: The majority of studies were conducted in the USA and in Europe, especially in the United Kingdom. Other countries were Australia, Belgium, Canada, China, Denmark, Finland, France, Germany, Hong Kong, India, Israel, Italy, Japan, Luxembourg, the Netherlands, New Zealand, Norway, Pakistan, Poland, Singapore, Spain, Sweden, Taiwan, Tanzania, Turkey.

Methods: Overall, several reviews were of comparatively low quality. Although there were three Cochrane reviews included, one did not include any suitable study. In sum, five meta-analyses were performed.

Table 7.1 *Evidence for skill-mix interventions in long-term care from the overview of reviews*

Skill-mix interventions				Outcomes		
Content of interventions and skill-mix changes	Profession(s) in intervention and in comparator group	Population	Countries (number)	Patient-related outcomes	Health-system-related outcomes	Profession-/Informal caregiver-specific outcomes
Case management in the community						
(i) For people with dementia and their caregivers [1–8]						
Case management interventions for people with dementia and their caregivers, including case identification, counselling, coordinating, multidimensional assessment, monitoring, educating	Intervention: case managers with advanced training [1, 4, 6] and background in nursing, social work, psychology, among others Comparison: not reported	People with dementia living at home and their caregivers	Europe, USA among others (not fully reported, but most studies were conducted in the USA (>60) and in Europe, especially in the United Kingdom (>25)	• No effects on mortality [1–3, 6, 7] • Mostly no effects on depressive symptoms [1–4, 6], only two RCTs showed positive effects [3] • Mostly no effects on functional status [1–3, 6], two RCTs [3] showed positive effects • No effects on cognition [1–4, 6] • No effects on quality of life [3–6], positive effects were shown in two studies only [3, 7] • No effects on ADL [2, 4]	• Most evidence on cost-effectiveness showed no effects [2, 3, 5, 6, 8] • Mixed evidence on ED-use with two RCTs showing positive and three RCTs showing no effects [2, 3, 8] • No evidence of effects on hospitalization-rates (>10 RCTs) [1–3, 6–8], only two RCTs showed intermediate effects [3] • Significant positive effect on length of hospital stay (two RCTs) [3] and reduction of days per month in a residential home or hospital unit at 6 months (one RCT) and at 12 months (one RCT) [6]	Professionals • Improved satisfaction (two RCTs) [2, 3] Informal caregivers • Greater satisfaction with social support and a decrease in symptoms of depression (one RCT) [5] • Significantly improved dementia-guideline adherence and/or medication management (seven RCTs) [2–4]

- Significant reduction of embarrassment, isolation and improved coping with memory problems or diagnosis of dementia, with additional effects for people with more severe impairment ($n = 1$) [2]
- Statistically significant improvement in patients' access to services ($n = 1$) [7]
- Modestly statistically significant improvements at 18 months in the intensity of behavioural problems ($n = 1$) [7]
- Modestly higher compliance with guideline recommendations ($n = 1$) [7]

- No differences in time to institutionalization in a residential home (five RCTs), only one RCT showed a significant impact [8]
- Many studies within the reviews showed significant positive effects on institutionalization rates ($n = 19$) [1–3, 6], but more studies showed no effects ($n = 42$) [1–3, 6–8]; a meta-analysis of 16 RCTs revealed a significant positive effect after stratification for time to follow-up less than 18 months [8]

Table 7.1 (cont.)

Skill-mix interventions		Outcomes				
Content of interventions and skill-mix changes	Profession(s) in intervention and in comparator group	Population	Countries (number)	Patient-related outcomes	Health-system-related outcomes	Profession-/Informal caregiver-specific outcomes

Case management in the community

(ii) For older adults and their caregivers [9, 10]

Case management interventions to support informal caregivers of older adults, including assessment, planning, coordinating, monitoring and counselling	Intervention: Case managers with various backgrounds, research assistants, nurses, dementia family nurse care coordinator. Comparison: not reported	Informal caregivers of adults aged 65 or older	FI (3), HK (1), ISR (1), IT (1), NL (1), UK (1), US (14)	• Improvements in emotional health (n = 1) [9] • Lower depression scores after 6 months (n = 2), but mixed results after 12 months [9] and no effect in psychiatric symptoms and associated behavioural problems (n = 2) [10] • No effects on quality of life (n = 1) [9] • Significantly improved health or well-being across different measures, such as self-perceived life satisfaction, morale, depression, mastery, and personal health status (n = 5) [10]	• Decreases in municipal care costs per family per year in Finland (n = 1) [9] • Significant reductions of admissions to long-term institutions in first (n = 1) and 18th month of intervention (n = 1), but no differences after 24 months (n = 2) [9]	Informal caregiver • No improvements in family caregivers emotional health, quality of life, sense of competence and mixed results regarding depressive symptoms (n = 2) [9] • Improved well-being (n = 1) vs no effects (n = 4) [10]

- Mixed results regarding functional status ($n = 4$ with positive, of which one only showed those effects in the long term rather than the short term and $n = 4$ with no or no clear effects) [9, 10]
- Significantly less pain and dyspnoea during the 12-month follow-up period ($n = 1$) while another study showed no difference in patients' health status [10]
- Mixed effects on patient satisfaction ($n = 5$) [9, 10]
- Significant effect on mortality ($n = 2$) vs no significant intervention-control group differences ($n = 5$) [10]
- Decreased unmet service needs ($n = 3$) [10]

- Mixed results on caregivers' stress or burden ($n = 5$): significant improvements in burden of caregiver ($n = 1$), significant reduced stress or burden ($n = 2$) vs no effect ($n = 2$) [10]
- Improved caregiver satisfaction ($n = 2$) [9, 10] vs no effects ($n = 1$) [9]

Table 7.1 *(cont.)*

Skill-mix interventions				Outcomes		
Content of interventions and skill-mix changes	Profession(s) in intervention and in comparator group	Population	Countries (number)	Patient-related outcomes	Health-system-related outcomes	Profession-/Informal caregiver-specific outcomes
Multidisciplinary team approach for the management of Parkinson [11]						
Multidisciplinary team approach, including group education activities specific to Parkinson's disease and individualized rehabilitation	Intervention: nurse, physical therapist, occupational therapist, speech therapist, dietician, neurologist, psychologist Comparison: not specified, but likely GPs or neurologist	Patients with Parkinson's disease	Japan (1), UK (1)	• Significant improvement in Parkinson's disease-related scores and patient mood ($n = 1$) • Improvements in health-related quality of life (e.g. 37% improvement), various function and mobility scores • Significant improvement in depression scores, voice articulation and speech ($n = 1$)		Informal caregiver • Caregiver mood did not significantly change

Abbreviations: ADL/EADL: activities of daily living/extended ADL; ED: emergency department; ER: emergency room; GP: general practitioner; IADL: instrumental ADL; MMSE: Mini–Mental State Examination; RCT: randomized controlled trial.

Country abbreviations: AU: Australia; FI: Finland; HK: Hong Kong; ISR: Israel; IT: Italy; NL: the Netherlands; UK: the United Kingdom, USA: the United States of America.

Sources: [1] Backhouse et al. (2017); [2] Goeman, Renehan & Koch (2016); [3] Khanassov, Vedel & Pluye (2014); [4] Khanassov & Vedel (2016); [5] Pimouguet, Lavaud & Dartigues (2010); [6] Reilly et al. (2015); [7] Somme et al. (2012); [8] Tam-Tham et al. (2013); [9] Berthelsen & Kristensson (2015); [10] You et al. 2012; [11] Prizer & Browner (2012).

their caregivers (Backhouse et al., 2017; Berthelsen & Kristensson, 2015; Goeman, Renehan & Koch, 2016; Khanassov, Vedel & Pluye, 2014; Khanassov & Vedel, 2016; Pimouguet, Lavaud & Dartigues, 2010; Reilly et al., 2015; Somme et al., 2012; Tam-Tham et al., 2013; You et al., 2012). This involved programmes integrating case managers into health care services for people specifically with dementia and their caregivers – covered by eight reviews (Backhouse et al., 2017; Goeman, Renehan & Koch, 2016; Khanassov, Vedel & Pluye, 2014; Khanassov & Vedel, 2016; Pimouguet, Lavaud & Dartiques, 2010; Reilly et al., 2015), and programmes targeting older patients with various conditions (including dementia) and their caregivers by introducing a case manager function, as in two reviews (Berthelsen & Kristensson, 2015; You et al., 2012). Regardless of the target group, the new tasks and skills covered by case management targeted various elements of care, ranging from counselling and coordinating care to assessing needs, planning care and support systems, monitoring and educating informal caregivers. Case managers had various backgrounds, in nursing, social work and psychology.

For people with Parkinson's disease, one review (Prizer & Browner, 2012) analysed a multidisciplinary team approach for the management of the condition. It included group education activities specific to Parkinson's disease and individualized rehabilitation. In this case, the multidisciplinary teams were composed of nurses, physical therapists, speech therapists, dieticians, neurologists and psychologists and were compared with usual care by GPs or neurologists. No example of skill-mix innovations involving new technologies or eHealth was identified.

Evidence on outcomes

Case management interventions for people with dementia and their caregivers were shown to reduce feelings of embarrassment and isolation, and to improve coping with memory problems or diagnosis of dementia, with additional effects for people with more severe impairment (one RCT) (Goeman, Renehan & Koch, 2016). The intensity of behavioural problems at 18 months follow up (one RCT) and adherence to guideline recommendations (one RCT) were also shown to be improved by introducing case management (Somme et al., 2012). Furthermore, patients' access to services was significantly improved compared with standard care (Somme et al., 2012). In terms of other patient-related outcomes, the majority of studies showed no impact of case management interventions, for example, regarding depressive symptoms (Backhouse et al., 2017; Goeman, Renehan & Koch, 2016; Khanassov, Vedel & Pluye, 2014; Khannassov & Vedel, 2016; Reilly et al., 2015), functional status (Backhouse et al., 2017; Goeman, Renehan & Koch, 2016; Khanassov, Vedel & Pluye, 2014; Reilly et al., 2015) and quality of life (Khanassov, Vedel & Pluye, 2014; Khanassov & Vedel, 2016; Pimouguet, Lavaud & Dartigues, 2010; Reilly et al., 2015; Somme et al., 2012). No effects were shown on mortality (Backhouse et al., 2017; Goeman, Renehan & Koch, 2016; Khanassov,Vedel & Pluye, 2014; Reilly et al., 2015; Somme et al., 2012), cognition (Backhouse et al., 2017; Goeman, Renehan & Koch, 2016; Khanassov, Vedel & Pluye, 2014; Khanassov & Vedel, 2016; Reilly et al., 2015), and activities of daily living (Goeman, Renehan & Koch, 2016; Khanassov & Vedel, 2016). In terms of health-system-related outcomes, the evidence for effects in the community was mixed. Significant positive effects were shown on length of hospital stay (two RCTs, Khanassov, Vedel & Pluye, 2014) and on the number of days per month in a residential home or hospital unit at 6 months (one RCT) and at 12 months (one RCT, Reilly et al., 2015). Most studies analysing costs or cost-effectiveness showed no effects (Goeman, Renehan & Koch, 2016; Khanassov, Vedel & Pluye, 2014; Pimouguet, Lavaud & Dartigues, 2010; Reilly et al., 2015; Tam-Tham et al., 2013). Several studies included in the reviews showed significantly reduced institutionalization rates ($n = 19$, Backhouse et al., 2017; Goeman, Renehan & Koch, 2016; Khanassov, Vedel & Pluye, 2014; Reilly et al., 2015), but more studies showed no effects ($n > 30$, Backhouse et al. 2017; Goeman, Renehan & Koch, 2016; Khanassov, Vedel & Pluye, 2014; Reilly et al. 2015; Somme et al., 2012; Tam-Tham et al., 2013). Mixed results were also shown for emergency department visits (Goeman, Renehan & Koch, 2016; Khanassov, Vedel & Pluye, 2014; Tam-Tham et al., 2013), for time to institutionalization to a residential home (Tam-Tham et al., 2013) and for hospitalization rates. For the latter, several RCTs showed no effects (Backhouse et al., 2017; Goeman, Renehan & Koch, 2016; Khanassov, Vedel & Pluye, 2014; Reilly et al., 2015; Somme et al., 2012; Tam-Tham et al., 2013) and only two RCTs reported intermediate effects (Khanassov, Vedel & Pluye, 2014). A meta-analysis of 16 RCTs revealed a significant positive effect after stratification for time to follow-up less than 18 months (Tam-Tham et al., 2013). In terms of profession-specific outcomes, the reviews found significantly improved guideline adherence and medication management (Goeman, Renehan & Koch, 2016; Khanassov, Vedel & Pluye, 2014; Khanassov & Vedel, 2016). In a few studies, satisfaction was shown to be improved for both professionals (Goeman, Renehan & Koch, 2016; Khanassov, Vedel & Pluye, 2014) and informal caregivers (Pimouguet, Lavaud & Dartigues, 2010). Moreover, receiving support from a case manager resulted in a decrease in depressive symptoms of caregivers (one RCT, Pimouguet, Lavaud & Dartigues, 2010).

Providing case management interventions to support older adults and their family caregivers (Berthelsen & Kristensson, 2015; You et al., 2012) was shown to improve patients' emotional health ($n = 1$) and depression 6 months after intervention ($n = 2$). However, after 12 months, results for depression were mixed (Berthelsen & Kristensson, 2015). Mixed results were also shown for functional status with four studies reporting positive and negative effects (Berthelson & Kristensson, 2015; You et al., 2012). One of the studies only showed positive effects on functional status in the long rather than the short term (You et al., 2012). Furthermore, one study showed no effects on quality of life and the results of five studies on effectiveness of case management for older adults and their caregivers were inconclusive in terms of patient satisfaction (Berthelson & Kristensson, 2015; You et al., 2012). The results on mortality were not clear either with two studies reporting significant positive effects and five studies reporting no significant differences. However, providing case management was shown to decrease unmet needs compared with standard care ($n = 3$, You et al., 2012). In terms of health system outcomes, some positive effects were shown, for example, decreased municipal care costs per family per year in Finland ($n = 1$) and significantly reduced admissions to long-term institutions in first ($n = 1$) and 18th month of intervention ($n = 1$). However, there were no differences after 24 months ($n = 2$). One study included in the review showed higher overall caregiver satisfaction, but two studies showed no improvements in emotional health, quality of life, sense of competence and mixed results in terms of caregivers' depression.

For people suffering from Parkinson's disease, integrating a multidisciplinary team approach in health care (Prizer & Browner, 2012) was shown to significantly improve Parkinson's disease-related scores and patient mood ($n = 1$), health-related quality of life as well as depression scores, voice articulation and speech ($n = 1$). Caregiver mood was not shown to be improved and no health-system-related outcomes were assessed.

Palliative care

Skill-mix interventions in palliative care
Generally, fewer skill-mix developments in palliative care were identified in the literature compared with long-term care, and as a consequence the evidence on their effectiveness is limited. Nevertheless, skill-mix interventions directed at patients in palliative situations and their caregivers included various models and were assessed by six reviews (Table 7.2).

A Cochrane review that aimed to analyse the effects of a systematic and organized approach to collaboration with a multidisciplinary team involving at least two professions from different disciplines and targeting adult home hospice patients could not identify any study that met the inclusion criteria (Joseph et al., 2016).

Another Cochrane review (Shepperd et al., 2016) assessed the effectiveness of any home-based end-of-life care interventions, including consultation, multidisciplinary care coordination, physiotherapy, informal help, nutrition and social care, and (if needed) 24-hour care, that provides active treatment for continuous periods of time by health care professionals, for example, specialist palliative-care nurses, qualified nurses, family physicians, palliative-care consultants, physiotherapists, occupational therapists, nutritionists and social care workers. In the majority of studies, the interventions were carried out by a multidisciplinary team.

Dy et al. (2013) analysed the effects of interventions that focus on continuity, coordination and transition, including (i) involvement of the patient, the family or the caregiver, for example, through education; (ii) coordination with an additional provider to provide care; (iii) conducting care plans or (iv) introducing palliative-care specialists. Professions involved in the interventions were palliative-care specialist, nurse case managers, physicians, GP, nurse specialist, social workers, case coordinators and case managers.

Furthermore, Carmont et al. (2018) analysed interventions designed to engage GPs with special secondary services in integrated palliative care, including shared consultations or case conferences. Professions in the intervention were GPs and at least one other profession, for example, nurses, medical specialists or allied health professionals.

Another skill-mix innovation in palliative care was pain medication management educational interventions for family caregivers of patients with advanced cancer (Latter et al., 2016). This included face-to-face

Table 7.2 *Evidence from the overview of reviews for skill-mix innovations in palliative care*

Skill-mix interventions				Outcomes		
Content of interventions and skill-mix changes	Profession(s) in intervention and in comparator group	Population	Countries	Patient-related outcomes	Health-system-related outcomes	Profession-/Informal caregiver-specific outcomes
Interventions mainly focusing on patients						
(i) Integrated palliative care involving GPs [1]						
Interventions designed to engage GPs with specialist secondary services in integrated palliative care, e.g. including shared consultations or case conferences	Intervention: GPs and at least one other profession, e.g. various, e.g. nurses, medical specialists, allied health professionals Comparison: GPs only, specialists only	Patients aged 18 years or older in a palliative situation receiving services through their GP, specialist hospital services or an integrated model of care	AU (4), CA (2), DK (1), NZ (1), NL (3), UK (1) and 5 with no country reported	• Significant improvements in patient functional status (n = 2) • Improved pain management, symptom control and safety for patients and family: from both GP (n = 1) and patient perspective (n = 2) • No effects on quality of life or symptom burden (n = 2)	• Significant decrease in number of hospital admissions (n = 3) • Case conferences and shared care were both effective in reducing the length of hospital stay (n = 2)	Professionals • Strengthening of service relationships, improved interprofessional communication and improvements in professional developments (n = 2)

Table 7.2 *(cont.)*

Skill-mix interventions			Outcomes			
Content of interventions and skill-mix changes	Profession(s) in intervention and in comparator group	Population	Countries	Patient-related outcomes	Health-system-related outcomes	Profession-/Informal caregiver-specific outcomes
Interventions mainly focusing on patients						
(ii) Structured interdisciplinary collaboration [2]						
Any systematic and organized approach to collaboration leading to the attainment of specific goals involving rules and guidelines	Intervention: at least two professions from different disciplines (not fully described) Comparison: not reported	Adult home hospice patients		no study met the inclusion criteria		
(iii) Home-based end-of-life care interventions [3]						
Any home-based end-of-life care intervention that provides active treatment for continuous periods of time by health care	Intervention: Specialist palliative-care nurses, qualified nurses, family physicians, palliative-care consultants, physiotherapist,	People, aged 18 years and over, who are at the end of life and require terminal care. Some had	USA (2), UK (1), Norway (1)	• Significant increased likelihood of dying at home compared with usual care ($n = 3$ RCTs)	• Significant reduction in health care costs ranging between 18% and 30% in the USA ($n = 2$ RCTs)	Informal caregivers • Higher caregivers' satisfaction only at 1-month, but not at 6-month, follow-up and caregivers of participants who had survived more than 30 days showed a decrease in psychological well-being (one RCT)

professionals in the patient's home for patients who would otherwise require hospital or hospice inpatient end-of-life care. Including: consultation, multidisciplinary care coordination, physiotherapy, informal help, nutrition and social care, if needed 24-hour care

occupational therapists, nutritionists, and social care workers; in three-quarters of studies working as a multidisciplinary team

Comparison: not reported

a diagnosis of chronic disease (like heart failure, obstructive pulmonary disease, cancer)

- Little difference to functional status (measured by the Barthel Index), psychological well-being, or cognitive status ($n = 1$ RCT)
- Slightly improved patient satisfaction at follow up after 1 month, but not after 6 months ($n = 2$ RCTs)
- Unclear effects on 6-month mortality ($n = 1$ RCT)

- Mixed results on admission to hospital ($n = 4$ RCTs)

- Little or no effect on caregiver bereavement response 6 months following death (one RCT)

Table 7.2 (*cont.*)

Skill-mix interventions				Outcomes		
Content of interventions and skill-mix changes	Profession(s) in intervention and in comparator group	Population	Countries	Patient-related outcomes	Health-system-related outcomes	Profession-/Informal caregiver-specific outcomes

Interventions mainly focusing on patients

(iv) Interventions that focus on continuity, coordination and transition [4]*

Interventions that focus on (i) patient/ family/caregiver involvement (e.g. through education); (ii) coordination with an additional provider to provide care; (iii) conducting care plans or (iv) introducing palliative-care specialists	Intervention: palliative-care specialist, nurse case managers, physicians, GP, nurse specialist, social workers, case coordinators, case managers Comparison: not reported	Adults with mixed illnesses or cancer patients. Those unlikely to be cured, recover or stabilize	Not reported	• Significant effects (*n* = 3) vs no effects on quality of life (*n* = 6) • Significant improved satisfaction (*n* = 6) vs no effects (*n* = 1)	• Only 5 out of 16 studies evaluating health care utilization, e.g. in terms of hospital admission and length of stay, found significant effects • No significant effects for most of the studies in each intervention component.	Informal caregivers • Significant effects on caregiver satisfaction (*n* = 4) vs no effects (*n* = 2) • No effects on caregiver burden (*n* = 3) • Significant quality of life improvements for caregivers (*n* = 1)

Interventions mainly focusing on family caregivers

(i) Pain medication management for family caregivers [5]

Pain medication management educational interventions for family caregivers of patients with advanced cancer, including face-to-face education or training sessions, opportunities for questions and discussion, and follow-up contacts for reinforcement or further coaching	Intervention: nurses, psychologists, researcher Comparison: not reported	Caregivers of patients with advanced cancer	NO (1), UK (1), USA (5), Taiwan (1)	• Significantly higher medication adherence at 2 and 4 weeks ($n = 1$ RCT) vs no reported data in a single-group pilot study • Significantly reduced pain ($n = 2$) vs no effects on significant effect on pain ($n = 4$)	Informal caregivers • Significant effects ($n = 3$) vs no effects on caregivers' knowledge and beliefs about pain management ($n = 4$) • Significant improvements on self-efficacy/perceived control over pain (one RCT)

Table 7.2 *(cont.)*

Skill-mix interventions					Outcomes		
Content of interventions and skill-mix changes	Profession(s) in intervention and in comparator group	Population	Countries		Patient-related outcomes	Health-system-related outcomes	Profession-/Informal caregiver-specific outcomes
Interventions mainly focusing mainly on family caregivers							
(ii) Psychosocially and/or psycho-educationally based interventions for family caregivers [6]							
Psychosocially and/or psycho-educationally based interventions for family caregivers including psychoeducation, psychosocial support, caregivers coping, symptom management, sleep promotion and family meetings	Intervention: not reported Comparison: not reported	Adult family caregivers of palliative care patients	Majority of the 14 studies were conducted in industrial countries				Informal caregivers • Positive effects on depression levels of caregivers of patients with Alzheimer's disease ($n = 1$) • Improvements in sleep quality and depression in the caregiver ($n = 1$) • No significant benefit to caregivers' psychosocial health or well-being ($n = 1$) • Significant favourable effects of a psycho-educational programme on caregivers' perceptions of positive elements of their role ($n = 1$); on family caregivers' quality of life ($n = 1$) as well as the perceived burden of patients' symptoms and their perceived burden of care tasks ($n = 1$) vs no significant benefit to caregivers through a separate psychosocial support intervention ($n = 1$)

- Significant positive effects on caregivers' preparedness, competence, reward ratings ($n = 1$)
- Reduction of unmet needs ($n = 2$)
- Positive caregivers' perception of the intervention ($n = 3$)
- Significant increased caregivers' levels of comfort, closure and satisfaction ($n = 1$)
- Psychological benefits for caregivers ($n = 1$)
- Significantly higher ratings of caregivers' self-efficacy for helping patients to control pain and other symptoms ($n = 1$)

Abbreviations: ED: emergency department; ER: emergency room; GP: general practitioner; RCT: randomized controlled trial.

Country abbreviations: AU: Australia; CA: Canada: DK: Denmark; NL: the Netherlands; NO: Norway; NZ: New Zealand; UK: the United Kingdom; USA: the United States of America.

Notes: * Evidence for different intervention components on patient/family/caregiver outcomes: improvement for patient or family-related outcomes with family/patient involvement (6/9); additional patient assessment was significantly improved in nine out of twelve studies; coordination showed significant improvements in six out of nine studies on either quality of life or satisfaction; improvements for palliative-care specialist involvement in three out of five studies.

Sources: [1] Carmont et al. (2018); [2] Joseph et al. (2016); [3] Shepperd et al. (2016); [4] Dy et al. (2013); [5] Latter et al. (2016); [6] Hudson, Remedios & Thomas (2010).

education or training sessions, typically supported by written and other resources, opportunities for questions and discussion, and follow-up contacts for reinforcement or further coaching. Professions covered in those interventions were nurses, psychologists and researchers.

Hudson, Remedios & Thomas (2010) assessed the effectiveness of psychosocially and/or psycho-educationally based interventions for family caregivers including psychoeducation, psychosocial support, caregivers' coping, symptom management, sleep promotion and family meetings. Professions involved in the interventions were not reported.

Examples of skill-mix innovations and new technologies/eHealth were not identified in the systematic reviews.

Evidence on outcomes

Interventions designed to engage GPs in integrated palliative care (Carmont et al., 2018) were shown to significantly improve patient functional status ($n = 2$), but to have no effects on patients' quality of life or symptom burden ($n = 2$). Results from qualitative studies included in the same review suggest improved pain management, symptom control as well as increased safety for patients and family from both GP ($n = 1$) and patient perspective ($n = 2$). In terms of health-system-related outcomes, the studies showed a significant decrease in the number of hospital admissions. Furthermore, case conferences and shared care were both effective in reducing the length of hospital stay. Outcomes related to professions were shown to be improved in terms of strengthened service relationships, a better interprofessional communication and professional development ($n = 2$).

In their Cochrane Review, Shepperd et al. (2016) showed that palliative patients receiving home-based end-of-life care were more likely to die at home than patients receiving usual care ($n = 3$ RCTs). In two RCTs, patient satisfaction was also shown to be slightly improved at follow up after 1 month. However, there was no difference after 6 months. Little effect on functional status (measured by the Barthel Index), psychological well-being or cognitive status ($n = 1$ RCT) was shown. The effects on 6-month mortality were unclear ($n = 1$ RCT). In terms of outcomes related to the health care system a significant reduction in health care cost between 18% and 30% in the USA was reported in two RCTs. But results on admission to hospital were mixed ($n = 4$ RCTs). Effects on informal caregiver outcomes are uncertain: Differences in caregivers' satisfaction were only reported at 1-month follow up, but not at 6-months. Furthermore, caregivers of participants who had survived more than 30 days showed a decrease in psychological well-being (n = 1 RCT). In terms of caregiver bereavement response little or no effect was shown 6 months following death (n = 1 RCT).

Interventions that focus on continuity, coordination and transition were shown to significantly improve satisfaction in six studies included in the systematic review from Dy et al. (2013). Only one study showed no effects. Effects on quality of life were more unclear with three studies showing positive effects and six studies showing no differences. The caregivers' quality of life was reported to be significantly improved (n = 1) while no effects on their burden were shown in three studies. In terms of caregiver satisfaction, the results were mixed. A significant positive effect on caregiver satisfaction was shown in four studies and no difference was reported in two studies. Evidence on effects of single intervention components revealed improvements for patient- or family-related outcomes with family/patient involvement in six of nine studies. Using additional patient assessment was found to be significantly improved in nine out of twelve studies. Furthermore, providing coordination showed significant improvements in six out of nine studies on either quality of life or satisfaction. Improvements for palliative-care specialist involvement were shown in three out of five studies. In terms of outcomes related to the health care system, most studies showed no effects of single components. Only 5 out of 16 studies evaluating health care utilization, for example in terms of hospital admission and length of stay, found significant effects.

Providing psychosocially and/or psycho-educationally based interventions for family caregivers resulted in positive effects on caregivers' depression (n = 2), on sleep quality (n = 1), as well as on their preparedness, competence and reward ratings (n = 1). Furthermore, a significantly increased level of comfort, closure and satisfaction was reported (n = 1). Another study showed significantly higher ratings of caregivers' self-efficacy for helping patients to control pain and other symptoms (n = 1). It was also reported that implementing such interventions resulted in a reduction of unmet needs (n = 2). In general, caregivers' perception of the intervention was shown to be positive (n = 3). A psycho-educational programme was shown to have significant favourable effects on caregivers' perceptions of positive elements of their role (n = 1) and on family caregivers' quality of life (n = 1). Effects on perceived burden of patients' symptoms and their perceived burden of care tasks were inconclusive with one study showing significant positive effects and one study showing no significant benefit to caregivers while receiving a separate psychosocial support intervention. Effects on psychological benefits for caregivers are also unclear with one study showing positive effects and another study showing no significant benefit to caregivers' psychosocial health or well-being. Hudson, Remedios & Thomas (2010) did not assess outcomes related to the patient or the health system.

In another review that aimed to analyse the effects of interventions focused on caregivers, providing pain medication management interventions to family caregivers of patients with advanced cancer (Latter et al., 2016) was shown to significantly improve medication adherence in one RCT. Mixed effects were found on pain and on caregivers' knowledge and beliefs about pain, although one study included in the review reported significant improvements in self-efficacy and perceived control over pain. Analyses are missing on health-system-related outcomes and outcomes related to professionals.

Education and training of the professions involved in the skill-mix changes

Most systematic reviews did not report details on the education and training of the professions covered in the studies. Only three studies on long-term care described the training in the skill-mix intervention groups, but not always in a systematic manner and they lacked details on the content, length and curricula. These studies reported that case managers received a specific advanced training (Backhouse et al., 2017; Khanassov & Vedel, 2016; Reilly et al., 2015). For example, Khanassov & Vedel (2016) described training of case managers in geriatrics/ geronto-psychiatry, communication with patients and their caregivers and dementia home care. Another review reported that case managers with advanced training in six RCTs received training ranging from a 1-week intensive course to advanced practice education (3½ years) and additional special education in dementia care with a duration of 1 year (Reilly et al., 2015).

Limitations and strength of evidence

A strength of this chapter is the comprehensive definition of skill-mix including not only all health professions but also explicitly including informal caregivers for people requiring long-term care and/or palliative care. However, several limitations exist. First, the number of reviews identified was low, particularly for palliative care. Second, the systematic reviews on long-term care presented an uneven coverage of conditions. Several systematic reviews exist for people with Alzheimer's disease. For people with other conditions, such as Parkinson's disease, the number of reviews was very low or non-existent, for example, for other functional impairments or mental health. Three Cochrane reviews were included of which two focused on palliative care. However, one of them did not identify studies that met the inclusion criteria. In sum, five meta-analyses were performed. The transferability of the findings across countries is limited as most studies were from the USA and there were only a small number of studies from Europe. Evidence on profession-related effects was limited across all reviews. The generally low quality of the evidence and heterogeneity of the interventions require cautious interpretation of the findings.

Summary of the evidence

The evidence suggests that case management for people with long-term care needs may result in some, albeit generally few, improvements for patients and their caregivers. For people with dementia, introducing case manager roles may be associated with reduced feelings of isolation and embarrassment of the condition, and may improve coping with memory problems. Furthermore, evidence provides indications that patients' access to services and their compliance with guideline recommendations is improved. On other outcomes, such as functional status, depression or mortality, the evidence was either inconclusive or showed no effect. The reason may be that improvements for this target group are more difficult to achieve and to measure than for other conditions, an issue that should be investigated in future research.

For case management provided to older people living at home and their caregivers, results were different; for example, regarding informal caregivers and also in terms of health-system-related outcomes, where the evidence suggests that municipal costs may decrease after implementing case management interventions. Interestingly, and similar to dementia-specific case management interventions, a decrease in unmet service need was found.

For patients with Parkinson's disease, introducing multidisciplinary teams may improve quality of life and other outcomes. Generally, the evidence was limited in terms of quantity and quality of effects.

On palliative care, the number of reviews covering people in their homes was low, but evidence suggests that home-based end-of-life care interventions may result in an increased likelihood of dying at home. Moreover, the majority of studies that analysed effects on patient satisfaction showed a positive impact. They also found improved caregiver satisfaction and a lower caregiver burden after introducing various skill-mix changes as well as a decrease in unmet needs. For patients' quality of life and pain management the results were inconclusive. There is also some evidence of enhanced efficiency gains for health systems (for example, decrease in hospital admissions, reduced length of stay) and improved profession-specific outcomes (such as strengthened communication and service relationships) with increased collaboration across disciplines in palliative care.

Given the rapid increase in the number of people requiring long-term and palliative care over the past decade in Europe, and future projections, there is an urgent need for more and high-quality research on skill-mix requirements to provide quality care for patients in their homes, also including new technologies/eHealth.

7.3   Skill-mix innovations and reforms: overview of trends across Europe

Long-term care

Skill-mix changes and reforms
Most debates on the workforce in long-term care at home have focused on increasing the quantity of staff, with little attention paid to their skill-mix. Nevertheless, two major trends can be noted. First, current and expected future workforce shortages generate a need to attract more health professionals in long-term care (De Klaver et al., 2013). To attract more health professionals, such as nurses or lay workers in long-term care, job opportunities are created for long-term unemployed, migrant populations or adults with disabilities (De Klaver et al., 2013). At the same time, especially as better-qualified staff are a scarce resource, specific tasks from better-qualified staff are re-allocated towards less-qualified staff. Second, due to the complexity in care and in delivery of coherent, high-quality care, a few European countries, for example, Austria, Bulgaria and Serbia, implemented new roles for better-qualified staff (specialized in the care of older adults) or introduced new

(multidisciplinary) teams or a new modality of teamwork to improve long-term care.

Examples specific to long-term care of creating job opportunities for unemployed or migrant populations are the introduction of geriatric home care assistants (Geronto service) in Serbia (Milicevic, forthcoming) (see Box 7.2), the 24-hour care workers in Austria (Habimana et al., forthcoming), or the assistants for disabled people in Bulgaria (De Klaver et al., 2013). Examples of task allocation are physicians that are partially substituted by registered nurses or registered nurses that are partially substituted by less-qualified assistants. In the Netherlands, nurse practitioners, physician assistants and registered nurses are legally allowed to partially substitute GPs or nursing home physicians. However, because of a shortage of nurses, this does not happen on a regular basis (Lovink et al., 2018). In Belgium, health care assistants were introduced, providing basic care under nurse supervision (Sermeus, forthcoming). In Austria, Belgium and Denmark, informal caregivers (often family members) receive (psychological) support (Burau, Doessing & Kuhlmann, forthcoming; Habimana et al., forthcoming; Sermeus, forthcoming). Supporting and investing in informal caregivers might be a solution to compensate for shortages in formal caregivers, as informal caregivers can take over parts of the tasks of formal caregivers.

Box 7.2 *Home care assistants – Geronto service in Serbia (Milicevic forthcoming)*

Over the past two decades a home care community-based care service for older people has been implemented in Serbia. The so-called Geronto service was introduced in 2007 as a 6-month project within the Poverty Reduction Strategy of the Serbian government with the aim of improving the economic and social position of socially vulnerable people such as older people and those with chronic illness and disabilities, by providing them with housekeeping and household maintenance services, personal hygiene services, preventive health care services, and psychosocial support services.

Contextual drivers
Serbia has one of the largest older population segments in the world (Sevo et al., 2009), so has a rising need for medical and social care and a reduced offer of informal care by family members. In order to implement

Box 7.2 (cont.)

a Geronto service, an accredited training programme for home care assistants was developed, including communication with older people, assistance with personal hygiene, nutrition, food procurement and taking medication (EU Delegation to the Republic of Serbia, 2017). The training enables people to work both in Serbia and abroad as qualified day-care assistants and also to carry out independent tasks in the field of nursing older and ill people living at home. In 2012 the Geronto services were provided in 85% of local governments.

Barriers to change and uptake in practice
Despite the development over the past two decades, the Geronto services are still insufficiently available. The number of beneficiaries covered only 1.2% of the population over 65 years of age, mostly females from urban areas (Center for Liberal-Democratic Studies and the Social Inclusion and Poverty Reduction Unit, 2013). The service was provided on a smaller scale or on a discontinuous basis in 122 out of 145 local governments, among which prevailed small and underdeveloped municipalities, while 15 local governments did not allocate any funds in their 2015 budgets for home care assistance (Matković & Stranjaković 2016).

To improve quality and coherence of long-term care, some countries introduced new roles for professionals specialized in the care of older adults or new (multidisciplinary) teams. In Norway, the role of advanced geriatric nurses, that is nurse practitioners specialized in the care of older adults, has been implemented (Henni et al., 2018). In the Netherlands, a new type of baccalaureate-educated registered nurses, specialized in gerontology and geriatrics, work in long-term care services (Huizenga, Finnema & Roodbol, 2016). To deliver coherent care at district level, the Visible Link programme (2009–2012) promoted the employment of district nurses (DeKlaver et al., 2013; Grijpsta et al., 2013) (Box 7.3). The new role of these district nurses was formalized in 2014 (Batenburg & Kroezen, forthcoming). In addition, there was a shift towards self-managing home care teams (Batenburg & Kroezen, forthcoming). Since 2016, a number of Dutch municipalities have introduced social district teams, aimed at connecting supply and demand of care in neighbourhoods, focusing on the residents' own capabilities (Batenburg & Kroezen, forthcoming). In Belgium, home-based occupational therapy was implemented to adapt the homes of patients to their conditions and to improve working conditions of home care professionals (Sermeus, forthcoming). In addition, nurses or social care workers received a case management role to allow older people to stay in their own home for as long as possible (Sermeus, forthcoming).

Box 7.3 The district nurse (the Netherlands)

With the aim to provide coherent care at district level, the role of district nurses in Dutch home care had a revival in 2009 (Grijpstra et al., 2013). District nurses were employed in Dutch home care in the 1960s, but their role disappeared later, when policy and economic development led to a reassignment of tasks to other home care workers (Cramm & Nieboer, 2017; den Boer, Nieboer & Cramm, 2017). The so-called new district nurse role is broader than the traditional role and is aimed at the integration of health care, housing, employment and integration (Grijpstra et al., 2013). The district nurse has achieved the lead role in care provision for frail people that live in the community (den Boer, Nieboer & Cramm, 2017).

Contextual drivers
The ageing of the population and the policy trend to enable vulnerable (older) people to stay in their own home for as long as possible, brought the Dutch government to organize support within people's informal networks (den Boer, Nieboer & Cramm, 2017; Grijpstra et al., 2013). Within the political climate in favour of community-based care, the district nurse is seen as a spearhead (Grijpstra et al., 2013). Between 2009 and 2012, the implementation of the new district nurse role took place at national level with the Visible Link initiative. This initiative was aimed at employing 250 extra district nurses (Grijpstra et al., 2013). In 2015, an ambassador programme for district nurses was launched, aimed at increasing the number of new district nurses that are capable of representing and lobbying for their profession at local, regional and national level (V & VN, 2018). Since 2015, district nurses are responsible for people's care needs assessments, which were formerly conducted by the Care Needs Assessment Centre, further strengthening their role (den Boer, Nieboer & Cramm, 2017).

Barriers to change and uptake in practice
The biggest barrier to change and uptake in practice is the shortage of district nurses. Attracting nurses to home care is a common problem in many countries (Drennan et al., 2018). Staff scarcity in Dutch home

---

Box 7.3 (cont.)

care leads to high work pressure, which might have a negative influence on quality of care and quality of work (Stuurgroep Kwaliteitskader Wijkverpleging, 2018). In recent years, the image of working in home care has suffered, as it has been associated with high work pressure, high administrative burden and a weak role of nurses. This image makes it difficult to attract sufficient district nurses (Zorginstituut Nederland, 2018).

Implementation of reforms

Across Europe older or disabled adults want to stay in their own home for as long as possible and the political climate is favourable to long-term care at home; this has brought several countries to implement skill-mix innovations in home care (De Klaver et al., 2013). There are differences in implementation between different roles, as some roles are more frequently implemented than others. In addition, the implementation of roles may differ across different regions within the same country. The introduction of new professional roles is usually supported by national governments. Incentives and facilitators to implement the skill-mix innovation may be (temporary) funding and legal changes. On the other hand, few large-scale reforms exist. Also, as most skill-mix innovations were implemented only recently, there is little evidence for the success of these innovations, though the formalization of the district nurse role in the Netherlands has shown positive results.

Palliative care

Skill-mix changes and reforms

Palliative home care is often delivered by the regular primary health care providers, such as family physicians and community nurses. Palliative care specialists are increasingly available in case of complex needs, yet some countries are still reporting a shortage of specialists in the field to ensure all people in need of palliative care receive it when needed. Overall, most skill-mix innovations identified have involved nurses more than health care professionals from other backgrounds. Task shifting has been introduced as a way to enhance teamwork and access to palliative care. The most frequent task shift identified was between doctors and nurses (Knaul et al., 2018). Often, new tasks were added to the job descriptions of professionals. Examples were coordination of services, case management and liaison functions between the patient, family and health care professionals (Sekse, Hunskar & Ellingsen, 2018; Thomas et al. 2014; van der Plas et al. 2016). Box 7.4 presents an example of the role of case managers in palliative care in the Netherlands, who are nurses with a specialization in palliative care. Other examples of nurses working in expanded roles in palliative care are nurses from specialized palliative home care teams in Belgium, whose task has been to advise and support other health care providers (for example, family physicians and community nurses) in caring for palliative patients. While performing specialist palliative care tasks in close collaboration with family physicians these nurses enhance the quality of care delivery and at the same time have a bed-side teaching role (Gomes et al., 2013; Seow et al., 2014). Workplace learning occurs through close collaboration with other professionals and as such can help professionals evolve and enhance quality of care delivery (Mertens et al., 2018; Pype et al., 2014, 2015).

Other examples of skill-mix innovations identified in palliative care were trainings for lay caregivers to get involved in the palliative care team by nurses, psychologists and social workers (Farquhar et al., 2016). Receiving training and support from the health care team has been shown to help family members and other informal caregivers to better manage the stress and burden in such complex situations.

Box 7.4 The case of case managers in primary palliative care in the Netherlands

Over the past decade, case managers have been introduced into palliative care in the Netherlands. These are nurses with expertise in palliative care who offer support to patients and their informal caregivers, collaborate with multiple health care providers, and provide continuity between professionals and organizations. A nationwide study investigated the implementation and outcomes of case management showed that compared with usual care, the GP is more likely to know the preferred place of death, the place of death is more likely to be at home, and there are fewer hospitalizations in the last 30 days of life (van der Plas et al., 2015a).

Contextual drivers
This model of case management relies on the principle that basic palliative care is provided by generalists and that specialist care is reserved for complex situations. Most patients are referred early to the

---

Box 7.4 (cont.)

palliative care trajectory and 62% of referrals are done by hospital staff. The majority (69%) of patients received a combination of curative or life-prolonging treatment and palliative care (van der Plas et al., 2013).

The organizational affiliation of the case managers in the Netherlands varies; case managers can be employed by a home care organization, by a hospice or by a collaborative venture between institutions (for example, a home care organization working together with a hospital). The organizational characteristics have been shown to add more to variability in the number and content of contacts than patient characteristics (van der Plas et al., 2015b).

Barriers to change and uptake in practice

Most patients referred are cancer patients, so broadening the scope to reach other patient groups is important (van der Plas et al., 2015c). The type and number of support actions offered is prompted by characteristics of the organization in which they work and not exclusively by the patients' needs, which could be considered as contradictory to patient-centred care (van der Plas et al., 2015b). Acceptance of and cooperation with providers is pivotal to the success of the intervention. In this context, a survey of general practitioners and community nurses showed that case managers should put more emphasis on building relationships with these providers (van der Plas et al., 2016).

The most frequent innovation however was the introduction of team collaboration through introducing specialized palliative home care teams into the primary care field, along with the regular health care providers. This was the case in 39 out of 46 European countries responding to a European Association for Palliative Care survey (Centeno Cea, 2013), for instance in Germany (Box 7.5). These palliative home care teams consist of specialized nurses, physicians specialized in palliative care, psychologists and administrative support. The palliative-care nurses perform home visits, whereas the other team members mostly have a supportive and supervisory role. In specific patient situations with complex problems, a patient–health care professional contact can be made with the physician or the psychologist. These teams often have a role to support and advise the regular health care providers, although in other countries they actually deliver care in collaboration with the existing health care providers. Another example of introducing collaboration

Box 7.5 Specialized ambulatory palliative care in Germany (SAPV)

Introduced in 2007, the SAPV aimed to improve palliative care in Germany and to give everyone the opportunity to stay at home for as long as possible in the last phase of life. Specifically, qualified teams are composed of specialized nurses, physicians specialized in palliative care, and psychosocial professions and work closely with the volunteer hospice aid. SAPV-Teams are targeting people with a time-limiting, non-curable and progressive diagnosis and complex symptoms, when the intensity or complexity of the conditions necessitates the use of a specialized palliative care team instead of, or in addition to, a general palliative care (AAPV) provided by GPs and other non-specialized providers. The services and skills offered by the teams include a broad range of interventions, from case management, coordination of care, comprehensive pain and symptoms management, psychosocial support, and is available with comprehensive 24/7 services (Kassenärztliche Bundesvereinigung (KBV), 2018). Although there is a clear structural, regulatory and financial division between institutional and ambulatory palliative care, services are provided at home and in home-like settings, such as nursing homes and hospices (Busse, Blümel & Spranger, 2017).

Contextual drivers
Before the introduction of SAPV, palliative care in the home, especially pain-management, was hardly realizable and left patients and informal caregivers more or less alone. Their demand for better support, together with a strong palliative movement that evolved in the past decades were some of the drivers (Enquete-Kommission, 2002; Jaspers & Schindler, 2005) of the introduction of SAPV.

Barriers to change and uptake in practice
SAPV teams are not yet implemented in every region of the country. Contrary to the European Association of Palliative Care's recommendation of 10 teams per million population (Radbruch et al., 2011a, 2011b), implementation rates in Germany range from 0.57 to 6.6 SAPV-Teams per million population (Melching, 2015). In order to counter those regional variations in implementation, quality and practice of SAPV, a national framework agreement has been concluded in 2019 (Deutscher Hospiz- und PalliativVerband e. V. (DHPV), 2018).

Other barriers for uptake of early integration of palliative care in practice is limited access due to tight criteria, for example a life expectancy <6 months (Kassenärztliche Bundesvereinigung (KBV), 2018), bureaucratic issues and workforce shortages (Richter-Kuhlmann, 2017).

was through initiating a network of volunteers (Woitha et al., 2015). These volunteers receive a basic training and their main task is to support the family caregivers.

Finally changing teamwork in existing multidisciplinary teams occurred through adding a palliative care leader, general practitioner and nurse, to a primary health care team (Llobera et al., 2017).

Implementation of reforms

Most innovations have been implemented at local level (in case of research projects or individual programmes, for instance case-manager projects) or at a national level (Arias et al., 2019). Yet, many countries are still reporting a gap in the supply of palliative care to provide timely care for those in need.

Some innovations have been spontaneous practice-based innovations driven by a strong sense of purpose for better patient care, for example, nurses taking up a coordinating role when observing a need. The recognition to improve the quality of patient care has been the main driver in these cases, in addition to the felt need to improve job satisfaction. Other innovations, such as the installation of specialized palliative home care teams or a network of volunteers, were supported by local or national governments. In the case of palliative home care teams, funding and official requirements towards professional qualifications were sometimes initiated and regulated by the government, which can be a policy lever to step up supply and standardize skills requirements.

The WHO recently initiated a pan-European programme that aims to strengthen palliative care competencies of and collaboration between involved health care professionals involved in palliative care (Box 7.6).

7.4   Conclusions

Long-term and palliative care services are expected to see a steep demand in the future. The current and expected future workforce shortages in both areas are likely to generate a need to attract more health professionals with a good mix of skills and educational levels.

For long-term care, a trend observed in many countries across Europe is the strengthening of informal caregivers and various skill-mix changes. Some countries have lowered the skill-sets of their health professionals towards a higher mix of lower qualified professions, such

---

Box 7.6 WHO collaboration for strengthening of palliative care education of all health care professionals (2016–2020)

The WHO is strongly committed to palliative care as a component of integrated treatment as it improves the quality of life of patients and their families who are facing problems associated with life-threatening illness, whether physical, psychosocial or spiritual (World Health Organization, 2014).

According to a WHO fact sheet (World Health Organization, 2018b), the lack of awareness among policy-makers, health professionals and the public about what palliative care is and the benefits it can offer patients and health systems, beliefs about death and dying, misconceptions about palliative care of being only for the last weeks of life, or misconceptions that improving access to opioid analgesia will lead to increased substance abuse, directly impact the access to palliative care services (WHO Collaboration Centre Paracelsus Medical University, 2018).

To remove this barrier and to ensure that palliative care needs are met together with training of volunteers and education of the public, education and training of health care professionals is of major importance. Therefore, the WHO European Region in collaboration with the newly proposed EAPC Reference Group on Palliative Care Education and Paracelsus Medical Private University (PMU) in Salzburg – a WHO Collaborating Centre – are working towards innovative solutions to cultivate and support interdisciplinary and intersectional collaboration across different health care sectors. The collaboration started in 2016 and aims to develop a matrix for a pan-European curriculum to assist in the promotion and embedding of palliative care into health care professional curricula at undergraduate and graduate level (WHO Collaboration Centre Paracelsus Medical University, 2018).

The goal is to break down the myths about palliative care and support health care professionals' collaborations across all fields of responsibility, for example, through provision of an online learning environment for strengthening palliative care education of all health care professionals by 2020 (WHO Collaboration Centre Paracelsus Medical University, 2018).

---

as health care assistants, or lay workers. Other countries have enhanced the skill-mix to improve the quality of care by introducing specialized professionals, such as the district nurse in the Netherlands (Box 7.3), or case management and multidisciplinary teamwork. The outcomes seem promising, at least for some outcome parameters, but are based on limited evidence.

Across Europe, in long-term care, several countries have changed the skill-mix towards lower-qualified professionals, with a focus on training informal caregivers. In other countries, job opportunities for unemployed or migrant populations were created, but with limited information on outcomes. On a small scale, tasks are allocated from better-qualified towards less-qualified staff. Until now, there was little evidence on the success of these innovations. However, for most countries in Europe, family members acting as informal caregivers should receive more support, both in their skills, competencies and coping strategies, including from professional teams, if they want to take up the caregiver role.

In terms of improving the quality and accessibility of long-term care at home, one promising large-scale reform is the formalization of the district nurse role in Dutch home care (see Box 7.3).

In long-term care, with the exception of case management interventions, especially for people suffering from dementia and their caregivers, there is in general little scientific evidence on the outcomes. In dementia care, case managers have shown promise in selected outcome parameters, for example, case manager roles may reduce feelings of isolation and embarrassment of the condition. It was also shown to improve coping with memory problems, to improve patient access to services and professionals' compliance with guideline recommendations. Yet, in long-term care for patients with conditions other than dementia, scientific research that examines the effects of different skill-mix models on specific outcome measures, health professionals and caregivers' roles is needed.

The same applies for palliative care, where evidence on effects of skill-mix changes is scarce. With the increased public attention on patient needs at the end of life, policy-makers across Europe are increasingly seeking strategies to improve the quality of care and ensure palliative services for all in need. Several countries have introduced palliative care skill-mix changes to teams, but in most cases they remain small in numbers and without ensuring everyone has timely access.

The most frequent skill-mix intervention in European countries is the introduction of palliative home care teams that bring specialized knowledge and skills to the patient's home and ease pain and suffering, often at the end of life. The evidence suggests that there are several benefits to patients and their caregivers and family from skill-mix changes that offer more specialized palliative care. Moreover, the professions involved in providing palliative care may also benefit, and there is some, but limited, evidence on reduced hospitalizations. To optimize the collaboration with each other and with the palliative home care teams, education and training of health care professionals should entail interprofessional collaborative competencies from the undergraduate level throughout the lifelong learning trajectory.

References

Arias-Casais N, Garralda E, Rhee JY et al. (2019). EAPC Atlas of Palliative Care in Europe 2019. Vilvoorde, EAPC Press.

Backhouse A, Ukoumunne OC, Richards DA et al. (2017). The effectiveness of community-based coordinating interventions in dementia care: a meta-analysis and subgroup analysis of intervention components. BMC Health Serv Res, 17(1):S717. DOI: 10.1186/s12913-017-2677-2.

Batenburg R, Kroezen M (forthcoming). Mobilising professionals, volunteers and patients in the Netherlands: shifting paradigms, tasks and skills. In: Wismar M, Glinos I, Sagan A eds. Skill-mix innovation in primary and chronic care. Mobilizing patients, peers, professionals. European Observatory on Health Systems and Policies. Volume 1. Copenhagen, WHO Regional Office for Europe on behalf of the European Observatory on Health Systems and Policies.

Berthelsen CB, Kristensson J (2015). The content, dissemination and effects of case management interventions for informal caregivers of older adults: a systematic review. Int J Nurs Stud, 52(5):988–1002. DOI: 10.1016/j.ijnurstu.2015.01.006.

Burau V, Doessing A, Kuhlmann E (forthcoming). New tasks and new demands on nurses and GPs in Denmark: a decentralised patchwork approach to innovation. In: Wismar M, Glinos I, Sagan A eds. Skill-mix innovation in primary and chronic care. Mobilizing patients, peers, professionals. European Observatory on Health Systems and Policies. Volume 1. Copenhagen, WHO Regional Office for Europe on behalf of the European Observatory on Health Systems and Policies.

Busse R, Blümel M, Spranger A (2017). Das deutsche Gesundheitssystem. Akteure, Daten, Analysen. 2. Aufl. Berlin, MWV.

Carmont S-A, Mitchell G, Senior H et al. (2018). Systematic review of the effectiveness, barriers and facilitators to general practitioner engagement with specialist secondary services in integrated palliative care. BMJ Support Pall Care, 8:385–399.

Centeno Cea IM (2013). EAPC Atlas of Palliative Care in Europe 2013 – Full Edition. Milan, European Association for Palliative Care.

Centre for Liberal-Democratic Studies and the Social Inclusion and Poverty Reduction Unit (2013). Mapping social care services within the mandate of local governments. Belgrade, Centre for Liberal-Democratic Studies and the Social Inclusion and Poverty Reduction Unit.

Colombo F, Llena-Nozal A, Mercier J et al. (2011). Help wanted? Providing and paying for long-term care. Paris, OECD Publishing (OECD Health Policy Studies).

Cramm JM, Nieboer AP (2017). Self-management abilities and quality of life among frail community-dwelling peoples; the role of community nurses in the Netherlands. Health Soc Care Commun, 25(2):394–401.

De Klaver P, van der Graaf A, Grijpstra D et al. (2013). More and better jobs in home-care services. Dublin, European Foundation for the Improvement of Living and Working Conditions (Eurofound).

den Boer J, Nieboer AP, Cramm JM (2017). A cross-sectional study investigating patient-centred care, co-creation of care, well-being and job satisfaction among nurses. J Nurs Manage, 25(7):577–584.

Deutscher Hospiz- und PalliativVerband e. V. (DHPV) (2018). Aktueller Stand zum Gesetzgebungsverfahren betreffend die Neuregelung der SAPV-Versorgung. (https://www.dhpv.de/aktuelles_detail/items/aktueller-stand-zum-gesetzgebungsverfahren-betreffend-die-neuregelung-der-sapv-versorgung.html, accessed 22 July 2020).

Drennan VM, Calestani M, Ross F et al. (2018). Tackling the workforce crisis in district nursing: can the Dutch Buurtzorg model offer a solution and a better patient experience? A mixed methods case study. BMJ Open, 8(6):e021931. DOI: 10.1136/bmjopen-2018-021931.

Dy SM, Apostol C, Martinez KA et al. (2013). Continuity, coordination, and transitions of care for patients with serious and advanced illness: a systematic review of interventions. J Palliat Med, 16(4):436–445. DOI: 10.1089/jpm.2012.0317.

Enquete-Kommission (2002). Schlussbericht: „Recht und Ethik der modernen Medizin". Deutscher Bundestag. Berlin (Drucksache 14/9020). (http://dip21.bundestag.de/dip21/btd/14/090/1409020.pdf, accessed 1 November 2018).

EU Delegation to the Republic of Serbia (2017). Project activities, success stories: Cuprija – provision of palliative care to terminally ill patients. Belgrade, EU Delegation to the Republic of Serbia.

European Commission (2007). Health and long-term care in the European Union (Eurobarometer, 283/Wave 67.3 - TNS Opinion & Social). (http://ec.europa.eu/commfrontoffice/publicopinion/archives/ebs/ebs_283_en.pdf, accessed 1 November 2018).

Farquhar M, Penfold C, Walter FM et al. (2016). What are the key elements of educational interventions for lay carers of patients with advanced disease? A systematic literature search and narrative review of structural components, processes and modes of delivery. J Pain Sympt Manage, 52(1):117–30.e27.

Goeman D, Renehan E, Koch S (2016). What is the effectiveness of the support worker role for people with dementia and their carers? A systematic review. BMC Health Serv Res, 16: 285. DOI: 10.1186/s12913-016-1531-2.

Gomes B, Calanzani N, Curiale V et al. (2013). Effectiveness and cost-effectiveness of home palliative care services for adults with advanced illness and their caregivers. Cochrane Database Syst Rev, 6:CD007760.

Grijpstra D, de Klaver P, Snijders J et al. (2013). More and better jobs in home-care services – The Netherlands. Dublin, European Foundation for the Improvement of Living and Working Conditions (Eurofound).

Habimana K, Bobek J, Lepuschütz L et al. (forthcoming). From solo practice to primary care health centres in Austria: innovating skill mix in a fragmented decision-making environment. In: Wismar M, Glinos I, Sagan A eds. Skill-mix innovation in primary and chronic care. Mobilizing patients, peers, professionals. European Observatory on Health Systems and Policies. Volume 1. Copenhagen, WHO Regional Office for Europe on behalf of the European Observatory on Health Systems and Policies.

Henni SH, Kirkevold M, Antypas K et al. (2018). The role of advanced geriatric nurses in Norway: A descriptive exploratory study. Int J Older People Nurs, 13:e12188.

Hudson PL, Remedios C, Thomas K (2010). A systematic review of psychosocial interventions for family carers of palliative care patients. BMC Palliat Care, 9:17.

Huizenga P, Finnema E, Roodbol P (2016). Learnt and perceived professional roles of a new type of nurse specialized in gerontology and geriatrics, a qualitative study. J Advanc Nurs 72(7):1552–1566.

Jaspers B, Schindler T (2005). Stand der Palliativmedizin und Hospizarbeit in Deutschland und im Vergleich zu ausgewählten Staaten. Gutachten im Auftrag der Bundestags-Enquête-Kommission Ethik und Recht der modernen Medizin. Berlin, Deutscher Bundestag.

Joseph R, Brown-Manhertz D, Ikwuazom S et al. (2016). The effectiveness of structured interdisciplinary collaboration for adult home hospice patients on patient satisfaction and hospital admissions and re-admissions: a systematic review. JBI Database Syst Rev Implement Rep 14(1):108–139. DOI: 10.11124/jbisrir-2016-2254.

Kassenärztliche Bundesvereinigung (KBV) (2018). Spezialisierte ambulante Palliativversorgung. (http://www.kbv.de/html/palliativversorgung.php, accessed 2 November 2018).

Khanassov V, Vedel I (2016). Family physician-case manager collaboration and needs of patients with dementia and their caregivers: a systematic mixed studies review. Ann Family Med, 14(2):166–177. DOI: 10.1370/afm.1898.

Khanassov V, Vedel I, Pluye P (2014). Barriers to implementation of case management for patients with dementia: a systematic mixed studies review. Ann Family Med, 12(5):456–465. DOI: 10.1370/afm.1677.

Knaul FM, Farmer PE, Krakauer EL et al. (2018). Alleviating the access abyss in palliative care and pain relief – an imperative of universal health coverage. Lancet, 391:1391–1454.

Latter S, Hopkinson JB, Richardson A et al. (2016). How can we help family carers manage pain medicines for patients with advanced cancer? A systematic review of intervention studies. BMJ Support Palliat Care, 6(3):263–275. DOI: 10.1136/bmjspcare-2015-000958.

Llobera J, Sanso N, Ruiz A et al. (2017). Strengthening primary health care teams with palliative care leaders: protocol for a cluster randomized clinical trial. BMC Palliat Care, 17(1):4.

Lovink M, Van Vught A, van den Brink G et al. (2018). Taakherschikking in de ouderenzorg: kansen, belemmeringen en effecten. Radboudumc, IQ healthcare & Eerstelijnsgeneeskunde. (http://www.iqhealthcare.nl/media/124512/20170908_eindrapportage-th-ouderenzorg_definitief.pdf, accessed 1 November 2018).

Matković G, Stranjaković M (2016). Mapping social care services within the mandate of local governments in the Republic of Serbia. Belgrade, Social Inclusion and Poverty Reduction Unit Government of the Republic of Serbia.

Melching H (2015). Palliativversorgung. Modul 2. Strukturen und regionale Unterschiede in der Hospiz- und Palliativversorgung. Bertelsmann Stiftung/ Deutsche Gesellschaft für Palliativmedizin. Gütersloh. (https://faktencheck-gesundheit.de/fileadmin/files/BSt/Publikationen/GrauePublikationen/Studie_VV__FCG_Versorgungsstrukturen-palliativ.pdf, accessed 1 November 2018).

Mertens F, de Groot E, Meijer L et al. (2018). Workplace learning through collaboration in primary healthcare: A BEME realist review of what works, for whom and in what circumstances. BEME Guide No. 46. Med Teacher, 40(2):117–134.

Milicevic MS (forthcoming). Top-down developments, short- and medium-term projects in Serbia: seizing the momentum for skill mix innovation. In: Wismar M, Glinos I, Sagan A eds. Skill-mix innovation in primary and chronic care. Mobilizing patients, peers, professionals. European Observatory on Health Systems and Policies. Volume 1. Copenhagen, WHO Regional Office for Europe on behalf of the European Observatory on Health Systems and Policies.

OECD/EU (2016). Health at a Glance: Europe 2016. State of Health in the EU Cycle. Paris, OECD Publishing.

Pimouguet C, Lavaud T, Dartigues JF (2010). Dementia case management effectiveness on health care costs and resource utilization: a systematic review of randomized controlled trials. J Nutr Health Aging, 14(8):669–676.

Prizer LP, Browner N (2012). The integrative care of Parkinson's disease: a systematic review. J Parkinson's Dis, 2(2):79–86. DOI: 10.3233/JPD-2012-12075.

Pype P, Mertens F, Deveugele M (2014). 'I beg your pardon?' Nurses' experiences in facilitating doctors' learning process - an interview study. Patient Educ Couns, 86(3):389–394.

Pype P, Mertens F, Wens J et al. (2015). Preparing palliative home care nurses to act as facilitators for physicians' learning: Evaluation of a training programme. Palliat Med, 29(5):458–463.

Radbruch L, Payne S, Bercovitch M et al. (2011a). Standards und Richtlinien für Hospiz- und Palliativversorgung in Europa: Teil 1. Weißbuch zu Empfehlungen der Europäischen Gesellschaft für Palliative Care (EAPC). Z Palliativmed, 12:216–227.

Radbruch L, Payne S, Bercovitch M et al. (2011b). Standards und Richtlinien für Hospiz- und Palliativversorgung in Europa: Teil 2. Weißbuch zu Empfehlungen der Europäischen Gesellschaft für Palliative Care (EAPC). Z Palliativmed, 12:260–270.

Reilly S, Miranda-Castillo C, Malouf R et al. (2015). Case management approaches to home support for people with dementia. Cochrane Database Syst Rev, 1: CD008345. DOI: 10.1002/14651858.CD008345.pub2.

Richter-Kuhlmann E (2017). Spezialisierte ambulante Palliativversorgung. Es geht langsam voran. Deut Ärztebl. 114(8):348–350.

Sekse RJT, Hunskar I, Ellingsen S (2018). The nurse's role in palliative care: a qualitative meta-synthesis. J Clin Nurs, 27(1-2):e21–e38.

Seow H, Brazil K, Sussman J et al. (2014). Impact of community based, specialist palliative care teams on hospitalisations and emergency department visits late in life and hospital deaths: a pooled analysis. BMJ 348:g3496.

Sermeus W (forthcoming). Interdisciplinary teams, new professions and new roles in Belgium: pilot projects in need of scaling up. In: Wismar M, Glinos I, Sagan A eds. Skill-mix innovation in primary and chronic care. Mobilizing patients, peers, professionals. European Observatory on Health Systems and Policies. Volume 1. Copenhagen, WHO Regional Office for Europe on behalf of the European Observatory on Health Systems and Policies.

Sevo G, Despotovic N, Erceg P et al. (2009). Aging in Serbia. Adv Gerontol 22(4):553–557.

Shepperd S, Gonçalves-Bradley DC, Straus SE et al. (2016). Hospital at home: home-based end-of-life care. Cochrane Database Syst Rev, 2:CD009231. DOI: 10.1002/14651858.CD009231.pub2.

Somme D, Trouve H, Dramé M et al. (2012). Analysis of case management programs for patients with dementia: a systematic review. Alzheimer's Dement 8(5):426–436. DOI: 10.1016/j.jalz.2011.06.004.

Stuurgroep Kwaliteitskader Wijkverpleging (2018). Kwaliteitskader Wijkverpleging. (https://www.zorginzicht.nl/bibliotheek/bestuurlijke-afspraken-kwaliteitsinformatie-wijkverpleging/RegisterKwaliteitsstandaardenDocumenten/Kwaiteitskader%20wijkverpleging%20(versie%201).pdf, accessed 9 October 2018).

Tam-Tham H, Cepoiu-Martin M, Ronksley PE et al. (2013). Dementia case management and risk of long-term care placement: a systematic review and meta-analysis. Int J Geriatr Psychiat, 28(9):889–902. DOI: 10.1002/gps.3906.

Thomas RE, Wilson DM, Birch S et al. (2014). Examining end-of-life case management: systematic review. Nurs Res Pract, 2014 (651681).

V & VN (2018). Ambassadeurs Wijk. (https://mgz.venvn.nl/Themas/Ambassadeurs-Wijk, accessed 9 October 2018).

van der Plas AG, Deliens L, van de Watering M et al. (2013). Palliative care case management in primary care settings: a nationwide survey. Int J Nurs Stud, 50(11):1504–1512.

van der Plas AG, Vissers KC, Francke AL et al. (2015a). Involvement of a case manager in palliative care reduces hospitalisations at the end of life in cancer patients; a mortality follow-back study in primary care. PloS One, 10(7):e0133197.

van der Plas AG, Francke AL, Vissers KC et al. (2015b). Case management in primary palliative care is associated more strongly with organisational than with patient characteristics: results from a cross-sectional prospective study. BMC Palliat Care, 14:31.

van der Plas AG, Onwuteaka-Philipsen BD, Francke AL et al. (2015c). Palliative care case managers in primary care: a descriptive study of referrals in relation to treatment aims. J Palliat Med, 18(4):324–331.

van der Plas AG, Onwuteaka-Philipsen BD, Vissers KC et al. (2016). Appraisal of cooperation with a palliative care case manager by general practitioners and community nurses: a cross-sectional questionnaire study. J Adv Nurs, 72(1):147–157.

WHO Collaboration Centre Paracelsus Medical University (PMU) (2018). About us. (http://whocc.pmu.ac.at/, accessed 10 October 2018).

Woitha K, Hasselaar J, van Beek K et al. (2015). Volunteers in palliative care – a comparison of seven European countries: a descriptive study. Pain Pract, 15(6):572–579.

World Health Organization (2014). Strengthening of palliative care as a component of integrated treatment throughout the life course. J Pain Palliat Care Pharmacother, 28(2):130–134.

World Health Organization (2017). Global strategy and action plan on ageing and health. Geneva. (http://www.who.int/ageing/WHO-GSAP-2017.pdf, accessed 1 November 2018).

World Health Organization (2018a). WHO definition of palliative care. (http:// www.who.int/cancer/palliative/definition/en/, accessed 9 October 2018).

World Health Organization (2018b). Palliative care – key facts. (http://www .who.int/news-room/fact-sheets/detail/palliative-care, accessed 9 October 2018).

You EC, Dunt D, Doyle C et al. (2012). Effects of case management in community aged care on client and carer outcomes: a systematic review of randomized trials and comparative observational studies. BMC Health Serv Res, 12(395).

Zorginstituut Nederland (2018). Kwaliteitsinformatie wijkverpleging. Kwaliteitsstandaard opgenomen in het Register. (https://www .zorginzicht.nl/bibliotheek/bestuurlijke-afspraken-kwaliteitsinformatie-wijkverpleging/Paginas/Home.aspx, accessed 10 October 2018).

8 Addressing the particular challenges of patients living in rural and remote areas and for disadvantaged groups: skill-mix innovations to improve access and quality of care

JAN DE MAESENEER, GIADA SCARPETTI,
HANNAH BUDDE, CLAUDIA B. MAIER

8.1 Introduction

The 2018 Declaration of Astana on Primary Health Care strengthens the importance of access to services (World Health Organization, 2018a). In the EU, the Council of Health Ministers had agreed in 2006 that "Equity relates to equal access according to need, regardless of ethnicity, gender, age, social status or ability to pay" (Council of the European Union, 2006). However, according to the data from the European Union Survey of Income and Living Conditions, in many countries up to 19% of the population report unmet needs for health care (EXPH, 2017).

Access can be defined as "the opportunity to reach and obtain appropriate health care services in situations of perceived need for care" (Levesque, Harris & Russel, 2013). There are different dimensions that contribute to access: geographical (distance, accessibility of infrastructure); financial (absence of out-of-pocket payments, especially important to enable access for vulnerable people); administrative (being insured, being registered, access for undocumented people); cultural (ethno-sensitive approaches, availability of translators and cultural mediators) and psychosocial (to what extent the patient experiences services as paying attention to their psychological and social condition). Worldwide, based on data in 174 countries, 56% of populations living in rural areas have shown not to be covered by basic health care, compared with 22% in cities and towns (World Health Organization, 2018b). Tackling gender, cultural, age and geographical issues is paramount to achieving equity of access for rural populations.

This chapter focuses on two population groups: those living in rural and remote areas and population groups that are described as vulnerable in accessing high-quality care, due to their ethnicity, or socioeconomic or other backgrounds. Both groups have in common that they have shown to be disadvantaged in their access to health care services compared with the majority of the population in a country, which may also impact on the quality of care. Definitions of rural and remote areas and vulnerable populations are provided in Box 8.1.

When it comes to strategies in relation to access of services, the Marmot Review (2010) *Fair Society, Healthy Lives* suggests starting from a universal approach, but implementing the principle of so-called proportionate universalism. This means that actions must be universal, but with the scale and intensity that is proportionate to the level of the disadvantage. Selective approaches targeting specific subgroups in society (according to socioeconomic status, ethnicity, disease), are not always sustainable and risk contributing to fragmentation of care and creating inequity by disease (De Maeseneer et al., 2011). The challenge for policy-makers, planners and health professionals alike is to identify the vulnerable population groups at risk of not seeking health care and offer services that are tailored to their specific needs and, to the extent that it is possible, integrated within health care services.

Box 8.1 Definitions: populations living in rural and remote areas and disadvantaged groups

Rural and remote areas populations:
For the purpose of this volume, rural and remote populations are defined as groups of persons who live in a non-urban area, which is scarcely populated and faces a shortage of health professionals. Definition of remote and rural populations varies according to country-specific context (World Health Organization, 2009).

Disadvantaged population groups:
There are various definitions of disadvantaged groups in the literature (Whiteman, 2014). For this volume, we focus on groups of persons that face higher levels of poverty, social exclusion, discrimination and violence than the general population, including, but not limited to, ethnic minorities, migrants, drug users, homeless and other groups, based on and modified from the definition of the European Institute for Gender Equality[1].

---

[1] European Institute for Gender Equality (website) N.D. (https://eige.europa.eu/thesaurus/terms/1083) [accessed 20/05/2019]

In addition to the overview of systematic reviews, we conducted a broad search on country reforms, programmes and experiences, drawing on PubMed and google scholar, to determine peer-reviewed as well as grey literature. In addition, we conducted manual checks of the reference lists of retrieved articles and citation searches. Individual webpages were also searched (OECD, WHO, DG Sante and other EU websites) and other institutions with a focus on rural health or vulnerable groups and health, moreover case studies from the European Observatory on Health Systems and Policies were included. In this chapter, we will explore which skill-mix strategies, used in various countries, have proven successful or seem to be promising for (i) rural populations and (ii) vulnerable population groups.

8.2 Skill-mix in relation to access to services and evidence on outcomes

The overview of reviews identified 13 systematic reviews that, taken together, summarized the results of 418 studies (see Box 8.2).

The population groups targeted by the skill-mix interventions were twofold: skill-mix innovations for rural populations; and skill-mix interventions for vulnerable, often socioeconomically disadvantaged population groups. Only one systematic review looked at rural populations, with a focus on mental health services (Table 8.1). The other 12 reviews focused on different vulnerable population groups, including

---

Box 8.2 Overview of the evidence

- Number of reviews: 13 systematic reviews covering a total of 418 studies were identified, focusing on improving access, quality of care and waiting time for rural or vulnerable population groups
- Country coverage: The majority of studies were conducted in the USA. Other countries were Australia, Austria, Canada, France, Italy, Ireland, New Zealand, Sweden and the United Kingdom, among others.
- Quality of the evidence: Overall, the reviews were based on limited evidence with mixed quality, and several studies showed limitations. One Cochrane systematic review was identified. Several systematic reviews included RCTs and two meta-analyses were conducted.

Table 8.1 *Skill-mix innovations in rural and remote areas*

Skill-mix interventions					Outcomes		
Description of intervention [Source]	Content of interventions and skill-mix changes	Profession(s) in intervention and in comparator group	Population	Countries	Patient-related outcomes	Health-system-related outcomes	Profession-specific outcomes
Task shifting and sharing in mental health care teams [1]	(i) CHWs (e.g. outreach, education, addressing stigma, cultural issues, mental health crisis management), (ii) non-mental health primary care providers collaboration with mental health specialists (e.g. shared consultations, telehealth)	Intervention: (i) CHWs or similar lay workers with some trainings, (ii) primary care providers, e.g. GPs, nurses, medical assistants, pharmacists, social workers; in collaboration with psychiatrists/ psychologists Comparison: n/r	Rural population/ mental health patients including at-risk groups	AU, NZ, UK, USA	Task shifting/sharing involving: CHWs • Improved knowledge about depression and how to seek treatment, decreased stigma • Partnerships with rural communities improved treatment Primary care providers • Improved mental health, treatment adherence and satisfaction	CHWs • Expanded access to (mental) health services and outreach Primary care providers • Improved communication between GP and psychiatrists • Teleconferencing improved delivery of collaborative care	CHWs • Increased knowledge, coping skill and perceived social support Primary care providers • Collaborative care models improved GP satisfaction

Abbreviations: CHW: community health worker; GP: general practitioner; n/r: not reported (for the majority of studies, no comparison groups available).

Country abbreviations: AU: Australia; NZ: New Zealand; UK: the United Kingdom; USA: the United States of America

Source: [1] Hoeft et al. (2018).

> **Box 8.3** *Definition of community health workers*
>
> The meaning of the term and profile of Community Health Workers (CHWs) varies in different countries. WHO defined CHWs as follows: "Community health workers should be members of the communities where they work, should be selected by the communities, should be answerable to the communities for their activities, should be supported by the health system but not necessarily a part of its organization, and have shorter training than professional workers" (World Health Organization, 1989).
>
> As the CHWs come from the community they serve, they act as a link between health and social services and the community, promoting trust and cultural competence. CHWs can be unpaid volunteers, or receive an allowance/salary.

ethnic minorities, socially deprived groups (such as mothers with low socioeconomic status, drug users) or young women at risk for unintended pregnancies.

Skill-mix innovations for rural populations and evidence on outcomes

In rural and remote regions, many countries face a shortage of primary care providers and certain specialties. One systematic review analysed mental health skill-mix models and the effects of task shifting and competency sharing in teams to improve access to mental health services in the USA, the United Kingdom, Australia and New Zealand (Hoeft et al., 2018) (Table 8.1). Interventions comprised task shifting and competency sharing from mental health specialists, first to community health workers (CHWs) and second, to primary care providers (for example, GPs, nurses) who are not mental health specialists. First, task shifting and competency sharing in teams that integrated CHWs or similar lay health workers were aimed at providing outreach, education, health literacy or personal assistance in rural areas. One example of CHWs working with predominantly Hispanic communities in the USA and offering tailored, culturally adapted services with a focus of health literacy was the *promotora* model, which addressed female migrant groups from Latin American origins. The review focusing on CHWs and task re-allocation to other providers, generally showed positive effects on several outcome parameters, namely improved patient access to mental health services, general health and knowledge about mental health. Moreover, CHWs' contributions were also associated with improved treatment outcomes for mental health patients. Most interventions actively reached out to communities or were fully community-based (Hoeft et al., 2018).

The second skill-mix model analysed included task-shifting and competency sharing between mental health specialists and primary care providers. Interventions included home visits, outreach at rural schools or universities, and collaborative care models between primary care providers in local clinics and remote expert teams. Often telepsychiatry and other new technologies were used as a means of communication and form of (co-)treatment (Hoeft et al., 2018). Collaborative care improved communication between GPs and psychiatrists and increased GP satisfaction. Yet, CHWs employed in clinic settings or added to Assertive Community Treatment showed no improved patient-related effects (Hoeft et al., 2018). Generally, the skill-mix models covering CHWs varied considerably across the regions and communities, suggesting that bottom–up, community grown models are effective. Yet, integrating CHWs showed to be effective in countries with very different health systems, such as the USA, but also in Australia, New Zealand and the United Kingdom. However, several studies highlighted the importance of ensuring the sustainability of CHW programmes and retention.

Skill-mix innovations for vulnerable populations

- Skill-mix interventions directed at vulnerable population groups included various models, ranging from patient navigation, CHW interventions, case management, shared care models to pharmacist-led care and were assessed in 12 reviews (Table 8.2).
  Patient navigation involved (former) patients, peers or other lay people with intense user knowledge by experience or professionals who act as navigators through the system (Bush, Kaufman & Shackleford, 2017; Genoff et al., 2016; Glick et al., 2012; Ranaghan et al., 2016, Roland et al., 2017).
- Patient navigation incorporated different components: facilitated communication between providers, outreach activities, cultural and

Table 8.2 *Skill-mix innovations with a focus on vulnerable populations and socially deprived populations*

Skill-mix interventions					Outcomes		
Description of intervention [Sources]	Content of interventions and skill-mix changes	Profession(s) in intervention and in comparator group	Population	Countries	Patient-related outcomes [Sources]	Health-system-related outcomes [Sources]	Profession-specific outcomes [Sources]
Patient navigation [1–5]	Facilitating communication with providers, outreach, assistance with appointments and scheduling, education, follow up, counselling	Intervention: CHWs, patient navigators (or other lay workers) and various professional backgrounds Comparison: Radiologists, physicians, breast surgeons	Cancer patients (incl. ethnic minority, [2–4] uninsured) [2, 3]; medically underserved populations [1], limited English proficient patients [5]	CA, KR, USA	• Improved patient satisfaction, statistically insignificant [2] • Improved adherence [3, 4]	• Mixed results on time to diagnosis: shorter [3], non-significant [2] • Earlier treatment and treatment initiation [3] • Increased screening rates [1, 4, 5] • Improved referral and follow up [1] • Improved completion of diagnostics [1] and completion of screening [4, 5] • Care coordination improved, statistically insignificant [2]	

| Lay health workers for child and maternity care and management of infectious diseases [6] | Various lay health worker interventions included home visits, reminders, education, referral and the facilitation of meetings | Intervention: Lay health worker (paid or voluntary) including CHW, birth attendants, peer counsellors, home visitors
Comparison: Not reported | Mothers and their children under the age of five with low socioeconomic status | AU, CA, NZ, UK, USA, IE, BR, CN, IN, MX, PH, TH, ZA, TR, BD, BF, ET, GH, IQ, JM, NP, PK, TZ, VN | • Positive effect on pulmonary TB cure rates (RR 1.22, 95% CI 1.13–1.31, $P < 0.0001$)
• May reduce child morbidity (RR 0.86, 95% CI 0.75–0.99, $P = 0.03$) and child mortality (RR 0.75, 95% CI 0.55–1.03, $P = 0.07$) and neonatal mortality (RR 0.76, 95% CI 0.57–1.02, $P = 0.07$) | • Effectiveness in promoting immunization childhood uptake (RR 1.22, 95% CI 1.10–1.37, $P = 0.0004$) and promoting initiation of breastfeeding (RR 1.36, 95% CI 1.14–1.61, $P < 0.00001$)
• Increase the likelihood of seeking care for childhood illness (RR 1.33, 95% CI 0.86–2.05, $P = 0.20$)
• Little or no effect on TB preventive treatment completion (RR 1.00, 95% CI 0.92–1.09, $P = 0.99$) |

Table 8.2 *(cont.)*

Skill-mix interventions					Outcomes		
Description of intervention [Sources]	Content of interventions and skill-mix changes	Profession(s) in intervention and in comparator group	Population	Countries	Patient-related outcomes [Sources]	Health-system-related outcomes [Sources]	Profession-specific outcomes [Sources]
CHW and other supplementary roles to improve the management of people with chronic conditions [7]	Education, counselling, case management, navigation assistance, facilitation to access social services and support delivered in collaboration with other health professionals or under their supervision	Intervention: CHW, primary care providers, nurse case managers, dieticians, social workers, psychologists Comparison: Physicians, CHWs, not consistently reported	Vulnerable population groups (incl. patients with cancer, CVD, diabetes, hypertension)	IN, PK, TW, USA	• Significant improvement for blood pressure and HbA1c • Significant improvement on CVD risk reduction, lipid profile and blood pressure control • Mixed results on self-reported physical activity and mental-health-related outcomes	• Improvement in cancer screening behaviours and mammogram and Pap test uptake • Positive effect on cost effectiveness	

| CHW interventions to improve screening rates [8] | Components of CHW interventions included education, referring to health care services, scheduling appointments, emotional and social support | Intervention: CHW
Comparison: Not reported | Women from ethnic minorities at risk for breast cancer | USA | • Statistically significant effect on mammography rates (RR 1.6, 95% CI 1.02–1.11, $P = 0.003$)
• An increase in statistically significant effects regarding mammography rates when the number of intervention components given by CHW increased
• Matching CHW interventions with population by race or ethnicity showed significant improvements in adherence to screening (RR 1.03, 95% CI 1.01–1.05, $P = 0.02$) |

Table 8.2 (cont.)

Skill-mix interventions

Description of intervention [Sources]	Content of interventions and skill-mix changes	Profession(s) in intervention and in comparator group	Population	Countries	Outcomes		
					Patient-related outcomes [Sources]	Health-system-related outcomes [Sources]	Profession-specific outcomes [Sources]
Various skill-mix changes in primary care for medication-assisted treatment [9]	Coordinated care models, multiprofessional models, shared care models, chronic care models, physician-centric models, coordinated care between specialized services and primary care, use of non-physician staff and home induction, use of technologies)	Intervention: Primary care providers, GP physicians, nurses, NP, LPN, pharmacists, psychologist, counsellors, social workers, mental health workers Comparison: Physicians, others not reported	Drug users/ opioid use disorder	AT, AU, CA, FR, IR, IT, UK, USA	• Patient retention • Positive health outcomes • Increased knowledge about comorbidities • Patient satisfaction	• Improved performance processes and collaborative work with nurses as liaison in coordination	• Increased provider confidence • Benefits of providing coordinated care
Community-based case management [10, 11]	Treatment planning, home counselling, comprehensive assessment, treatment coordination, referral	Intervention: Case managers with background in nursing, social work and mental health care	Patients with substance use disorder (incl. women and court judgements [10])	CA, SE, USA	• Reduced substance use [11] • Improved patient satisfaction [10, 11]	• Improved access to health care and linkage between providers [10] • Increased treatment initiation [10]	

		Comparison: Not reported [10] compared with clinical case management and usual care [11]			• Improved health related outcomes, socioeconomic factors [10] and retention rates [10, 11]	• Mixed results on hospitalization [10] • Reduction in mental health service use, but no effect on health service use [11]
Pharmacists in expanded roles providing access to emergency contraceptives [12]	Expanding scope of practice: providing access to emergency contraception; partnerships between pharmacists, clinics and physicians	Intervention: Pharmacists Comparison: Not reported	Women (incl. young women at risk for unintended pregnancy, diverse ethnicities)	USA	• Increased patient satisfaction • No effect on health-related outcomes and pregnancy rates • 700 prevented pregnancies in one (pilot) study	• Improved access to emergency contraceptives • Pharmacists feel comfortable providing service

Abbreviations: CHW: community health worker; CI: confidence interval; CVD: cardiovascular disease; GP: general practitioner; HbA1c: glycated haemoglobin; NP: nurse practitioner; RR: relative risk.

Country abbreviations: AU: Australia; AT: Austria; BR: Brazil; CA: Canada; CN: China; BD: Bangladesh; BF: Burkina Faso; ET: Ethiopia; FR: France; GH: Ghana; IN: India; IR: Ireland; IT: Italy; IQ: Iraq; JM: Jamaica; MX: Mexico; NZ: New Zealand; NP: Nepal; KR: Korea; PH: The Philippines; PK: Pakistan; SE: Sweden; TH: Thailand; TR: Turkey; TW: Taiwan; TZ: Tanzania; UK: the United Kingdom; USA: the United States of America; VN: Vietnam; ZA: South Africa.

Sources: [1] Roland et al. (2017); [2] Ranaghan et al. (2016); [3] Bush, Kaufman & Shackleford (2017); [4] Glick et al. (2012); [5] Genoff et al. (2016); [6] Lewin et al. (2010); [7] Kim et al. (2016); [8] Wells et al. (2011); [9] Lagisetty et al. (2017); [10] Penzenstadler et al. (2017); [11] Joo et al. (2015); [12] Farris et al. (2010).

linguistic support, education and follow up. Patient navigators from the same community, same language and similar patient experience were reported to be well placed to reach out to at-risk populations in the community (Bush, Kaufman & Shackleford, 2017; Genoff et al., 2016; Glick et al., 2012; Ranaghan et al., 2016; Roland et al., 2017). Three reviews focused on cancer patients, including ethnic and other minorities, uninsured individuals and medically underserved and socioeconomically deprived population groups (Bush, Kaufman & Shackleford, 2017; Glick et al., 2012; Ranaghan et al., 2016), uninsured individuals (Bush, Kaufman & Shackleford, 2017; Ranaghan et al., 2016) and population groups with limited English proficiency (Genoff et al., 2016). One review included a wide range of different patients from medically underserved rural, suburban and urban areas (Roland et al., 2017). Across all systematic reviews, overcoming language barriers through the introduction of a patient navigator was considered very important (Bush, Kaufman & Shackleford, 2017; Genoff et al., 2016; Glick et al., 2012; Ranaghan et al., 2016; Roland et al., 2017).

- Other skill-mix interventions for vulnerable population groups included pharmacist-led services, case management in the community and various other interventions, for example for opioid users. The latter specifically targeted buprenorphine or methadone treatment for opioid use disorder linked with psychosocial care. Most interventions were shared care models between primary care and specialized services, but also task re-allocation (for example, care coordination, counselling or supervision of medication dispensing) from physicians to other professions such as nurses or pharmacists (Lagisetty et al., 2017).

- One Cochrane review focused on lay health workers providing support and delivering child and maternity care and being responsible for the management of infectious diseases for mothers and their children with low socioeconomic status. Intervention components varied widely and included home visits, reminders and education, among others (Lewin et al., 2010).

- Interventions by CHWs were the focus of two reviews. While the components of CHW interventions were similar, one review included CHWs along with other professionals and interventions were delivered in collaboration with or with the supervision of health professionals such as nurse case managers or psychologists. The review included components such as education, counselling, case management and navigation assistance (Kim et al., 2016). The other review, targeting women from ethnic minorities who were at risk for breast cancer, covered education, referral, scheduling and emotional and social support (Wells et al., 2011).

- Two systematic reviews assessed the outcomes of case management in the community for patients with substance use disorder, including individuals with court judgements. The interventions often used a combination of services and treatment planning, counselling, treatment coordination and home visits performed by nurses, social workers or mental health professionals (Joo et al., 2015; Penzenstadler et al., 2017). The comparator was either not reported (Penzenstadler et al., 2017) or covered usual care or clinical case management (Joo et al., 2015).

The pharmacist intervention focused on the expansion of their clinical role. It involved providing access to emergency contraceptives to prevent unintended pregnancies or administering re-injection of depot medroxyprogesterone acetate and providing other contraceptives in collaboration with clinics and physicians. Studies included women at different ages, adolescents at risk for unintended pregnancy and various ethnic minorities (Farris et al., 2010).

Outcomes on skill-mix innovations for vulnerable population groups
Involving patient navigators in outreach, education and coordination for patients with cancer, primarily for ethnic minorities and other vulnerable groups, was shown to improve access to screening (Genoff et al., 2016; Glick et al., 2012; Roland et al., 2017), and earlier treatment and treatment initiation (Bush, Kaufman & Shackleford, 2017). In terms of patient-related outcomes, the studies showed improved adherence rates in two systematic reviews (Bush, Kaufman & Shackleford, 2017; Glick et al., 2012). Results on patient satisfaction were mixed (Ranaghan et al., 2016). One systematic review reported improved care coordination (Ranaghan et al., 2016) and another reported improved completion of diagnostics (Roland et al., 2017). Improved completion of screening (Genoff et al., 2016; Glick et al., 2012) and referral and follow up (Roland et al., 2017) were also demonstrated. Mixed effects

were found for time to diagnosis (Bush, Kaufman & Shackleford, 2017; Ranaghan et al., 2016).

Introducing lay health workers in child and maternity care and management of infectious diseases for mothers and their children showed significantly improved patient and health system outcomes in a Cochrane review. Concerning the latter, effectiveness in promoting immunization uptake during childhood and initiation of breastfeeding was reported. Likelihood of seeking care for childhood illness significantly increased but little or no effect was shown on preventive tuberculosis (TB) treatment completion. In terms of patient outcomes, lay health worker interventions showed a positive effect on cure rates for pulmonary TB. The review reported reduction in child morbidity and child and neonatal mortality (Lewin et al., 2010).

Use of CHWs in combination with other supplementary roles to improve the management of people with chronic conditions in vulnerable populations showed significant improvement for blood pressure control, HbA1c, lipid profile and cardiovascular disease risk reduction. Although there were mixed results for self-reported physical and mental health, cancer screening behaviour and mammogram and Papanicolau test uptake improved. Positive effects on cost effectiveness were reported (Kim et al., 2016).

Interventions that only included CHWs showed statistically significant effects on mammography rates. Moreover, this effect increased when the number of intervention components increased and when CHWs were matched by population, race or ethnicity screening adherence was positively impacted (Wells et al., 2011).

Most of the included studies that targeted skill-mix interventions to drug users and patients with opioid use disorder, showed enhanced patient adherence to buprenorphine or methadone treatment. Some studies in the review showed improved health outcomes and knowledge about comorbidities for patients with opioid use disorder. Patients reported to be satisfied with the treatment models. Providers reported increased confidence and benefits from providing coordinated care (Lagisetty et al., 2017).

The studies that included case management in the community for populations with substance use disorders showed generally improved access to health care services, treatment initiation and linkage between providers (Penzenstadler et al., 2017). Although there was a reduction in mental health service use, the intervention showed no effect on the use of health services (Joo et al., 2015). There were mixed results for the effect on hospitalization rates. Health outcomes and socioeconomic factors ameliorated for patients benefiting from case management (Penzenstadler et al., 2017). A reduction in substance use (Joo et al., 2015) and increased patient satisfaction and treatment retention were found (Joo et al., 2015; Penzenstadler et al., 2017).

The systematic review analysing the effect of pharmacists in expanded roles, providing women direct access to contraceptives, reported improved access to contraceptives. Although some studies showed other improved patient- and profession-related outcomes, the reported effects were limited to individual studies (Farris et al., 2010).

Education and training of the professions involved in the skill-mix changes

Several reviews described the training in the skill-mix intervention groups, but not always in a systematic manner and they lacked details of the nature, length and curricula/contents changes. The education and training of the professions in the comparator groups were very rarely reported.

The CHWs and patient navigators received some additional training, for example, skills-based training covering motivational interviewing and communication (Hoeft et al., 2018; Kim et al., 2016; Roland et al., 2017; Wells et al., 2011). Kim et al. (2016) included bilingual CHWs; the training received varied between 4 and 240 hours. Patient navigators supporting cancer patients received information relating to cancer and health, screenings guidelines and patient support (Roland et al., 2017). Yet, detailed information was lacking.

In the review of patient navigators for underserved population groups, training covered health education, public speaking, and observing a mammography unit (Ranaghan et al., 2016). The review on access to medication-assisted treatment reported more specific details about the duration of training for their counsellors in some studies (Lagisetty et al., 2017). For instance, primary care providers received a 1-day training in methadone induction guidelines and procedures in one study, a drug misuse training twice a year in another study and 8 hours of didactic methadone maintenance training for nurse practitioners and community pharmacists in a third study.

> **Box 8.4 Examples of skill-mix innovations and new technologies/eHealth**
>
> - In rural and remote areas, a large number of interventions were highlighted that supported skill-mix changes and task shifting. Telepsychiatry was used in rural schools and universities with off-site mental health specialists. It was also suggested to support home visit models for patients with mental health conditions. Televideo conferencing showed to support the delivery of collaborative care. Telemedicine was suggested to be an important means for education, support and supervision particularly for staff in rural areas (Hoeft et al., 2018)
> - In the skill-mix interventions targeting patients with opioid use disorder, the use of electronic medical records facilitated treatment, communication and helped update patient information. Panel management structure was used to monitor patient level data (Lagisetty et al., 2017)

Training for pharmacists to work in expanded roles offering emergency contraception covered contraceptive management, injection techniques and 12 hours of continuing education addressing reproductive physiology and practice guidelines (Farris et al., 2010). Concluding, the training and educational background were not systematically reported and the education and professional training in the interventions differed to a large extent.

Limitations and strength of the evidence

The overview of reviews identified a limited number of systematic reviews on the topic, particularly when compared with other themes covered in this volume, for example, chronic care (see Chapter 6). The quality of the included reviews was mixed, which limits the attribution of causality. While several RCTs were covered in the systematic reviews, only two meta-analyses were performed and one of them was a Cochrane review. Furthermore, most of the included studies were based in the USA. Due to the variety of interventions and population groups covered in the systematic reviews and the non-systematic reporting of outcome measures, transfer of the findings has to be made with caution. Moreover, evidence on profession-related effects is very limited across all reviews.

Conclusions

The systematic reviews showed a positive effect of expanding teams to incorporate CHWs, lay workers or other professions into teams as an important strategy towards improving access for vulnerable groups. Promising effects were also reported for rural and disadvantaged populations for mental health. The roles of patient navigators and CHWs were identified as one policy option to overcome obstacles in accessing primary care services. Moreover, case management in the community for drug users seems important to assist with accessing services and seems to positively affect the course of treatment. Community-based strategies and partnerships were considered critical in supporting the expanded skill-mix teams and outreach activities.

8.3 Skill-mix innovations and reforms: country skill-mix examples for vulnerable and rural populations

Several skill-mix innovations have been evaluated for their effectiveness and access (Tables 8.1 and 8.2). While reviews are important to assess the potential impacts of different skill-mix strategies in various country contexts, additional evidence on country developments and reforms is required to complement the picture.

Several reforms have emerged across Europe to tackle the challenges in accessing care faced by disadvantaged groups and remote/rural populations. Elaborating on the review of the literature, this section presents several examples of innovations from Europe, North America and some high-income countries identified in the grey literature and single case studies.

Remote and rural populations

Recruitment and retention of health care providers in rural and remote areas is a well-established challenge (World Health Organization, 2010). Monetary incentives alone are not sufficient to convince health care personnel to settle in remote areas (European Commission, 2015). There is increasing evidence that local recruitment for primary care careers, early exposure to primary health care, embedding training in health services that reach those most in need, an emphasis on more generalist competencies (Strategic Advisory Board, 2015) in undergraduate training and ensuring a curriculum guided by social

---

Box 8.5 Delivering on social accountability: Canada's Northern Ontario School of Medicine (Strasser, 2016)

- The Northern Ontario School of Medicine (NOSM) opened in 2005 with a social accountability mandate to contribute to improving the health of the people and communities of Northern Ontario, which is a vast underserved rural part of Canada. NOSM recruits students from Northern Ontario or similar backgrounds and provides distributed community engaged learning in over 90 clinical and community settings located in the region.
- The curriculum was developed through a community consultative process and emphasizes learning at the local level, exposing students to different health service settings.
- After 10 years, outcomes suggest that NOSM has been successful in fulfilling its social accountability mandate: 92% of all students are from Northern Ontario, including 7% indigenous and 22% francophone students; 62% of all NOSM medical graduates have chosen family practice (predominantly rural) training; 69% of the graduates of NOSM's postgraduate education are practising in Northern Ontario; 94% of the doctors who completed undergraduate and postgraduate education with NOSM are practising in Northern Ontario.
- Because of its social accountability mandate, NOSM has also monitored its socioeconomic impact on the communities, which included new direct and indirect economic activity; enhanced retention and recruitment for the universities and hospitals/health services; and a sense of empowerment among community participants attributable in large part to NOSM.

---

accountability are strategies to increase appropriate human resources for primary health care in rural and remote areas (Strasser & Neusy, 2010). Some of the providers at primary care level will also require a broader scope of practice (with a specific skill-mix), when secondary care services are far away or transport is problematic. Box 8.5 illustrates the successful trajectory at Canada's Northern Ontario School of Medicine.

In addition to recruitment and retention strategies, a common skill-mix response to geographical and health workforce shortage is task shifting from physicians to nurses and other health professionals. Several countries in Europe (including Finland, Hungary, Latvia, Germany), and from outside Europe, (for example, Australia and Canada), have introduced reforms to instigate the expansion of roles for health professionals and task shifting. This is most commonly found affecting the nursing profession. In Finland, nurses lead consultations in remote areas and can prescribe medicines, supported by e-consultations with physicians if needed (Delamaire & Lafortune, 2010; World Health Organization, 2015). In Australia, the so-called Scheduled Medicines registered nurses administer and supply a limited set of medicines in rural and remote settings to improve access to medicines (Nursing and Midwifery Board of Australia, 2010)[2]. Nurses also play an increasing role in outreach services. In certain provinces of Canada, nurse practitioners employed in rural practices perform outreach activities (for example, in British Columbia) and prescribe medications (Maier, Aiken & Busse, 2017). In Hungary, the role of health visitors – also called public health nurses – was expanded to include carrying out cervical cancer screening in rural areas, which improved participation rates for cervical cancer screening (Döbrőssy et al., 2015). The project was initially implemented as a pilot and then extended nationally, using a train-the-trainer approach to educate about 1400 volunteer health visitors on effective communication and support, as well as in smear taking, which was then included as part of the traditional undergraduate training for health visitors.

Other examples of task shifting and roles expansion include *feldsher* or midwives, who still provide a considerable share of primary care in rural areas in Latvia, in which about a third of the population lives (OECD, 2016). In Canada, the role of physician assistants was introduced to improve care in rural and remote areas in four provinces (New Brunswick, Alberta, Manitoba and Ontario). There are about 500 physician assistants practising in Canada (300 of them in Ontario), with plans for further expansion (Canadian Association of Physician Assistants, n.d)[3]. Further, in line with the literature review highlighting the role of pharmacists in providing emergency contraception for vulnerable groups (Farris et al., 2010), evidence of the expanded role

---

[2] Nursing and Midwifery Board of Australia (website): https://www
.nursingmidwiferyboard.gov.au/registration-and-endorsement/endorsements-
notations/registration-standard-for-endorsement.aspx [accessed 20/05/2019]
[3] Canadian Association of Physician Assistants (website), N.D: https://capa-acam
.ca/about-capa/strategic-plan-2015–2018/ [accessed 20/05/2019]

of pharmacists was also found in remote areas of Australia, where pharmacists administer influenza and other vaccines (OECD, 2015).

There are several country examples of skill-mix strategies that have been introduced in conjunction with service re-design to enhance health services outreach in remote and rural areas. One example is the increased use of mobile facilities to reach people in countries where geographic distances are particularly challenging, for example, Finland, Romania, Australia and New Zealand. Examples include a 3-year pilot in eight communities in rural Finland. In these communities, a bus with a planned route was covering 100 000 potential patients, staffed by nurses, in which health monitoring services, influenza vaccines and small operations were carried out (European Network for Rural Development, n.d). In Romania, every month, the Caravana cu' medici NGO's mobile unit brings a multiprofessional team of doctors (20–30 specialists, residents and medical students) to one of Romania's remote villages (Caravana Cu Medici, n.d)[4]. They engage with the local authorities, the local GP and the community, to raise awareness and examine the health status of about 150–250 people, providing specialist consultations and medical equipment that are often missing in remote areas, as well as educating patients on their health. This initiative started in 2014, and had reached 3000 people in 25 villages by 2017. The Heart of Australia project includes three mobile units staffed by a team of cardiologists and respiratory specialists who, on a rotating roster, bring cardiology, neurology, endocrinology and respiratory services to 16 rural and outback communities (Heart of Australia, n.d)[5]. In New Zealand, mobile health bus units deliver low-risk elective day surgery to rural New Zealanders, and have provided continuing education to rural health professionals via a telepresence network since February 2002. Teams of surgeons, anaesthetists and nurses are transported to and from the bus location on the day of surgery bookings, and so far the service has treated about 24 000 patients in rural New Zealand, and provided over 50 000 hours of education (Mobile Health, n.d)[6].

[4] Caravana cu Medici (website), N.D: https://www.caravanacumedici.ro/en/mobile_unit.html [accessed 20/05/2019]

[5] Heart of Australia website, N.D: https://www.heartofaustralia.com/services-2/ [accessed 20/05/2019]

[6] Mobile Health (website), N.D: http://www.mobilesurgical.co.nz [accessed 20/05/2019]

Vulnerable groups

Several systematic reviews highlighted changes in the skill-mix of individual professions and teams to address the specific needs of vulnerable population groups. These groups vary considerably and include ethnic minorities, drug users, uninsured individuals and socioeconomically disadvantaged or other medically underserved populations. Moreover, a further search of the grey literature and individual country case studies identified skill-mix innovations concerning immigrants, homeless people, alcohol users, minorities, men who have sex with men (MSM), people who have been in prison and seasonal agricultural workers.

Overall, there is evidence that an increasing number of high-income countries have implemented strategies to employ CHWs, following similar experiences with CHWs in low- and middle-income countries. Among high-income countries, most programmes exist in the USA, Canada, New Zealand and Australia. CHWs can act as an effective bridge between communities and providers to reach vulnerable populations. A specific enabler is the cultural sensitivity component, particularly relevant for CHWs among First Nations in Canada, Maori communities in New Zealand, and Aboriginal and Torres Strait Islander health workers across Australia. Similarly, in the USA (North Carolina), Latino MSM were recruited and trained as part of a behavioural intervention to serve as lay health advisors (known as *Navegantes*) to promote sexual health among Spanish-speaking MSM groups of Latin-American origin. The intervention was found to be efficacious in reducing risk behaviour among study participants (Rhodes et al., 2017). Another example is the role of *promotores* who act as important support figures contributing to health care delivery and health outreach services among immigrants (Frank et al., 2013).

In Europe, one training for CHWs working with LGBTQ communities in Europe is the *European Surveys and Training to Improve MSM Community Health* (ESTICOM). The programme aims to develop a toolbox-training package suitable for CHWs, to improve access, quality of prevention, diagnosis of HIV and other sexually transmitted infections and viral hepatitis, and health care for MSM. The programme was piloted in 2018 in Training of Trainer Workshops and National Pilot Trainings involving participants from 29 European countries. In Germany, the ESTICOM programme defined CHWs as all people providing sexual health support to gay, bisexual and other MSM in a community setting, and they were referred to as peer CHWs (ESTICOM, n.d)[7]. In Belgium, CHWs have been employed as part of multidisciplinary teams in community health centres (Box 8.6).

Box 8.6 Community Health Centre Botermarkt – Ledeberg in Ghent (Belgium)[8]

- The CHC Botermarkt is a not-for-profit organization, operating since 1978 in Ledeberg, at the time a deprived area of the city of Ghent. The interprofessional team is composed of family physicians, nurses and assistant nurses, social workers, dentists, nutritionists, specialists in tobacco addiction, psychologists, receptionists and health promoters, which put the preventive function of CHWs in practice. The CHC takes care of 6200 patients, representing 95 nationalities, and of 250 undocumented persons. Further, it is responsible for health promotion activities for a community of 10 000 people.
- The main purpose of the Centre is to deliver integrated primary health care, including promotion, prevention, curative care, rehabilitation, palliative care and social care (De Maeseneer, 2017). The service delivery invests in universal accessibility (no financial, geographical or cultural threshold, but so-called proportionate efforts, for example through interpreters, Webcam-translation) and quality, using a comprehensive eco-bio-psycho-social frame of reference. Special focus is on the empowerment of patients and enhancing social cohesion.
- Participation of the population and the community is of utmost importance. CHC Botermarkt implements community-oriented primary care and regularly, local stakeholders meet on the platform of Society–Welfare–Health. Using epidemiological, sociological and practice-based information, they perform a community diagnosis and develop interprofessional and intersectoral programmes that tackle the upstream causes of ill-health (for example, poverty, traffic safety, lack of playgrounds, bad housing conditions, epidemics, oral health).
- All patients are registered on a patient-list, open to all people living in the defined geographical area. Payment is through a monthly integrated needs-based capitation (taking into account sociodemographic, epidemiological, contextual and income variables). This financing mechanism stimulates task-shifting and

---

[7] ESTICOM website, N.D: https://www.esticom.eu/Webs/ESTICOM/EN/about-project/consortium-partners/About_DAH_rev.html [accessed 20/05/2019]
[8] *www.wgcbotermarkt.be/eng/*

Box 8.2 (cont.)

competency sharing and strengthens prevention and the self-reliance of people. An interprofessional goal-oriented electronic health record (Tange, Nagykaldi & De Maeseneer, 2017), accessible to all health care providers as well as the patient, documents the episodes of care (encoded using the International Classification of Primary Care-2, developed by the WONCA International Classification Committee, n.d).

• An analysis of the performance of CHCs (compared with usual practices in fee-for-service settings) in Belgium concluded that the centres score excellently on access, especially for vulnerable groups; they demonstrate good quality of prevention, antibiotic prescription and other indicators; and patients in CHCs cost less than usual practices in utilization of secondary care services (Annemans et al., 2008).

In Europe, CHWs are less well-known than in other regions of the world and the terminology overlaps with a variety of other titles, such as community advocates, outreach workers and peer counsellors. This may explain why a search of the literature reported only a few CHW programmes in Europe. Further, similar groups such as peers or other groups that emanate from the same community may take up roles that are similar to those of CHWs. It may also be that informal caregivers, relatives or other volunteers implicitly assume this role.

Spearheaded by the USA (Valaitis et al., 2017), the role of patient navigators has slowly emerged in Europe (for example, Belgium, Austria), and have been shown to overlap with the CHWs' role. For example, a pilot project in Belgium recruits patient navigators for Dutch-speaking cancer patients receiving treatment (Anticancer Fund, n.d)[9]. Another example in Belgium is the establishment of the roles of patient navigators as well as cultural mediators who help to guide migrants across a new health care system (European Commission, 2018). In Austria, although on a small scale, cultural mediators or trained patient navigators are available to help migrants in accessing health care (International Organization for Migration, 2015). However, the exact tasks and roles

---

[9] Anticancer fund (website), N.D: https://www.anticancerfund.org/nl/my-cancer-navigator [accessed 20/05/2019]

of these new health workers are not described in sufficient detail, nor evaluated, which limits the assessment of their contribution.

An example of skill-mix changes as part of larger service re-design is the use of mobile units for outreach, also identified specifically for vulnerable populations. Examples include units in Romania, the United Kingdom and the USA. In Romania, a mobile medical unit staffed by a team specifically trained on the use of equipment for diagnostics offers screenings for early detection of TB for homeless people, drug users and minorities such as Roma, who may have limited access to health care (E-detect TB, n.d)[10]. Similarly in London (the United Kingdom), the Find & Treat outreach service promotes early detection of TB for homeless people, drug or alcohol users, vulnerable migrants and people who have been in prison. It screens almost 10 000 high-risk people annually using a mobile digital X-ray unit. The programme also recruits TB patients who have experienced homelessness to support others through treatment and out of homelessness in a peer advocate role similar to that of patient navigators identified in the literature review; this is now expanding outside London (UCLH, n.d)[11]. The United Kingdom also presents a particular case of cross-professional collaboration and outreach activities, where firefighters work together with NHS England to perform home checks to identify health risks such as loneliness and isolation among the older population. Health and local authority colleagues support fire and rescue services in training and raising the awareness of their staff if deemed necessary (NHS England, n.d)[12]. In the USA, in some states (for example, California, Maine) there are medical mobile programmes staffed with primary care providers, nurses and CHWs providing primary and preventive care, oral health, mental health and substance abuse services especially for migrant and seasonal agricultural workers (Central City Health, n.d)[13].

There is evidence that an effective way to address the needs of vulnerable populations is through a primary health care multi-level approach,

[10] E-detect TB (website): https://e-detecttb.eu/2018/03/24/e-detect-factsheets-available-now/ [accessed 20/05/2019]
[11] University College London Hospitals (website) N.D: https://www.uclh.nhs.uk/ourservices/servicea-z/htd/pages/mxu.aspx [accessed 19/05/2019]
[12] National Health Service England (website), N.D: https://www.england.nhs.uk/ourwork/clinical-policy/older-people/working-together/ [accessed 20/05/2019]
[13] Central City Health website: https://centralcityhealth.org/migrant-seasonal-agricultural-worker-program-msaw/

such as that observed in Norway and Slovenia. In Norway, a new team model consisting of a GP, a nurse and a health secretary is being implemented to provide multi-level care for vulnerable patients, for example, patients suffering from substance or alcohol abuse. To date, the project is run as a pilot until March 2021, and so far, eight municipalities with 80 teams are participating (the companion volume; Wismar, Glinos & Sagan, forthcoming). In Slovenia, a new model of Health Promotion Centres focuses on integrating different health prevention and promotion services, targeting mostly the unemployed, homeless and socially and economically disadvantaged groups. The pilot project concluded in 2016 with plans to introduce the new model to at least 25 additional Health Promotion Centres by 2020, supported by €15 million from the European Union cohesion funds (World Health Organization, 2018c).

This trend in promoting a multiprofessional approach targeted to local needs also applies to Community Health Centres (CHCs). Accountable for a defined population (for example, based on empanelment or patient-lists, or geographic areas), CHCs are community-oriented primary care organizations that deliver health and social services through interprofessional teams, focusing on the specific health and social needs of local communities. CHCs involve members of the community in planning and programming, and implement an intersectoral approach to address social determinants of health. CHCs currently exist in dozens of countries around the world (Susic et al., forthcoming), and the International Federation of Community Health Centres is in the process of scaling-up CHCs worldwide. Examples in North America and Europe include over 300 CHCs across Canada (101 in Ontario alone), which offer services by a range of primary care providers (GPs, nurse practitioners, social workers, dieticians) and cover mainly individuals from disadvantaged backgrounds (the companion volume; Wismar, Glinos & Sagan, forthcoming). There are about 1400 CHCs in all 50 states and United States territories. CHCs also exist in Europe, such as the CHC Botermarkt in Ledeberg, Ghent, Belgium (Box 8.6).

CHCs present an opportunity to contribute to the attainment of the Universal Health Coverage and health-related Sustainable Developments Goals. Moreover, CHCs contribute to the growing expertise on skill-mix innovations in interprofessional teams, especially concerning vulnerable populations.

In addition, investment is needed in the recruitment of future health professionals from the communities they will serve. More resources should be invested in interprofessional training modules (International Organization for Migration, 2013) for all students in health and welfare professional education, teaching students to address the social determinants of health (The National Academies of Sciences-Engineering-Medicine, 2013) and enhancing community participation. Some institutions have integrated interprofessional community-based learning activities, where students of the second Bachelor year participate in a community-oriented primary care exercise (Art et al., 2008).

8.4 Conclusions

A variety of different skill-mix strategies have been implemented across Europe and other Anglophone countries to improve the access to care for populations living in rural and remote areas. While certain recruitment and retention strategies hold some promise, they have been shown to be insufficient. Additional skill-mix strategies include task shifting and re-allocation within teams to share workloads effectively and expand access to care. Other strategies involve skill-mix changes within teams combined with activating outreach to remote regions, for example, via mobile units. There is limited evidence on the effectiveness of these different skill-mix strategies in underserved regions, which also affects the transferability across regions and countries. However, several countries have shown that in very remote regions, mobile units staffed by multiprofessional teams and clear division of work, supported by e-technology, may be promising for expanding outreach activities.

For vulnerable population groups, several innovative skill-mix strategies have been implemented across Europe and other countries. These include the establishment of community-based workers or other, similar roles, such as patient navigators, who are close to and understand the needs of these vulnerable communities. Community-based strategies and partnerships among stakeholders are considered critical in supporting the expanded skill-mix teams and outreach activities. In order to enhance the contribution of new disciplines (CHWs or other community-based roles) that will improve the access to care for vulnerable groups, investment in a strong comprehensive team-based primary care model is critical, with appropriate financing-mechanisms, such as CHCs.

Despite a relative lack of scientific evidence, there is a move in the field towards an optimized skill-mix approach in improving access in rural and remote areas and for vulnerable groups. To an extent, evidence from high-income countries points to skill-mix innovations that are also mirrored in low- and middle-income countries. At the same time, other countries may not have the education and regulatory prerequisites for adopting similar models or may not apply them in the same ways. On the other hand, there is a lot of practice-based expertise, for example, in low- and middle-income countries, that could contribute to innovation. The creation of global so-called learning communities could be a way forward.

There is a recognized need to promote a community-oriented focus that spans across sectors. Such an approach should be mirrored in the education and curricula that prepare the next generation of health care professionals, to include skills training in shared decision-making, social determinants of health, intercultural communication and interprofessional cooperation, ideally complemented by more training facilities and more placements in disadvantaged and remote areas. Increased dissemination of community diagnosis, facilitated by multiprofessional teams, could further enhance health care and health promotion tailored to specific community contexts. Finally, there is a need for integration of public health services and primary care (Allen at al., 2018) to be responsive to today's challenges that require both a person- and population-centred approach.

References

Allen LN, Barkley S, De Maeseneer J et al. (2018). Unfulfilled potential of primary care in Europe. BMJ, 363:k4469 doi: 10.1136/bmj.k4469

Annemans L, Closon JP, Closons MC et al. (2008). Comparison of cost and quality of two financing systems for primary care in Belgium. Health Services Research. Brussels, Federal Knowledge Centre for Health Care (KCE); KCE report 85A (D/2008/10.273/49) (https://kce.fgov.be/en/comparison-of-the-cost-and-the-quality-of-two-financing-systems-of-primary-health-care-in-belgium accessed 17 May 2019)

Art B, De Roo L, Willems S et al. (2008). An interdisciplinary community diagnosis experience in an undergraduate medical curriculum: development at Ghent University. Acad Med, 83(7):675–683.

Bush M, Kaufman M, Shackleford T (2007). Adherence in the cancer care setting: a systematic review of patient navigation to traverse barriers. J Cancer Educ, 33(6):1222–1229.

Council of the European Union (2006). Council conclusions on common values and principles in European Union health systems. Official Journal of the European Union (2006/c 146/01).

De Maeseneer J (2017). Family medicine and primary care at the crossroads of societal change. Leuven, LannooCampus Publishers. ISBN 978 94 014 4446 0

De Maeseneer J, Roberts RG, Demarzo M et al. (2011). Tackling NCDs: a different approach is needed. Lancet, 379:1860–1861.

Delamaire M, Lafortune G (2010). Nurses in advanced roles: a description and evaluation of experiences in 12 developed countries. OECD Health Working Papers, No. 54. Paris, OECD Publishing (http://dx.doi .org/10.1787/5kmbrcfms5g7-en).

Döbrőssy L, Kovács A, Budai A et al. (2015). Education and training of health visitors to undertake cervical screening. J Nurs Educ Pract 5:28.

European Commission (2015). Recruitment and retention of the health workforce in Europe. Final Report. (https://ec.europa.eu/health/sites/health/ files/workforce/docs/2015_healthworkforce_recruitment_retention_frep_ en.pdf, accessed 20 May 2019).

European Commission, European website on Integration (2018). Migrant health across Europe: little structural policies, many encouraging practices. (https://ec.europa.eu/migrant-integration/feature/migrant-health-across-europe, accessed: 17 May 2019).

European Network for Rural Development (website) (n.d). (https://enrd .ec.europa.eu/sites/enrd/files/fi-mallu-does-the-rounds-gp_web.pdf, accessed 17 May 2019).

Expert Panel on Effective Ways of Investing in Health (EXPH) (2017). Opinion on benchmarking access to health care in the EU. Brussels, European Commission.

Expert Panel on Effective Ways of Investing in Health (EXPH) (2019). Task shifting in healthcare systems. Brussels, European Union.

Farris K, Ashwood D, McIntosh J et al. (2010). Preventing unintended pregnancy: pharmacists' roles in practice and policy via partnerships. J Am Pharm Assoc, 50(5):604–612.

Frank A, Liebman A, Ryder B et al. (2013). Health care access and health care workforce for immigrant workers in the agriculture, forestry, and fisheries sector in the southeastern US. Am J Indust Med, 56:960–974. DOI 10.1002/ajim.22183

Genoff M, Zaballa A, Gany F et al. (2016). Navigating language barriers: a systematic review of patient navigators' impact on cancer screening for limited English proficient patients. J Gen Intern Med, 31(4):426–434.

Glick S, Clarke A, Blanchard A et al. (2012). Cervical cancer screening, diagnosis and treatment interventions for racial and ethnic minorities: a systematic review. J Gen Intern Med, 27(8):1016–1032.

Hoeft T, Fortney J, Patel V et al. (2018). Task-sharing approaches to improve mental health care in rural and other low-resource settings: a systematic review. J Rural Health, 34(1):48–62.

International Organization for Migration (IOM) (2015). Country Report: Austria. Migrant Integration Policy Index Health Strand. (https://eea.iom .int/sites/default/files/publication/document/AUSTRIA_MIPEX_Health .pdf, accessed: 17 May 2019).

Joo JY, Huber DL (2015). Community-based case management effectiveness in populations that abuse substances. Int Nurs Rev, 62:536–546.

Kim K, Choi J, Choi E et al. (2016). Effects of community-based health worker interventions to improve chronic disease management and care among vulnerable populations: a systematic review. Am J Public Health, 106(4):e3-e28.

Lagisetty P, Klasa K, Bush C et al. (2017). Primary care models for treating opioid use disorders: What actually works? A systematic review. PLOS One, 12(10):p.e0186315.

Levesque JF, Harris M, Russel G. (2013). Patient-centred access to health care: conceptualising access at the interface of health systems and populations. Int J Equity Health, 12(18), (https://doi.org/10.1186/1475-9276-12-18).

Lewin S, Munabi-Babigumira S, Glenton C, et al. (2010). Lay health workers in primary and community health care for maternal and child health and the management of infectious diseases. Cochrane Database Syst Rev, 2010(3):CD004015.

Maier C, Aiken L, Busse R (2017). Nurses in advanced roles in primary care: policy levers for implementation. OECD Health Working Papers, No. 98. Paris, OECD Publishing. (https://dx.doi.org/10.1787/a8756593-en).

Marmot Review (2010). Fair Society, Healthy Lives. Strategic review of health inequalities in England, post-2010. London, University College London.

OECD (2015). Reviews of health care quality: Australia, 2015. Raising standards. Paris, OECD Publishing. (https://doi.org/10.1787/9789264233836-en).

OECD (2016). Reviews of health systems: Latvia 2016. Paris, OECD Publishing. (https://doi.org/10.1787/9789264262782-en).

Penzenstadler L, Machado A, Thorens G et al. (2017). Effect of case management interventions for patients with substance use disorders: a systematic review. Front Psychiat. 8(51).

Ranaghan C, Boyle K, Meehan M et al. (2016). Effectiveness of a patient navigator on patient satisfaction in adult patients in an ambulatory care setting. JBI Database Syst Rev Implement Rep, 14(8):172–218.

Rhodes SD, Alonzo J, Mann L et al. (2017). Small-group randomized controlled trial to increase condom use and HIV testing among Hispanic/ Latino gay, bisexual, and other men who have sex with men. Am J Public Health, 107(6):969–976. DOI: 10.2105/AJPH.2017.303814

Roland K, Milliken E, Rohan E et al. (2017). Use of community health workers and patient navigators to improve cancer outcomes among patients served by federally qualified health centers: a systematic literature review. Health Equity, 1(1):61–76.

Strasser R (2016). Delivering on social accountability: Canada's Northern Ontario School of Medicine. Asia Pacific Scholar, 1(1):3–9.

Strasser R, Neusy AJ (2010). Context counts: training health workers in and for rural and remote areas. Bull WHO, 88:777–782.

Strategic Advisory Board Wellbeing, Health, Family (2015). Vision Statement: New professionalism in Care and Support as a Task for the future. Brussels, Flemish Community, 2015. (http://www.sarwgg.be/sites/default/files/documenten/SARWGG_20151217_New%20Professionalism_Vision%20statement_DEF.pdf, accessed 17 May 2019).

Susic AP, De Maeseneer J, Wolfe SW et al. (forthcoming). Community Health Centres: a century of "Alma-Ata" in practice. Europanorama.

Tange H, Nagykaldi Z, De Maeseneer J (2017). Towards an overarching model for electronic medical-record systems, including problem-oriented, goal-oriented, and other approaches. Eur J Gen Pract, 23(1):257–260.

The National Academies of Sciences-Engineering-Medicine (2013). A framework for educating Health Professionals to address the Social Determinants of Health. Washington DC, The National Academies Press. 2013. ISBN 978 0 309 39262 4

Valaitis R, Carter N, Lam A et al. (2017). Implementation and maintenance of patient navigation programs linking primary care with community-based health and social services: a scoping literature review. BMC Health Serv Res, 17(116): (https://doi.org/10.1186/s12913-017-2046-1).

Wells K, Luque J, Miladinovic B et al. (2011). Do community health worker interventions improve rates of screening mammography in the United States? A systematic review. Cancer Epidemiol Biomarkers Prevent, 20(8):1580–1598.

Whiteman J (2014). Tackling socio-economic disadvantage: making rights work. Equal Rights Rev, 12:95–108.

Wismar M, Glinos I, Sagan A (forthcoming). Skill-mix innovation in primary and chronic care. Mobilizing patients, peers, professionals. Copenhagen, WHO Regional Office for Europe on behalf of the European Observatory on Health Systems and Policies.

WONCA International Classification Committee (n.d) International Classification of Primary Care. Wonca (World Organisation of Family Doctors) (https://www.globalfamilydoctor.com/site/DefaultSite/filesystem/documents/Groups/WICC/International%20Classification%20of%20Primary%20Care%20Dec16.pdf, accessed 17 May 2019).

World Health Organization (1989). Strengthening the performance of community health workers in primary health care. Report of a WHO Study Group. Tech Rep Ser 780:1–46.

World Health Organization (2009). Increasing access to health workers in remote and rural areas through improved retention. Background paper draft. 2009: (https://www.who.int/hrh/migration/background_paper .pdf?ua=1, accessed 17 May 2019).

World Health Organization (2010). Increasing access to health workers in remote and rural areas through improved retention: global policy recommendations. (https://apps.who.int/iris/bitstream/handle/10665/ 44369/9789241564014_eng.pdf?sequence=1&isAllowed=y, accessed 17 May 2019).

World Health Organization (2018a). Global Conference on Primary Health Care. Declaration of Astana. (https://www.who.int/docs/default-source/ primary-health/declaration/gcphc-declaration.pdf, accessed 17 May 2019).

World Health Organization (2018b). The Delhi Declaration: Alma Ata revisited. (https://www.who.int/hrh/news/2018/delhi_declaration/en/, accessed 17 May 2019).

World Health Organization (2018c). Health promotion centres in Slovenia: Integrating population and individual services to reduce health inequalities at community level. (http://www.euro.who.int/en/countries/slovenia/ publications/health-promotion-centres-in-slovenia-integrating-population- and-individual-services-to-reduce-health-inequalities-at-community- level-2018, accessed 17 May 2019).

World Health Organization Regional Office for Europe (2015). Nurses and midwives. A vital resource for health. European compendium of good practices in nursing and midwivery towards Health 2020 goals. (http:// www.euro.who.int/__data/assets/pdf_file/0004/287356/Nurses-midwives- Vital-Resource-Health-Compendium.pdf?ua=1, accessed 20 May 2019).

9 Education and planning: anticipating and responding to skill gaps, changing skill needs and competencies

RONALD BATENBURG, MARIEKE KROEZEN

9.1 Introduction

Most European countries are faced with a chain of challenges in health care. Due to the ageing of the population and a growing number of chronically ill patients with multimorbidity, the demand for health care is higher than ever. At the same time, countries are confronted with current and forecasted health workforce shortages and maldistribution. Many countries have turned to interprofessional work and task substitution in response to these challenges (De Bont et al., 2016). Both concepts are interconnected and imply changes in the skills of health care professionals (OECD Health Division Team, 2018) as well as in the skill-mix of health care organizations (Dussault & Buchan, 2018). A key requirement for these changes to successfully take place, is that education and planning systems effectively and rapidly respond to the changing skill requirements at the workplace (Frenk et al., 2010).

Education and health workforce planning

When defining education, this chapter refers to the range of learning opportunities provided throughout a health professional career; from basic professional education to advanced education and lifelong learning opportunities within the workplace, including in-service training and continuous professional development. Health workforce planning is defined as the process concerned with ensuring that the right number of people, with the right skills, are at the right place at the right time to deliver the right services to those in need of them (Maxtrix Insight Centre for Workforce Intelligence, 2012; OECD, 2016). The main aim of planning is to achieve an optimal balance of demand and supply of health workers in both the short and long term (Kroezen, Van

Hoegaerden & Batenburg, 2018; Ono, Lafortune & Schoenstein, 2013; Scheffler et al., 2018).

The linkages between education, health workforce planning and skill-mix

As the main source of health workforce development, education can contribute to meeting demographic challenges by preparing the appropriate number of professionals to enter the health workforce. Apart from influencing the quantity of health workers, education can also address issues of quality and relevance in order to address population health needs (World Health Organization, 2013). For example, where new skills are required in practice, such as for nurses in advanced roles, educational systems are (partly) responsible for equipping health professionals with these skills.

Currently, the link between training and practice requirements is suboptimal. A recent OECD study showed that doctors and nurses report high rates of skills mismatch (Schoenstein, Ono & Lafortune, 2016). Defined as the inadequacy or over-adequacy of a worker's skills relative to the requirements of the job they are currently doing, more than three-quarters of all doctors and nurses reported over-skilling in their current job, and nearly half reported under-skilling. Especially advanced nurses (Master's degree or above) appear to face a high level of over-skilling whereby their skills exceed those required by the job. Although partly related to organizational, institutional and regulatory barriers, which prevent them from using their skills to the maximum (Schoenstein, Ono & Lafortune, 2016). This also demonstrates that the responsiveness of education systems to the changing skill requirements in health care can be improved. Various examples of this can be found across Europe. In some cases, educational systems appear to be too slow in responding to changing skill demands. For example in the Netherlands and Spain, nurses have learned the skills to prescribe medicines in practice, but actually performed this task illegally (or in legally grey areas) for a long time. This was related to the fact that the required educational basis was missing (Kroezen et al., 2013). In other cases, educational reforms were only implemented after the required legislative changes for the new role or task substitution were made, again creating a mismatch between practice and education (Delamaire & Lafortune, 2010). Often, these challenges are complicated by the fact that some professions, particularly medical doctors, have a monopoly over some skills through regulations and legislation (Andrew, 1988).

The challenges faced by health workforce planning systems in response to skill-mix innovations are naturally linked to the challenges that confront the educational system. Just as the responsiveness of education systems to the changing skill requirements in health care can be improved, so can the responsiveness of planning systems to bottom–up developments concerning skill-mix be improved (Fraher & Brandt, 2019). This includes not only the response to new skill-mix developments from practice, but also educational reforms implemented by universities or other training institutions. One of the reasons that proactively planning skill-mix changes is challenging for many planning systems, is that workforce planning often misses essential and structural connections to other policy areas, such as general health policy and education (Kuhlmann & Larsen, 2015). If these linkages were in place, it would allow a more efficient response to future health needs of the population. Currently, however, many European countries are faced with health workforce shortages (Kroezen et al., 2015). These shortages and maldistributions only seem to grow, even if a great variety of planning models are used in European countries (Batenburg, 2015; Ono, Lafortune & Schoenstein, 2013). This urges the question of what type of education and health workforce planning is best suited to support the challenges in the health services and its change in demand.

In this chapter, we describe how and what types of education and health workforce planning models can anticipate and respond to observed skill gaps, changing skill needs and competencies, and thereby support the design and implementation of effective skill-mix interventions. We first present evidence from a systematic review that was identified through the overview of systematic reviews (see section 9.2). Next we discuss strategies, frameworks and tools in the field of (i) basic professional education of health professionals, (ii) postgraduate training and continuing professional development, and (iii) health workforce planning systems. In our concluding section (9.4), we synthesize these three fields, and propose further steps that can be taken to improve the role of education and health workforce planning in skill-mix innovation in health care.

9.2 Overview of the evidence on education, planning and skill-mix

The overview of reviews identified one systematic review on education and none on workforce planning (Table 9.1). The identified review (Reeves et al., 2013) focused on the effectiveness of interprofessional education (IPE) interventions and included 15 studies. The groups targeted were health professionals, teams and patients who were involved in an IPE intervention. It was shown that IPE interventions vary in content and length. Examples of learning methods used in the IPE interventions included interprofessional learning sessions, role plays, discussions, practical exercises, videos, homework and phone calls by the instructors. The length and intensity of the IPE interventions also varied considerably, with some interventions comprising 1-day sessions only, while other interventions had sessions that ran over a period of 18 months. Seven of the 15 studies included in the review reported positive outcomes on clinical care and collaboration, such as improved teamwork, improved development of competencies, improved information sharing and adherence to guidelines. Improved patient or quality-related outcomes were reported in six studies. Four studies reported a mixed set of outcomes and another four reported that the IPE interventions had no impact on either processes or patient-specific and other related outcomes.

9.3 Role of education and health workforce planning in the implementation of skill-mix innovations

In this section, we discuss some of the main trends related to skill-mix innovation that are visible in education and health workforce planning. We do so by successively discussing strategies, frameworks and tools that are used in the field of basic professional education of health professionals, postgraduate training and continuing professional development, and health workforce planning systems.

Skill-mix implementation by basic professional education

A significant part of the health workforce of tomorrow is in school or at university today. In view of the current levels of skills mismatch, and of the trend towards multiprofessional work and skill-mix (OECD Health Division Team, 2018), basic professional education is being adapted, and needs to be further adapted to respond to these changing skill needs

Table 9.1 *Overview of evidence on interprofessional education from included systematic review*

Intervention					Outcomes		
Description of intervention	Content of interventions and skill-mix changes	Profession(s) in intervention & comparator group	Population	Countries	Patient-related outcomes	Health-system-related outcomes	Profession-specific outcomes
Interprofessional education, including all types of educational, training, learning or teaching initiatives, involving more than one profession in joint, interactive learning	Various forms of IPE, including workshops, role plays, discussions, practical exercises, videos	Intervention: Health and social care professionals Comparator: Teams without IPE or same team as before intervention	Professionals or patients that are involved in IPE intervention	USA, UK	• Improved patient outcomes (6/15 studies) • Improved patient satisfaction (2/15 studies)	• IPE leads to changes in the use of guidelines or standards (3/15 studies) • IPE might lead to changes in clinical process (1/15 studies)	• Improved teamwork, development of competencies, orientation to patient groups and information sharing (no adequate assessment possible)

Abbreviations: IPE: interprofessional education.

Country abbreviations: UK: the United Kingdom; USA: the United States of America.

Source: Reeves et al. (2013)

and competencies. Most notably, the following trends can be discerned in basic education in relation to skill-mix innovations:

- development of interprofessional education
- development of competency-based education
- academization of health professions.

Development of interprofessional education

In order to prepare future health professionals for multiprofessional and interprofessional work, to advance teamwork and to increase the understanding of roles across health care, it is important to instil students with a multiprofessional and interprofessional perspective from an early stage onwards (Rossler & Kimble, 2016). Therefore, a relatively small but steadily growing number of health care educational institutions are modernizing their curricula to include IPE collaborative experiences. This happens in university-based medicine, nursing and allied health curricula (Olson & Bialocerkowski, 2014). IPE, often used interchangeably with multiprofessional education, is defined as educational initiatives that incorporate interactive learning methods between different professionals to foster collaborative practice (Hale, 2003). It has been recognized by the World Health Organization as an innovative strategy that can play an important role in mitigating global health workforce challenges (World Health Organization, 2010). However, most of the evidence so far comes from Anglophone OECD countries.

A number of key factors have been identified as crucial for the development of interprofessional education, namely: having a shared culture, support and leadership, strategic facilitation and planning, and effective feedback and evaluation of curriculum intent (Gum et al., 2012). In terms of the design of IPE courses or modules, there seems to be a trend to extend the format of didactic lectures to include other forms of education (Rossler & Kimble, 2016). High-fidelity human patient simulations and practice-based learning experiences have been argued to be more meaningful to students, as the links between IPE and interprofessional work become more apparent (Joseph et al., 2012). Findings showed that students had more positive attitudes about interprofessional learning following simulation and practice-based learning (Joseph et al., 2012; Rossler & Kimble, 2016).

There are a number of factors that limit the potential effectiveness of IPE. One of the main barriers to IPE is the logistical difficulty of coordinating academic calendars and student timetables (Hermann et al., 2016; O'Carroll, McSwiggan & Campbell, 2016). A possible solution for this, is to limit the contact teaching time and make more extensive use of other learning methods, such as self-directed learning and asynchronous e-learning (Holland et al., 2013). A related problem is the way in which schedules are devised. For example programmes operating under a credit hour ratio, may be limited in the number of hours that they can free up for IPE.

Also, deciding what to teach in the IPE module has proven to be a difficult task, especially as duplication of content must be avoided if students are to view the IPE experience as adding value to their education. In the development of an interdisciplinary curriculum for oncology palliative care education, for example, it was found that nursing, medicine, social work and chaplaincy had dramatically different views on the amount of content related to palliative care principles and teamwork (Hermann et al., 2016).

Finally, negative attitudes and uncertainty about the value of IPE, both among students and teaching staff, have repeatedly been reported (Hermann et al., 2016; O'Carroll, McSwiggan & Campbell, 2016). For staff, the problem is partly related to the fact that many health professionals had no exposure to IPE during their own training, and development of faculty members has been identified as a key factor supporting the success of IPE initiatives (Hall & Zierler, 2015).

A number of facilitating factors have also been identified that can positively influence views on IPE. Among others, it is advised to use vectors such as improving patient safety as the explicit IPE curriculum and teamwork as the implicit curriculum. In this way, students can be taught the importance of teamwork in ways that resonate with their professional goals. Also, it is important to develop information resource centres to support those teaching IPE (Hall & Zierler, 2015). The report by Frenk et al. (2010) also argued that adapted educational resources, such as syllabuses and didactic material, are needed to equip teachers to teach interprofessional care. Finally, it is clear that a substantial amount of resources should be devoted to facilitate coordination among the educators and curriculum developers, and that making attendance compulsory and developing flexible schedules can increase participation rates among students (World Health Organization, 2013). The main conclusion, however, is that evidence is poor overall, that the impact, if measured, is often small and that it is difficult to demonstrate the benefits of IPE, also for patients (Jackson et al., 2016).

Development of competency-based education

While a number of definitions of competency-based education exist, most explain it as an approach "in which the student demonstrates the attainment of certain learning outcomes prior to progressing in their course of study" (Gravina, 2017). The basic focus is on learning concrete skills rather than only abstract notions. Instead of courses or modules, individual skills and competencies are the single units of a training programme or education. The principles of competency-based education are that:

- students work on one competency at a time, which is a 'component' of a larger learning goal;
- students are evaluated on the individual competency and can only move on to other competencies after they have mastered the current skill being learned;
- students are able to skip learning modules on competencies if they demonstrate mastery by learning assessment or formative testing.

Competency-based education promotes flexibility in the time and sequence of what is to be learned, which is regulated by the needs of the learner. It is designed to allow an individualized learning process rather than the traditional one-size-fits-all curriculum (Murad et al., 2010). The uptake and diffusion of competency-based education are not only driven by the need to adapt to societal changes and changing health care needs, they also fit the existing need of health care professionals to extend their education and lifelong learning, in balance with their career and private life. For instance, competency-based education specifically enables nurses to attain their Bachelor's degree in nursing science at their own pace. Most nurses begin their career after graduation working full-time and find returning to school difficult because of time and financial constraints (Gravina, 2017) (see also the section below on Advanced practice).

Competency-based education and skill-mix interventions

In theory, competency-based education is well-suited to contribute to skill-mix innovations. Frenk et al. (2010) have noted that the adoption of competency-based curricula and the promotion of interprofessional education can break down professional silos and enhance collaboration in the field. However, while (core) competency-based education has the potential to typically support skill-mix relevant behaviour and hence skill-mix interventions, its implementation is confronted with obstacles. For example, in a review paper on orthopaedic trauma education in the USA, the United Kingdom and Canada, the authors illustrate this by noting that "moving towards competency-based frameworks will place emphasis on technical skills which are easy to assess and measure, while other essential abilities of a competent clinician, including professional judgement, compassion, communication and collaboration skills, may not be so easily defined and the tools to assess these skills are lacking" (Nousiainen et al., 2016). Another illustration is the example from the Netherlands, where curricula for medical specialists and nurses have become competency-based (Box 9.1).

Competency-based education and CanMEDS

Probably the best known example of competency-based learning in the medical domain is CanMEDS; a contraction of Canadian Medical Education Directives for Specialists. CanMEDS is an educational framework that "describes the abilities physicians require to effectively meet the health care needs of the people they serve" (Frank, Snell & Sherbino, 2015). The CanMEDS Framework defines professional values and competencies of medical experts in six intrinsic roles: communicator, collaborator, leader, health advocate, scholar and professional. Skill-mix-related competencies are specifically addressed in the collaborator role, such as:

- negotiate overlapping and shared responsibilities with physicians and other colleagues in the health care professions in episodic and ongoing care
- engage in respectful shared decision-making with physicians and other colleagues in the health care professions
- implement strategies to promote understanding, manage differences, and resolve conflicts in a manner that supports a collaborative culture
- determine when care should be transferred to another physician or health care professional.

While the CanMEDS approach and framework has been adopted in several high-income countries (in particular Anglophone countries and some European countries), studies of its effects on skill-mix innovation (teamwork, task-shifting and interprofessional collaboration) are

Box 9.1 Competency-based curricula in the Netherlands

Dutch health professional schools and specialist training institutes have thoroughly changed their curriculum and educational approach over the last years. The innovations in both medical specialist and nursing training clearly show that required skill-mix changes provide a more coordinating and **competency-based** role to the respective health professionals. Moreover, a number of competency areas defined in both curricula overlap.

A programme of modernization labelled *The medical specialist 2025* was initiated by the Dutch Federation of Medical Specialists (Federatie Medisch Specialisten, 2017). The programme implies individualization of training duration and a **competency-based** curriculum. This curriculum emphasizes interprofessional collaboration, patient safety, medical leadership, shared decision-making, substitution and efficiency. The programme clearly resonates with developments towards additional professional requirements such as flexibility of medical positions and roles, being open for substitution, changing hierarchies, patient orientation and team or group collaboration.

Likewise, the Dutch Nurses' Association developed its new strategic vision towards *Future-proof professions in nursing and caring* (Stuurgroep Verpleging & Verzorging 2020, 2015). Occupational profiles were redesigned and renamed. The general job title "nurse" was re-categorized into:

- Coordinating nurse (trained at higher vocational educational level)
- Basic nurse (trained at intermediate vocational educational level 4)
- Health care assistant (trained at intermediate vocational educational levels 1–3).

At the same time, a number of **competency** areas were defined for the coordinating nurse. These include support of self-management for patients/clients, their relatives and social network, initiating and developing quality systems, innovation, research and evidence-based professionalism, and coordinating the full-care processes for patients and clients into an interdisciplinary and integrated care provision. Because of the relative novelty of these curricular changes, no results can yet be reported on the implementation of the acquired competencies in practice, how they influence multiprofessional working and what wider health system outcomes have occurred.

scarce. In Canada, the effectiveness of a core-competency-based care of elderly diploma programme was evaluated by comparing it with a diploma programme based on learning objectives. The study showed that Family Medicine residents who followed the core-competency-based programme achieved significantly higher scores on the CanMEDS roles Communicator, Collaborator, Manager and Scholar (Charles et al., 2016). While other frameworks exist, such as the Accreditation Council for Graduate Medical Education framework (Educational Commission for Foreign Medical Graduates, 2019), there is great consistency between the frameworks, and their effects on skill-mix innovation are largely unknown.

Academization of health professions

A third trend that can be discerned, next to the development of interprofessional and competency-based education, is the upskilling and academization of health professions. Over recent decades, health professions in multiple countries have undergone a process of academization. For example, in Germany, a fast-paced development can be observed in terms of a growing number of graduate courses in the care sciences, with principal areas in nursing science and nursing education (Friedrichs & Schaub, 2011), although the share of nurses with a Bachelor degree is still low compared with most other countries in Europe. This evolution of advanced roles for nurses can be observed on a global scale. In many instances, the development of advanced roles occurred in parallel to other sociopolitical changes, such as the need for nursing unmet and more complex health issues, and as a response to the desire for a clinical career path for nurses, instead of only a managerial one (Lowe et al., 2012; O'Connor et al., 2018). Naturally, the academization of nurses and other health professionals has clear links to skill-mix innovations. It is a driver of new roles, leading to changes in the labour market. After all, professional groups are made up of a larger number of roles and job qualifications, which translate into different career paths (Friedrichs & Schaub, 2011). The other way around, (new) extended roles for nurses and other health professionals, such as pharmacists, are being used as a vehicle for academization (Giam, McLachlan & Krass, 2011). However, so far, it is not clear to what extent the academization of health professions contributes to the implementation of skill-mix innovations. This is partly due to the fact that academization often occurs in conjunction with other developments, such as the introduction of new professional roles or changes in curricula, which makes it difficult to separate the effects of the academization process itself.

Skill-mix implementation by postgraduate training, continuing professional development and competency-based frameworks

Adaptations in basic education alone will not be sufficient to respond to current skill gaps, changing skill needs and competencies. After all, skills and competencies needed in a certain job tend to change during the course of careers and may be different for people in the same profession. This becomes especially important when external factors are changing – such as demographic changes and changing demands from patients, clients, organizations and systems – but also in view of internal factors – such as intrinsic motivation of health workers to foster their career and personal development. Important trends in this regard are:

- developments in postgraduate training for advanced practice
- developments in continuing professional development
- developments in competency-based frameworks.

Developments in postgraduate training for advanced practice
The concept of advanced practice is particularly applied to nursing, but it is also a feature of other health care professions (Barton & Allan, 2015). Where health professionals take up new roles and tasks and engage in advanced practice, additional (postgraduate) training is often required to ensure that they are equipped to do so. However, it has been noted for a long time that this is not always the case. For example, both new pharmacy graduates and experienced pharmacists were found not to be always adequately prepared to perform the new roles that were expected of them by new pharmaceutical care models. These required pharmacists to collaborate with other health professionals, engage in problem solving and communicate through both oral and written reports (Schommer & Cable, 1996). Providing health professionals with the necessary education and training can prevent this and ensure that they are adequately prepared to perform new tasks and assume new roles

and responsibilities. However, additional courses are not always taken by professionals. For example in the United Kingdom, 20% of nurses with an advanced respiratory care role had not undertaken accredited training, and in Australia, similar findings were reported for nurses involved in chronic disease care (Dennis et al., 2009). This occurs even if robust education programmes are in place, for example within courses such as nonmedical prescribing (Barton & Allan, 2015; Maier & Buchan, 2018).

A number of persistent barriers have been reported, not only for nurses, but also for other health professionals to engage in advanced practice education. Time constraints, scheduling difficulties, costs and geographic accessibility are among the most often mentioned (Kovner et al., 2012; Salyers, 2005). Suggested solutions to remove these barriers include web-enhanced courses (instead of classroom-based learning), as it is likely that those who return to school will (partially) need to continue to work (Kovner et al., 2012; Salyers, 2005). At the same time, employers should also be supportive in allowing health professionals to have days off and flexible scheduling in order to follow advanced practice education. A proper arrangement of postgraduate education for advanced practice has been identified as a key trigger for effective advanced practice (Maier & Buchan, 2018). However, the degree of effectiveness that can be achieved is strongly related to the regulatory arrangements that are in place in a country. As explained in more detail in Chapters 11 and 12 of this volume, there is a need to address regulation, education and legislation in a co-ordinated manner to enable the introduction of advanced practice roles (Maier & Buchan, 2018).

Developments in continuing professional development

It has been stated that lessons learned during initial basic education are often out of date within 10 years of practice. Moreover, knowledge, skills and competencies are not static. Hence, it is important that structured learning continues to take place after graduation from initial education. This learning should be based on up-to-date knowledge and developments in health service delivery, including new tasks, roles and skill-mix innovations. Hence, continuing professional development (CPD) forms one of the most important educational tools when discussing the implementation of skill-mix interventions in health care practice. CPD refers to learning opportunities during the health professional's career (Langins & Borgermans, 2015) and includes:

- continuing medical education: generally used to designate continued professional education for physicians
- continued professional education: used to refer to continued professional education for other professionals
- setting-based in-service training: a brief learning opportunity that happens directly in the clinical setting during a health worker's work time.

In order to support skill-mix innovations, it has increasingly been argued that health professionals' education and training institutions should implement CPD and in-service training relevant to the evolving health care needs of their communities (World Health Organization, 2013). Health professionals should be provided with the necessary in-service training and development to support them in their constantly evolving roles. This positively influences the quality of care that is provided. For example, in Australia, it was found that specifically the exposure of nursing home staff to in-service training, one of the various measures of skill-mix, positively affected the quality of care (Pearson et al., 1992). In France, recent reforms have put CPD at the forefront of supporting interprofessional working and enabling skill-mix interventions (Box 9.2).

Box 9.2 Continuing professional development in health professions in France

For the past 20 years, France has followed a bumpy road of various arrangements for the CPD system intended for its 1.9 million health care professionals (Maisonneuve, 2014). In 2016, a new CPD system was put in place to respond to those challenges. Despite barriers and limits to the implementation of this new scheme and in the context of the launch of a health system reform, CPD has been identified as a potential driver for the development of new forms of collaboration and cooperation in primary care.

As in most countries, CPD in France is two-sided: it is grounded in the individual ethical duty of the health care professionals to maintain and develop their skills and competencies, but it is also thought of and used as a policy instrument to implement changes in health systems.

Box 9.2 (cont.)

In 2009, a mandatory CPD system extended to all health professions was established. However, the model of governance and regulation of CPD were not clarified until 2016, when legislation was introduced and the National Agency for CPD (*Agence Nationale du DPC*) was established, a public body that oversees the CPD system for all health professions at national level.

The new CPD system has yet to be fully rolled out and the implementation is meeting barriers of several types:

• there is still a lack of engagement and awareness among the majority of health professionals;
• at this stage, no compliance enforcement is in place;
• the professional organizations have yet to define frameworks of CPD within the specific scope of each profession or specialty that would allow the development of high-quality CPD curricula;
• there are still unsolved and heated debates on questions such as the respective roles of professional and public bodies in the governance of CPD.

Despite these difficulties, the establishment of a national governance body acting as single platform for all health professions has been an opportunity to raise awareness of the need to leverage collaboration between professions through CPD. In 2017, the *Haut Conseil du DPC* – an advisory body to the Agency that involves high-level stakeholders from the health care field, including professional councils, unions and learned societies – identified the promotion of interprofessional learning to sustain coordination of care as a strategic priority.

In 2018, the same imperative stemmed from another source: one of the key measures of the health system reform *Ma santé 2022* is the development of innovative and collaborative organizations in primary care. A clear mandate is given to the National Agency for CPD and its professional stakeholders to support this objective. A national programme on continuing interprofessional practice and education is now being devised. It includes direct commission of CPD programmes supporting skill-mix innovation in primary care. The National Agency for CPD will select and fund CPD programmes targeted at multiprofessional primary care teams or networks using team-based and interprofessional learning methodologies in order to improve coordination of care. Whether this programme will fulfil its promises and effectively support the development of skill-mix innovations is unknown, as no other comparable programme has been deployed as of this date. The effectiveness of the programme will be assessed by research teams.

Developments in competency-based frameworks for health professionals

So far, the focus on competency consolidation has mainly been limited to looking at the professional education of health professionals, that is, college- and university-based education where initial exposure to competencies takes place (Langins & Borgermans, 2015). Recently, efforts have been made to develop health workforce competency compilations that are more closely related to developments in health care practice. This is also recommended by WHO, who urges health professionals' education and training institutions to consider adapting curricula to population needs through defining the competencies that are required to meet the evolving needs of populations (World Health Organization, 2013). For example, compilations have been identified for disease-specific programmes such as sexual health in primary care (World Health Organization, 2011) and competencies for integrated behavioural health and primary care (Hoge, Pomerantz & Farley, 2014). In 2015, five clusters of health workforce competencies were developed to provide integrated care to people with multiple or complex health problems (Langins & Borgermans, 2015), namely: patient advocacy, effective communication, teamwork, people-centred care and continuous learning. In addition to the health workforce competency cluster itself, a number of tools were identified that can be helpful in establishing competency-based continuing professional development:

- engaging staff to develop and select priorities for CPD
- staff information boards that include reminders and teaching aids
- engaging professional associations to develop CPD and in-service training opportunities
- engaging patients and patient associations in CPD activities to ensure patient needs and perspectives are included
- learning plans designed between managers/clinical leaders and staff
- online quizzes and certification courses
- continuous medical education
- regular staff-led in-service training on relevant topics provided during working hours.

Skill-mix implementation by health workforce planning

Apart from the skills and competencies that the various health professionals (should) possess, a structural concern at the policy level is the matter of health workforce planning. Health workforce planning can (and should) take account of changes in the skills and competencies of health professionals, and assess in an integrated way the impact this has on health care delivery. In this way, health workforce planning can support policies for expanding or reducing student numbers and postgraduate training posts, to achieve an optimal balance between the required and available capacity of various health workers (Fraher & Brandt, 2019; Ono, Lafortune & Schoenstein, 2013).

Types of workforce projection models

Health workforce planning can be organized in many different ways and by many different models. As the main aim is to control so-called pork-cycles (that is unwarranted cyclical fluctuations of supply and demand), workforce projections play a central role in these models. Projection models can be supply-based, demand-based or needs-based (Batenburg, 2015; Kroezen, van Hoegaerden & Batenburg, 2018; Malgieri, Michelutti & Hoegaerden, 2015; Ono, Lafortune & Schoenstein, 2013; Roberfroid, Leonard & Stordeur, 2009).

Supply-based models are mainly designed to project the inflow and outflow of professionals, and optimize their replacement by increasing or decreasing training inflow to sustain the workforce at its current level. Supply-based models do not take changing health care demands into account. Hence, supply-based models have little relationship with skill-mix innovations. Demand-based models on the other hand do take into account changing health care demands. Demand-based models therefore seem to be preferred, but their application can also lead to overestimations of the required work-force capacity and hence an oversupply in training and employment (Birch et al., 2013).

The third type of projection models, needs-based models, aim to project supply and demand in parallel, taking as many trends at both sides of the labour market into account (Murphy, Birch & Mackenzie, 2007). These models require – next to demographic data about the patient and professional population – epidemiological data as well as data on sociocultural, sectoral, organizational and policy changes that influence the required and available supply of health workers in the near future. Currently, therefore, needs-based models seem most fit to take skill-mix innovations into account.

Obviously, needs-based models are more complex, require more data, higher data quality, as well as more assumptions to quantify the impact of sociocultural, sectoral, organizational and policy development (Ono, Lafortune & Schoenstein, 2013). One factor that draws a lot of attention in this regard is technology and its influence on the number of required health workers. Often, technological progress is included in projection models under the factor productivity growth (Ono, Lafortune & Schoenstein, 2013), assuming that technology will reduce the demand for health workers. However, it should be noted that the capacity effect of productivity growth (including technology) is actually an arbitrary assumption reflecting high uncertainty, as many other factors may be driving productivity growth in health care services as well (Cruz-Gomes et al., 2018).

The professional scope of health workforce policies and projection models

In relation to skills and competencies, health workforce policies and models differ in their professional scope. Traditionally, health workforce planning models are developed independently for each professional group, without taking into account possible (future) interactions between different health professionals (Fraher & Brandt, 2019; Kroezen, van Hoegaerden & Batenburg, 2018; Ono, Lafortune & Schoenstein, 2013). Moreover, most countries focus their planning models on doctors only and do not plan for other health professions (Maxtrix Insight Centre for Workforce Intelligence, 2012; Ono, Lafortune & Schoenstein, 2013). This focus can be understood from the so-called lead time to train health professionals, with doctors having the longest training time. Another important reason is that many countries are lacking the required information systems and data on the number of active health care workers, at least for those other than doctors, and their distribution in the health system (Kroezen, van Hoegaerden & Batenburg, 2018). Moreover, in some countries, not all health professionals are regulated. For example in England and Finland, advanced practice nurses are not specifically regulated – although nurse prescribers are – (Maier et al., 2018) and in Ireland, Malta and the United Kingdom, health care assistants are not regulated (Kroezen et al., 2018). Hence, where registration or regulation data are to be used as source of planning data, routine data are not available or not complete (Maier et al., 2018).

The advantage of planning professions in silo is that for each occupation, the training inflow is optimally forecasted and the profession-specific conditions are taken into account. The disadvantage, however, is that interprofessional collaboration, education and task shifting can only be partially captured in planning. Moreover, where only physicians are being planned, skill-mix innovations can hardly be taken sufficiently into account in health workforce policies and models. For example, if the skill-mix innovation is for nurse practitioners to take up additional medical tasks, planning should be aimed at having a sufficient capacity of nurse practitioners in the pipeline to perform the increasing number of tasks that is required of them (Maier et al., 2018). This requires data and a planning model on nurse practitioners. This also applies the other way around; planning systems should also ensure that fewer of the professionals who see their role decreasing as a result of skill-mix innovations are being trained, to prevent an oversupply. So far, this is not the case.

From silo to multiprofessional health workforce planning
In a context of changing patient needs and increased interprofessional work and task substitution, the current silo approach to health workforce planning hampers the possibility of analysing health workforce requirements in a more integrated way, taking into account possible new roles and responsibilities of different providers (Fraher & Brandt, 2019). In an overview of 26 health workforce planning models in 18 OECD countries, only five countries were found to have multiprofessional workforce projection models in place: the Netherlands, Norway, Switzerland, Japan and the USA (Maier et al., 2018; Ono, Lafortune & Schoenstein, 2013). The level of integration in these models varies. Models with an intermediate level of integration look at the demand for different providers by taking into account some possible task sharing and substitutions between different providers, such as the models in the Netherlands and Switzerland. Models with a higher level of integration require that the current and possible future demand and supply of different providers are taken more fully into account, based on alternative scenarios on the demand side and on the supply side. The overview by the OECD did not identify any model that already reached such a high level of integration, but mentioned that one of the models from the USA moved in that direction (Ono, Lafortune & Schoenstein, 2013).

There are hardly any studies that describe the integration of skill-mix changes into health workforce planning, or integrated health workforce planning. A recent study, one of the few on this topic, found that out of eight participating countries that have introduced the new professional roles of nurse practitioners and physician assistants, only three included these professions partially or fully in their health workforce projections. Canada, the Netherlands and the USA did so, with Canada testing new projection methods while the Netherlands and the USA fully integrated nurse practitioners and physician assistants in their planning system. Results from these two last countries showed that this can result in considerable differences in the projected numbers of GPs or medical specialists required in the future. Hence, this suggests that physician-only models are likely to overestimate the number of required physicians (Maier et al., 2018).

9.4   Conclusions

In this chapter, we described how education and health workforce planning models are responding to meet the changing skill demands, competencies and identified skill gaps in the health workforce, and thereby support the design and implementation of effective skill-mix interventions. We did so by discussing strategies, frameworks and tools that can be found in the fields of (i) basic professional education of health professionals, (ii) postgraduate training and continuing professional development, and (iii) health workforce planning systems. Naturally, all of these fields are strongly interconnected.

Basic professional education

Interprofessional education and competency-based education are being introduced in a relatively small but steadily growing number of health care educational institutions, mostly in Anglophone countries and some European countries. The aim of these forms of education is to train new generations that are oriented towards multiprofessional education in open, adaptive and collaborative cultures. However, studies on the effect of these new types of education on skill-mix innovations are scarce, as was also shown by the results from the overview of reviews. Another trend visible in basic education is the academization process taking place in several professions, most notably nursing. As of now, however, empirical studies are still lacking to show how and to what extent the academization of health professions contributes to the implementation of skill-mix innovations.

Postgraduate training, continuing professional development and competency-based frameworks

Additional (postgraduate) training is often required for health professionals to take up new roles and tasks. However, this training is not always followed or completed. Identified barriers include time constraints, scheduling difficulties, costs and geographic accessibility. The introduction of web-enhanced courses (instead of classroom-based learning) may be a solution to overcome some of these barriers, as are supportive attitudes by employers, by allowing health professionals days off and flexible scheduling. As knowledge, skills and competencies are not static, CPD and in-service training (with relevance to the evolving health care needs of communities) were identified as other educational tools with high relevance to skill-mix innovations. An example of this can be found in France, where CPD has been at the forefront of supporting interprofessional working and enabling skill-mix interventions. A final trend that could be discerned is the introduction of competency frameworks for the HWF, which can be more closely related to developments in health care practice and hence can bridge the skills gap between education and practice.

Health workforce planning

The way in which health workforce policies and planning systems are organized, reflects the way in which (and extent to which) changes in the skills and competencies of health professionals (as well as their impact on health care delivery) can be taken into account. Differences can be found in the type of projection model in place and in the professional scope of these models. Supply-based projection models do not take changing health care demands into account and have the least connection to skill-mix innovations. Needs-based models on the other hand include both supply and demand trends, and are therefore most fit to take skill-mix innovations into account. In the majority of countries, health workforce planning models are developed independently for each professional group, without taking into account possible (future) interactions between different health professionals. Most countries focus their planning models on doctors only and do not plan for other health professions, which are often important actors in skill-mix innovations. An important barrier in this regard is the lack of available data, complicated by the fact that not all professions are regulated in all countries. As a result, in most planning models, interprofessional collaboration, education and task shifting can only be partially captured. Multiprofessional health workforce planning is attempted in a small number of countries, but so far the level of integration is limited and there are hardly any studies on the effectiveness in terms of skill-mix innovation.

Identified trends, effects and the future

This chapter shows that to effectively implement skill-mix interventions in health care practice, basic and postgraduate education and health workforce planning systems are essential and closely interlinked vehicles. A number of trends were identified in these areas. Some of the trends take place on a larger scale, such as the academization of nursing, whereas most others are relatively smaller and younger, such as the introduction of interprofessional learning. For all trends, it can be concluded that evidence about the effectiveness from the point of view of skill-mix innovations is still lacking. This is partly due to a lack of studies on this subject (see also the limited results that came out of the overview of reviews on education and health workforce planning), but also to the difficulty in demonstrating a causal effect. After all, there are many confounding factors that influence the relationship between educational systems, health workforce planning systems and skill-mix innovations.

As many countries are re-organizing the way health services are provided by new professional roles, task substitution and increased interprofessional working, it is safe to say that educational institutions in many countries will have to strengthen health professionals' competencies. This can be done by revising and updating curricula on a regular basis, and increasing the competencies of existing staff (World Health Organization, 2013). Moreover, in view of the skill-mix changes taking place in health care practice, health workforce planning systems should incorporate these changes and adapt their projections based on current and future skill-mix changes in the health workforce. To achieve the full potential of skill-mix interventions as well as education innovations, planning systems should therefore include more professions in their models and broaden the silo planning approach. However, changes in educational and planning systems will not deliver quick wins. There can be a significant time lag before the innovations in basic professional education show effect, which also applies for health workforce planning, in particular when it is institutionalized in health systems.

References

Andrew A (1988). The system of professions: an essay on the division of expert labor. Chicago, University of Chicago Press.

Barton TD, Allan D (2015). Advanced nursing practice: changing healthcare in a changing world. London, Macmillan International Higher Education.

Batenburg R (2015). Health workforce planning in Europe: creating learning country clusters. Health Policy, 119:1537–1544.

Birch S, Mason T, Sutton M et al. (2013). Not enough doctors or not enough needs? Refocusing health workforce planning from providers and services to populations and needs. J Health Serv Res Policy, 18:107–113.

Charles L, Triscott J, Dobbs B et al. (2016). Effectiveness of a core-competency-based program on residents' learning and experience. Can Geriat J, 19:50–57.

Cruz-Gomes S, Amorim-Lopes M, Almada-Lobo B (2018). A labor requirements function for sizing the health workforce. Hum Resour Health, 16:67.

De Bont A, Van Exel J, Coretti S et al. (2016). Reconfiguring health workforce: a case-based comparative study explaining the increasingly diverse professional roles in Europe. Bmc Health Serv Res, 16:637.

Delamaire M-L, Lafortune G (2010). Nurses in advanced roles. OECD Health Working Papers. Paris, OECD.

Dennis S, May J, Perkins D et al. (2009). What evidence is there to support skill mix changes between GPs, pharmacists and practice nurses in the care of elderly people living in the community? Aust NZ Health Policy, 6:23.

Dussault G, Buchan J (2018). Noncommunicable diseases and human resources for health: a workforce fit for purpose. In: Jakab M, Farrington J, Borgermans L et al. (eds) Health systems respond to NCDs: time for ambition. Copenhagen, WHO Regional Office for Europe; 182–199.

Educational Commission For Foreign Medical Graduates (2019). Acgme Core Competencies [Online]. (http://Www.Ecfmg.Org/Echo/Acgme-Core-Competencies.html, accessed 2 May 2019).

Federatie Medisch Specialisten (2017). Visiedocument Medisch Specialist 2025 Ambitie, Vertrouwen, Samenwerken [Vision Document Medical Specialist 2025 Ambition, Trust, Cooperation]. Utrecht, Federatie Medisch Specialisten.

Fraher E, Brandt B (2019). Toward a system where workforce planning and interprofessional practice and education are designed around patients and populations not professions. J Interprof Care, 33:389–397.

Frank J, Snell L, Sherbino J (2015). Canmeds 2015 physician competency framework. Ottawa, Royal College of Physicians and Surgeons of Canada.

Frenk J, Chen L, Bhutta ZA et al. (2010). Health professionals for a new century: transforming education to strengthen health systems in an interdependent world. Lancet, 376:1923–1958.

Friedrichs A, Schaub H-A (2011). Academisation of the health professions – achievements and future prospects. GMS Z Med Ausbild. 28(4):Doc50. DOI: 10.3205/zma000762, URN: urn:nbn:de:0183-zma0007625.

Giam JA, Mclachlan AJ, Krass I (2011). Community pharmacy compounding – impact on professional status. Int J Clin Pharm, 33:177–182.

Gravina EW (2017). Competency-based education and its effect on nursing education: a literature review. Teaching Learning Nurs, 12:117–121.

Gum LF, Richards J, Bradley SL et al. (2012). Preparing interprofessional clinical learning sites: what the literature tells us. Focus Health Prof Educ: Multi-Disc J, 13:55.

Hale C (2003). Interprofessional education: the way to a successful workforce? Br J Ther Rehab, 10:122–127.

Hall LW, Zierler BK (2015). Interprofessional education and practice guide no. 1: developing faculty to effectively facilitate interprofessional education. J Interprof Care 29:3–7.

Hermann CP, Head BA, Black K et al. (2016). Preparing nursing students for interprofessional practice: the interdisciplinary curriculum for oncology palliative care education. J Prof Nurs, 32:62–71.

Hoge MA, Pomerantz A, Farley T (2014). Core competencies for integrated behavioural health and primary care. Washington, Samhsa – HRSA Centre For Integrated Health Solutions.

Holland C, Bench S, Brown K et al. (2013). Interprofessional working in acute care. Clin Teacher, 10:107–112.

Jackson M, Pelone F, Reeves S et al. (2016). Interprofessional education in the care of people diagnosed with dementia and their carers: a systematic review. BMJ Open, 6:E010948.

Joseph S, Diack L, Garton F et al. (2012). Interprofessional education in practice. Clin Teacher, 9:27–31.

Kovner CT, Brewer C, Katigbak C et al. (2012). Charting the course for nurses' achievement of higher education levels. J Prof Nurs, 28:333–343.

Kroezen M, Van Hoegaerden M, Batenburg R (2018). The joint action on health workforce planning and forecasting: results of a European programme to improve health workforce policies. Health Policy, 122:87–93.

Kroezen M, Van Dijk L, Groenewegen PP et al. (2013). Knowledge claims, jurisdictional control and professional status: the case of nurse prescribing. PLOS One, 8:E77279.

Kroezen M, Dussault G, Craveiro I et al. (2015). Recruitment and retention of health professionals across Europe: a literature review and multiple case study research. Health Policy 119:1517–1528.

Kroezen M, Schäfer W, Sermeus W et al. (2018). Healthcare assistants in EU member states: an overview. Health Policy, 122:1109–1117.

Kuhlmann E, Larsen C (2015). Why we need multi-level health workforce governance: case studies from nursing and medicine in Germany. Health Policy, 119:1636–1644.

Langins M, Borgermans L (2015). Strengthening a competent health workforce for the provision of coordinated/integrated health services. Working Paper. Copenhagen, WHO Regional Office For Europe.

Lowe G, Plummer V, O'Brien AP et al. (2012). Time to clarify – the value of advanced practice nursing roles in health care. J Advanc Nurs, 68:677–685.

Maier CB, Buchan J (2018). Integrating nurses in advanced roles in health systems to address the growing burden of chronic conditions. Eurohealth, 24:24–27.

Maier CB, Batenburg R, Birch S et al. (2018). Health workforce planning: which countries include nurse practitioners and physician assistants and to what effect? Health Policy.

Maisonneuve H (2014). How France messed up CPD/CME for healthcare professionals. BMJ, 349:g6171.

Malgieri A, Michelutti P, Hoegaerden M (2015). Handbook On Health Workforce Planning Methodologies Across EU Countries. Joint Action On Health Workforce Planning And Forecasting. Bratislava, Ministry of Health of Slovak Republic.

Matrix Insight Centre For Workforce Intelligence (2012). EU level collaboration on forecasting health workforce needs, workforce planning and health workforce trends – a feasibility study. Brussels, European Commission.

Murad MH, Coto-Yglesias F, Varkey P et al. (2010). The effectiveness of self-directed learning in health professions education: a systematic review. Med Educ, 44:1057–1068.

Murphy GT, Birch S, Mackenzie A (2007). Needs-based health human resources planning: the challenge of linking needs to provider requirements. Ottawa, Canadian Nurses Association.

Nousiainen M, McQueen SA, Hall J et al. (2016). Resident education in orthopaedic trauma. Bone Joint J, 98-B:1320–1325.

O'Carroll V, McSwiggan L, Campbell M (2016). Health and social care professionals' attitudes to interprofessional working and interprofessional education: a literature review. J Interprof Care, 30:42–49.

O'Connor S, Deaton C, Nolan F et al. (2018). Nursing in an age of multimorbidity. BMC Nursing, 17:49.

OECD (2016). Health workforce policies in OECD countries – right jobs, right skills, right places. Paris, OECD Publishing.

OECD Health Division Team (2018). Feasibility study on health workforce skills assessment: supporting health workers achieve person-centred care. Paris, OECD.

Olson R, Bialocerkowski A (2014). Interprofessional education in allied health: a systematic review. Med Educ, 48:236–246.

Ono T, Lafortune G, Schoenstein M (2013). Health workforce planning in OECD Countries: a review of 26 projection models from 18 countries. OECD Health Working Papers, No. 62. Paris, OECD Publishing. (https://doi-org.eur.idm.oclc.org/10.1787/5k44t787zcwb-en).

Pearson A, Hocking S, Mott S, Riggs A (1992). Skills mix in Australian nursing homes. J Adv Nurs, 17:767–776.

Reeves S, Perrier L, Goldman J et al. (2013). Interprofessional education: effects on professional practice and healthcare outcomes (update). Cochrane Database Syst Rev, 3.

Roberfroid D, Leonard C, Stordeur S (2009). Physician supply forecast: better than peering in a crystal ball? Hum Res Health, 7:10.

Rossler KL, Kimble LP (2016). Capturing readiness to learn and collaboration as explored with an interprofessional simulation scenario: a mixed-methods research study. Nurse Educ Today, 36:348–353.

Salyers VL (2005). Web-enhanced and face-to-face classroom instructional methods: effects on course outcomes and student satisfaction. Int J Nurs Educ Scholarship, 2.

Scheffler RM, Campbell J, Cometto G et al. (2018). Forecasting imbalances in the global health labor market and devising policy responses. Hum Resour Health, 16:5.

Schoenstein M, Ono T, Lafortune G (2016). Skills use and skills mismatch in the health sector: what do we know and what can be done. In: Lafortune G, Moreira L, eds. Health workforce policies in OECD countries: right jobs, right skills, right places. OECD Health Policy Studies. Paris, OECD Publishing.

Schommer JC, Cable GL (1996). Current status of pharmaceutical care practice: strategies for education. Am J Pharm Educ, 60:36–41.

Stuurgroep Verpleging & Verzorging 2020 (2015). Toekomstbestendige beroepen in de verpleging en verzorging rapport stuurgroep over de beroepsprofielen en de overgangsregeling [Future-proof professions in nursing and caring. steering committee report on the professional profiles and the transitional arrangement]. Utrecht, Verpleegkundigen & Verzorgenden Nederland.

World Health Organization (2010). Framework for action on interprofessional education & collaborative practice. Geneva, World Health Organization.

World Health Organization (2011). Sexual and reproductive health core competencies in primary care: attitudes, knowledge, ethics, human rights, leadership, management, teamwork, community work, education, counselling, clinical settings, service, provision. Geneva, World Health Organization.

World Health Organization (2013). Transforming and scaling up health professionals' education and training: World Health Organization Guidelines 2013. Geneva, World Health Organization.

10 | Implementing skill-mix innovations: role of policy and financing

GIADA SCARPETTI, CLAUDIA B. MAIER,
HANNAH BUDDE, DHEEPA RAJAN, ERICA
RICHARDSON, WALTER SERMEUS

10.1 Introduction

This chapter analyses the role of policies and financing and their implications for the uptake of skill-mix changes in routine care. In particular, it addresses if and how regulatory or nonregulatory policies can facilitate the skill-mix innovation shift (and so act as a facilitator) or rather hinder the shift from taking place (and so act as a barrier). Further, this chapter addresses the role of financing and payment policies and identifies related common barriers and facilitators to skill-mix reforms. The chapter first presents the evidence from the overview of reviews, and then complements these findings by presenting trends and country examples from different sources.

According to the WHO, health policy refers to "decisions, plans, and actions that are undertaken to achieve specific health care goals within a society" (WHO website, n.d). Effective health policy is based on a vision, specific aims or targets, it involves stakeholders and the wider public and sets out an implementation plan to steer change.

When it comes to implementing skill-mix changes, there are several governance instruments that countries can consider in the process. These include policies and strategies, changes to regulation and nonregulatory mechanisms. Establishing specific policies on the health workforce or skill-mix can range from broad, comprehensive health workforce policies (for example, strengthening the primary care workforce in a country) to specific skill-mix policies or strategies (for example, policies on scopes-of-practice). With regard to health professionals and skill-mix, regulation is described as legally binding policy instruments, which limit entry to a profession or a practice (Maier, Aiken & Busse, 2017). The government itself can take charge of regulatory mechanisms, or it may delegate them to a professional body or association in accordance with set laws, thereby resulting in self-regulation (Baron, 2015; Bauchner, Fontanarosa & Thompson 2015; Maier, 2015).

Health financing refers to the "function of a health system concerned with the mobilization, accumulation and allocation of money to cover the health needs of the people" (WHO, 2000). Further, reimbursement for health services includes a number of payment mechanisms, for example fee-for-service, capitation, salary and global budget. In this chapter, the literature will be summarized as to the impact of financing and payment policies on the implementation of skill-mix reforms. To the extent possible, it will also address if and which countries have made available additional financial resources, such as start-up funding and financial incentives for skill-mix and outcomes (Struckmann et al., 2016).

10.2   Review of the evidence

Characteristics of included reviews

The overview of systematic reviews, the methodology of which is described in Chapter 1, resulted in seven articles which fit the inclusion criteria. The reviews were largely qualitative in nature, with a focus on Anglophone countries and Western Europe. Only two reviews specifically addressed health policy per se, whereas the other reviews covered health policy and other influencing contextual drivers, which limits the generalizability of the findings. Most reviews addressed several barriers and facilitators, of which some were of policy relevance. Several articles focused on challenges to skill-mix changes, rendering the conclusions skewed towards elements acting as potential barriers rather than potential facilitators to policy implementation.

One systematic review focused on pharmacists in expanded roles (Farris et al., 2010), two on nurses in expanded roles (Joo & Huber, 2017; Kroezen et al., 2011), one on midwives (Colvin et al., 2013), and one on task shifting from specialist physicians to primary care providers for HIV/AIDS services (Mapp, Hutchinson & Estcourt, 2015). Moreover, two reviews focused on multiprofessional, team-based care (Carter et al., 2016; Karam et al., 2018). An overview of the included systematic reviews is provided in Table 10.1.

Evidence on impact of policy interventions on skill-mix innovation

Four main themes emerged from the overview of reviews with regards to barriers and facilitators for policy implementation: (i) policies, laws

Table 10.1 *Characteristics of the seven systematic reviews on policy related to implementation*

Authors	Year	Skill-mix intervention	Description of intervention	Country coverage	No. of included studies
Farris et al.	2010	Pharmacists expanding their role in sexual and reproductive health services	Systematic review of the empirical literature focusing on US pharmacist practices in reducing unintended pregnancy	USA	38
Kroezen et al.	2011	Nurses taking on a prescribing role	124 documents (75 from the UK) examining views of nurses, doctors and other parties on nurse prescribing	UK, USA, NZ, NL, IE, SE, CA, AU	124
Joo & Huber	2017	Nurses becoming case managers	10 qualitative studies on barriers perceived by nurse case managers when implementing case management	USA, SE, UK, AU, DK, BE	10
Colvin et al.	2013	Task shifting to and from midwives	37 qualitative studies on task shifting between midwives and other health workers/other birth attendants/community-based health volunteers	AU, CA, USA, SE, UK, AO, DO, GT, JO, KE, ID, MX, ZA	37
Mapp et al.	2015	HIV care partly shifting from specialist to primary care providers	8 studies detailing 9 models of shared care from 5 countries	AU, CH, DE, CA, UK	8
Carter et al.	2016	Team-based primary care provider practices	14 studies looking at primary care reform towards team-based practices in Canada with its effects on (i) health service utilization (ii) processes of care, (iii) physician costs and productivity	CA	14
Karam et al.	2018	Interprofessional/interorganizational collaboration with emphasis on nurses	16 qualitative studies describing a conceptual framework of interprofessional or interorganizational collaboration in health care	USA, UK, DE, CA	16

Country abbreviations: AO: Angola; AU: Australia; BE: Belgium; CA: Canada; CH: Switzerland; DE: Germany; DK: Denmark; DO: Dominican Republic; GT: Guatemala; IE: Ireland; ID: Indonesia; JO: Jordan; KE: Kenya; MX: Mexico; NL: the Netherlands; NZ: New Zealand; SE: Sweden; UK: the United Kingdom; USA: the United States of America; ZA: South Africa.

Sources: Carter et al. (2016); Colvin et al. (2013); Farris et al. (2010); Joo & Huber (2017); Karam et al. (2018); Kroezen et al. (2011); Mapp, Hutchinson & Estcourt (2015).

and policy frameworks; (ii) professional regulation linked with education; (iii) professional legal and liability issues, and (iv) policy context
and political force field. Additionally, some systematic reviews covered
aspects of payment mechanisms. Table 10.2 provides an overview on
the evidence about barriers and facilitators covered in the systematic
reviews structured according to policy-related and financing/payment-
related factors.

Theme 1: Policies, laws and policy frameworks

Despite country differences concerning legislative approaches, a clear
policy and legal framework for new mix of health professional skills
was cited in several reviews as facilitator to successful skill-mix implementation and as barrier, if not in place, or insufficiently in place (Farris
et al., 2010; Joo & Huber, 2017; Karam et al., 2018; Kroezen et al.,
2011) (see Table 10.2). If scope-of-practice laws did not take account
of skill-mix changes, this was identified as an important bottleneck for
implementation.

Farris et al. (2010) deplored the legal ambiguity for pharmacists to
provide contraceptive counselling in several states in the USA where
conscience clauses existed alongside patient rights legislation to access
medication. They unequivocally stated that this controversy should be
addressed through profession-targeted policy statements and in public
in order to enable pharmacists to use their health counselling skills to
increase patient access to sexual health services.

Kroezen et al. (2011) assessed nurse prescribing in Anglophone
countries and showed that in those countries where nurse prescribing
was introduced, there have often been (initial) legal restrictions on the
new task, acting as barriers to implementation. After changes to laws
and bylaws in line with the new prescribing skills of nurses, these barriers were transformed into enablers. Moreover, limited formularies as
well as restrictions on the types of patients that nurses are allowed to
prescribe to were barriers to implementation. Several Australian and US
states, Canada and the Netherlands have used protocols to enable nurse
prescribing. Similarly, Joo & Huber (2017) identified unclear scopes-
of-practice as an important barrier for nurses to perform effective case
management roles. Examples were uncertainty over the official tasks
and responsibilities due to the nonregulation of the scope-of-practice,
with implications for role clarity, the case managers' identity and

Table 10.2 *Overview of the evidence on policy implementation barriers and facilitators on skill-mix innovation*

Innovation	Countries	Barriers	Facilitators
Pharmacists in expanded roles (Farris et al., 2010)	USA	**Policy:** • Lack of adequate training • Lack of clarity on liability issue • Lack around the issue of conscience clauses and right to access legal medications reflecting political and public controversy, which needs to be addressed in policy and public arena **Financing:** • Lack of reimbursement model	**Policy:** • To improve access and enable pharmacies to provide emergency contraceptives requires working together with state programmes • State-regulated collaborative practice agreements authorizing pharmacists to initiate and modify medication therapy **Financing:** • Partnerships with payers through coalitions of pharmacists, pharmacy organizations and faculties • Pharmacist reimbursement must be sufficient to meet time, costs and liability, and payment needs to go beyond contraceptive product
Nurse prescribing (Kroezen et al., 2011)	UK, US, NZ, NL, IE, SE, CA, AU	**Policy:** • Restrictions on the types of patients nurses can prescribe for • In Australia, Spain and the USA, professional medical organizations have mainly opposed nurse prescribing, explaining limited prescribing rights **Financing:** • Lack of payers covering nurse prescriptions in some US states	**Policy:** • Formal responsibilities and accountabilities were widely used to establish clarity around the issue of liability • Prescriptive authority for nurses in Canada, New Zealand and the USA followed the development of advanced practice nurse roles, which clearly connects their prescribing privileges with internal developments within the nursing profession • The aim of task reallocation in the health care sector and more particularly the undesirable situation in which nurses prescribe medicines on an illegal basis, have been the main driving force behind the introduction of nurse prescribing in the Netherlands

Table 10.2 *(cont.)*

Innovation	Countries	Barriers	Facilitators
Nurses as case managers (Joo & Huber, 2017)	US, SE, UK, AU, DK, BE	Policy: • Unclear scope and boundaries of practice • Lack of clarity around the role of case managers • Lack of training, education and adequate skills • Challenges by contractual requirements • Influence of policies on case manager's practice	Policy: • Clear practical guidelines with role clarification need to be provided by policy-makers • Practical training consistent with the case manager role
Task shifting (to/ from midwives) (Colvin et al., 2013)	AU, CA, USA, SE, UK, AO, DO, GT, JO, KE, ID, MX, ZA	Policy: • Midwives in one study who were not used to working in a team were slow to build trust, especially when individual versus group liability was unclear • Lack of adequate training and educational preparation for midwives • Unclear regulatory framework and policies for midwifery care and fear around liability • Pressure from medical professionals for midwives to do either more or less than the law allows • Lack of specificity around the role of midwives in nursing policies • Ambivalent role clarification between midwives and traditional birth attendants	Policy: • Ongoing training, support and clinical supervision critical for the effectiveness of task shifting

Task shifting (from specialist to GP care for HIV) (Mapp et al., 2015)	AU, CH, DE, CA, UK	Policy: • Maintaining the skill set of the clinical workforce as a potential threat to the long-term feasibility of shared care • Vulnerable political situation challenging the long-term feasibility of shared care Financing: • Funding and financially unsustainable programmes were a significant issue for services Policy: • Small professional networks facilitated to coordinate care effectively and to build relationships • Adequate training
Team-based primary care provider practices (Carter et al., 2016)	CA	Policy: • Clear definition of roles, processes and activities intended by the changes need to be provided by policy-makers and researchers to inform future efforts Financing: • Blended capitation instead of enhanced fee-for-service may be favourable for team-based services • Concerning pay-for-performance incentives, a reward system that avoids incentive for patient risk selection by physicians needs to be considered

Table 10.2 *(cont.)*

Innovation	Countries	Barriers	Facilitators
Interprofessional/ interorganizational collaboration (Karam et al., 2018)	USA, UK, DE, CA	**Policy:** • Lack of clarification of one's own professional role and those of others as a significant barrier to interorganizational collaboration • Broader cultural, political, social and economic issues frame collaboration: private health care systems with high competition for profit, financial limitations and lack of reimbursement and the image of a profession can be a barrier to interprofessional collaboration • Power struggles between professions and confusion due to lack of role clarification • Infrastructural arrangements including governance structure, resources and information management systems **Financing:** • Fee-per-service payment as barrier to collaboration	**Policy:** • Professional role and responsibility clarification, definition of task characteristics and practice parameters • Formalizing collaboration through policies and procedures • Formalization and professional role clarification are more difficult to achieve in interprofessional collaboration than in interorganizational collaboration and need to receive more attention when planning or implementing interorganizational collaboration • For interprofessional collaboration, professional roles and the scope of practice should be clearly understood including clinical paradigms, education and training as well as of their own limitations • Adequate resource allocation, education and training • A formal collaborative leadership as a decision-making authority for interprofessional collaboration

Country abbreviations: AO: Angola; AU: Australia; BE: Belgium; CA: Canada; CH: Switzerland; DE: Germany; DK: Denmark; DO: Dominican Republic; GT: Guatemala; IE: Ireland; ID: Indonesia; JO: Jordan; KE: Kenya; MX: Mexico; NL: the Netherlands; NZ: New Zealand; SE: Sweden; UK: the United Kingdom; USA: the United States of America; ZA: South Africa.

Sources: Carter et al. (2016); Colvin et al. (2013); Farris et al. (2010); Joo & Huber (2017); Karam et al. (2018); Kroezen et al. (2011); Mapp, Hutchinson & Estcourt (2015).

boundaries compared with other professions. Likewise, Karam et al. (2018) suggested to overcome the unclear legal ground on which health professionals who have re-skilled sometimes practice and to clarify the scope-of-practice of each actor and organization in a collaboration through formal legal instruments. They suggested that formalization of roles and scopes-of-practice of individuals is particularly crucial for interorganizational collaboration and needs to receive more attention from policy-makers.

Regulation can be a facilitator to role clarification. Joo & Huber (2017) in their examination, mainly of nurses taking on a new case manager job, noted that several of the studies they reviewed confirmed that case managers "struggled because there was lack of clarity over [...] roles". The need for clear tasks, roles and responsibilities as well as clear regulatory and accountability frameworks seemed to be especially critical due to the novel nature of the case manager role for many, both for those taking on the new roles and those collaborating with them. Hence, the authors suggested that a clear policy or practical guideline clarifying the roles should be provided by policy-makers. Similarly, Carter et al. (2016), Colvin et al. (2013) and Karam et al. (2018) also identify a clear definition and understanding of roles, tasks and scopes-of-practice as an important measure to enable skill-mix changes (see Table 10.2).

Theme 2: Professional regulation and education

Four of the reviews demonstrated from a policy perspective the importance of training and educational preparation for the implementation of skill-mix changes (Colvin et al., 2013; Farris et al., 2010; Joo & Huber, 2017; Mapp, Hutchinson & Estcourt, 2015) (see Table 10.2). The lack of adequate training, education and skills for pharmacists to provide emergency contraception (Farris et al., 2010), for task shifting to/from midwives (Colvin et al., 2013) and for nurses as case managers (Joo & Huber, 2017) was considered an important barrier. Colvin et al. (2013) indicated that midwives were reluctant to undertake complex tasks for which they had received limited training. Mapp, Hutchinson & Estcourt (2015) considered maintaining the skill set of the clinical workforce as a potential threat to long-term feasibility of shared HIV care. Case managers in Joo & Huber (2017) reported insufficient training as a main barrier wherein nurses did not receive the practical training that was consistent with their case manager role. Hence, adequate training and education were suggested as enabling factors for skill-mix interventions (Joo & Huber, 2017; Karam et al., 2018; Mapp, Hutchinson & Estcourt, 2015) (see Table 10.2). Legal and non-regulatory policies can support this process, for instance through the regulation of professions or roles and their education to ensure minimum educational standards.

When it comes to implementing skill-mix changes, it is important to align the education standards within and across the professions undertaking these new roles (see also Chapter 9). Policy processes and (minimum) regulation of education can support that process.

Theme 3: Legal and liability issues

Concerns around liability were also reported as a barrier to implementation (see Table 10.2) (Colvin et al., 2013; Farris et al., 2010; Kroezen et al., 2011). Colvin et al. (2013) refer to a lack of clarification in job descriptions, policy and legal frameworks. The authors underscored the fear of liability, which hindered health professionals from accepting new tasks. In addition, unclear individual versus group liability interfered negatively with relationship building and trust between health workers. The fear of liability stemmed from a blurry regulatory and legal environment where criteria for undertaking or not undertaking certain tasks were ambiguous and clear accountability frameworks were missing. In the case of nurse prescribing, Kroezen et al. (2011) showed that formal responsibilities and accountabilities were widely used to establish clarity around the issue of liability.

The review by Karam et al. (2018) suggested clarification of the scope-of-practice of each actor and organization through formal legal channels. While the reviews suggested the need to clarify liability and jurisdictional accountability when implementing skill-mix changes, they remained vague on the policy options of how to achieve this in practice.

Theme 4: Policy context and political forcefield

The policy contexts are highly country-specific and influence implementation as does the political forcefield in which policy-making occurs. Two systematic reviews (see Table 10.2) pointed out the influence of broader political environments on implementation (Karam et al., 2018; Mapp, Hutchinson & Estcourt, 2015). For instance, a vulnerable political situation can challenge the long-term feasibility of the implementation of a skill-mix project, for example, shared care arrangements (Mapp, Hutchinson & Estcourt 2015). Moreover, the broader political contexts such as the governance structure next to cultural and economic issues were considered critical to the uptake of skill-mix changes (Karam et al., 2018).

One review (Karam et al., 2018) brought to the fore the dilemma of skill-mix interventions shaking up the established interprofessional hierarchy and power relations, reinforcing preconceived notions of each other's abilities, attitudes and tasks, and exposing differing views on patient care. As seen in how regulation can facilitate role clarification, an explicit description of team members' new and specific tasks, roles and lines of responsibilities was suggested. How this is being achieved in practice was largely dependent on the policy contexts and stakeholder engagements. The review on nurse prescribing (Kroezen et al., 2011) suggested that the role of medical associations was strong in opposing laws on nurse prescribing (for example, in Australia, Spain, USA) and, as the result of a compromise between the stakeholders, led to limited prescribing rights for the nurses. Conversely, in the United Kingdom, the involvement of the British Medical Association and their support for nurse prescribing has proved to be a facilitator in the policy process and its implementation (Kroezen et al., 2011) (see Table 10.2).

Evidence on financing and payment mechanisms

No reviews were found with a main focus on the impact of health financing on skill-mix. However, five systematic reviews on skill-mix touched partially on health financing or payment mechanisms and are dealt with in more detail in this section (see Table 10.2).

The systematic review by Karam et al. (2018) found fee-for-service payments to be a particular threat to collaboration. Therefore, adequate resource allocation was considered an essential aspect in the implementation of interprofessional and interorganizational collaboration. Carter et al. (2016) in their study about team-based primary care services and new payment models in Canada indicated that using blended capitation (that is, a mix of capitation payments based on the list of registered patients and fee-for-service-based on the services provided) instead of fee-for-service, reduced the number of patients seen per day. They suggest that a blended capitation may be more efficient as it contributes to better quality of care. The review also assessed pay-for-performance payment schemes and demonstrates some positive findings; however, the overall evidence was mixed on its contribution to enabling team-based primary care services. The authors put forward that a reward system that avoids patient risk selection by physicians should be considered.

Another review (Kroezen et al., 2011) describes how the skill-mix intervention of nurse prescribing is not taken up in some states in the USA because payers do not cover nurse prescriptions (see Table 10.2). On the other hand, in the Netherlands, patients are reimbursed for a prescription written by a nurse, facilitating intervention uptake. Indeed, several studies emphasized the fundamental need for recognition by payers of the new roles, and an adequate level of reimbursement. Farris et al. (2010) in their study on pharmacists taking on additional sexual health counselling tasks reported the lack of reimbursement models as a barrier in the context of the USA and similar findings were reported by Karam et al. (2018). Farris et al. (2010) went so far as to say that "the single most critical aspect of these initiatives is payment for pharmacists' services". Moreover, they state that pharmacist reimbursement must also consider professionals' time, costs and liability issues. Mapp, Hutchinson & Estcourt (2015) also mentioned insufficient funding and financially unsustainable programmes as a significant challenge to delivering primary care-based HIV care.

No evidence was found on countries in which staff are salaried, levels of salary, incentive structures and implications on skill-mix changes.

An important methodological challenge while reviewing the literature on health financing for skill-mix innovations is the impossibility of disentangling the contribution made by a single policy, for example, financing or payment policy vis-à-vis the cumulative effects of the various policy levers used together. This shows that focusing on a single (payment) policy or law is likely to be too short-sighted or result in unintended consequences. An integrated policy on skill-mix and the health workforce should revisit all relevant policies, laws, financing and payment mechanisms as to potential barriers and unintended consequences and adapted in a way that facilitates the implementation process at the policy level.

10.3 Policy and implementation: trends and country examples

This section complements the information from the overview of reviews with selected country examples from a broader literature search, including grey literature and mini case studies. Different countries were selected with the aim to portray examples from different financing schemes (for example, social health insurance, tax-based). Discerning trends was a challenge. The evidence from the reviews was not suitable for this purpose, and ~~although~~while the country examples identified are important, they are by no means a systematic mapping exercise, and certainly cannot claim to identify trends. Nevertheless, these examples reveal that countries are trying to draw together the four themes described in the previous section, and that they aim to simultaneously or sequentially tackle all the complexities. The examples discussed in this section mirror the main trends in skill-mix change identified in the companion volume (Wismar, Glinos & Sagan, forthcoming), which include the strengthening of multiprofessional practices in primary care, nonmedical prescribing and the role of nurse practitioners[1] and other professions.

First, this section looks at examples in the context of policies, followed by examples on financing and payment mechanisms.

Policies to strengthen the health workforce and skill-mix for primary care

Several policies focusing on strengthening the health workforce in primary care were found in Europe, for example: Austria, with recent reforms on establishing 75 primary health care units by 2021 staffed with multiprofessional teams; Estonia, with strategies implemented to strengthen primary care practices with expanded roles for family nurses; Slovenia, with a focus on primary care and health promotion through nurses in advanced roles; and the United Kingdom, with new elements to improve capacity and care coordination.

In 2017, Austria established the foundations for a new primary health care system paradigm. With the aim to improve accessible, multiprofessional and interdisciplinary primary care, the government announced that a total of 75 new primary health care units will be established by

---

[1] Also referred to as advanced nurse practitioners in some countries

2021 and earmarked €200 million for this purpose. Six primary health care units were already operational at the beginning of 2018, and three more were in progress (BMASGK, 2019). The multiprofessional team consists of at least a core team of GPs and qualified nurses but also includes other health professionals. The reform aims to reinforce access to primary care by ensuring longer opening hours in an effort to reduce the burden on hospital outpatient departments (BMGF, 2017 in OECD/ European Observatory on Health Systems and Policies, 2017).

Estonia is also taking steps to strengthen primary health care by setting up health centres. The traditional family doctor and nurse model moves towards a multidisciplinary collaboration to increase access and improve management of chronic diseases, in which family nurses play a key role. In 2016, after 5 years of consultation among interest groups, the Estonian Parliament adopted an amendment to the Health Service Organization Act enabling family nurses to prescribe a limited number of medicines, mainly for chronic conditions. Prescriptions by family nurses have to be regularly validated. Family nurses are required to attend a training in clinical pharmacology before being granted the right to prescribe medicine. Further, family nurses have also taken over responsibilities from GPs such as managing chronically ill patients, pregnant women and healthy newborns.

Similarly, in Slovenia in 2011 the Ministry of Health piloted a new approach to strengthen primary care and management of patients with chronic diseases through the GP model practices. The main innovation is adding a 0.5 full-time equivalent qualified nurse with specific training in noncommunicable disease prevention to the core team of the practice (traditionally a GP and a nurse). This nurse is responsible for assessing the condition of stable chronic patients and coordinating care, carrying out preventive counselling and screening for risk factors. Nurses undergo specific training consisting of eight modules (with a focus on prevention and chronic diseases) for carrying out protocols in the follow up of chronic patients. This new role is also meant to ease GPs' workload by undertaking the monitoring of patients with certain chronic diseases and preventive activities, supporting a multidisciplinary approach to patient care. The full conversion of GP practices into model practices was expected by 2018, but budgetary constraints postponed the deadline to mid-2020. In 2017, 75% of all GP practices nationwide employed an additional 0.5 full-time equivalent nurse (OECD/European Observatory on Health Systems and Policies, 2019c).

Another initiative to improve coordination of care in Slovenia is the integration of public health and primary health care through a network of health promotion centres within primary care. In these centres, multidisciplinary teams promote a healthy lifestyle and provide disease prevention programmes, among other services. Although originally health promotion centres focused on providing lifestyle interventions for patients at risk for noncommunicable diseases, the programme evolved to tackle inequalities, and extended its scope to include the healthy population across Slovenia (OECD/European Observatory on Health Systems and Policies, 2019c).

Against the backdrop of chronic workforce shortages in primary care in the United Kingdom, the National Health Service (NHS) introduced the long-term plan in 2019. The reform is aimed at improving capacity, coordination and integration of care. To this end, GPs are required to join Primary Care Networks of between 30 000 and 50 000 patients. Moreover, to reduce health inequalities the NHS Long-Term Plan promotes the use of digital solutions: so-called digital first general practices will be strengthened, where patients will have the right to online and video consultations by April 2021. Further, a component of the NHS Long-Term Plan's effort to strive towards universal personalized care, which has gained attention as an innovative skill-mix element, is social prescribing. Also known as community referral, social prescribing is a means for local agencies to refer people to a link worker. Link workers are also known as health advisors, social prescribing coordinators and community navigators, and are generally nonclinically trained individuals who work in a social prescribing service and receive people who have been referred to them (University of Westminster, n.d). Key responsibilities of the link workers are: to provide personalized support to individuals to take control of their well-being, live independently and improve their health outcomes; to co-produce a simple personalized care and support plan to improve health and well-being, introducing or reconnecting people to community groups and using local resources and statutory services to tackle loneliness; and to evaluate the individual impact of a person's wellness progress. Social prescribing can involve a number of activities, which are generally provided by voluntary and community sector organizations (Public Health England, 2019). The NHS estimates that by 2023–2024, social prescribers will be handling around 900 000 patient appointments a year, which will require new skills and (re-)training of existing health professionals to assess the need for and issue social prescriptions (NHS England, 2019). Hence, the reform aims to improve the integration and coordination of care, and has added social prescribing to the health coverage basket, with available additional funding to make primary care more attractive and to kick-start new skill configurations among its workforce. Due to the recent introduction of reforms, it is too early to analyse the effects.

Having looked so far at large reforms (for example, for primary care) that entail changes in health service delivery and teams, Box 10.1 focuses on reforms of nonmedical prescribing, which although more limited in scope, have nevertheless important implications on health systems.

Overview of the regulation of health professionals: strategies to improve access and quality of health services and protect populations

The scope of regulation for certain health professionals varies among countries, and we now present some examples from nurse practitioners, physician assistants and other professions. As discussed in Section 10.2, regulation can facilitate role clarification and provide a frame of reference to deal with liability.

A number of countries, such as Ireland, the Netherlands, Australia, Canada and the USA, enforce national regulation of advanced nurse practitioner titles, practice and registration (Maier, 2015). The United Kingdom and Finland followed a different path and used local governance mechanisms of the advanced nurse practitioner's role, although prescriptive authority is regulated nationally (Maier, 2015). In the United Kingdom, the decision not to regulate nurse practitioners was taken on the basis of proportionality of risk, through an evaluation that concluded that additional regulation would not be necessary given the (limited) potential threat to public safety. However, it remains to be seen whether the lack of national role regulation for nurse practitioners in the United Kingdom has impacted discrepancy in practice, challenges in role clarity, and difficulties in tracking workforce data (Maier, 2015).

In Canada, physician assistants are regulated in Alberta, Manitoba and New Brunswick, but remain unregulated in Ontario. In 2012 the Ministry of Health and Long-Term Care decided against regulation of the physician assistant profession. This decision was based on the Health Professions Regulatory Advisory Council's recommendation that public safety and quality of care are sufficiently upheld at this

Box 10.1 Reforms on nonmedical prescribing with implications on health systems

As of 2019, there were 13 European countries with laws on nurse prescribing adopted, most of which have introduced laws over the past decade (Maier, in review). All countries adopted changes to pre-existing laws to officially and legally authorize nurses and other health professions (such as pharmacists, midwives, physiotherapists) to prescribe certain medications. Hence, adaptations to existing laws were the precondition to implementing change in routine care for this specific expanded role. Due to the highly country-specific nature, several country examples are provided below to highlight how policy processes were steered. All countries had in common that these policy processes were usually lengthy and controversial.

In Finland, successful pilots in nurse prescribing produced positive evidence accepted by all stakeholders, which led to legislation on nurse prescribing being implemented in 2010, followed by regulations on postgraduate education in 2011. Nurse prescribers receive this title after completing specific education and meeting other requirements. These nurses work in health centres in close collaboration with doctors, and perform routine visits for patients with chronic conditions. Since 2011, nurse prescribers are allowed to prescribe medications on a continued basis for patients with hypertension, type 2 diabetes and asthma (Maier et al., 2017).

In Ireland, nurse and midwife prescribing was successfully established after protracted advocacy efforts from health professional associations, providers and other groups, as well as pilots supporting the evidence of safety and effectiveness of nurse/midwife prescribing. In 2007 the government passed legislation that allowed licenced registered nurses and midwives (certified after successfully passing a 6-month postgraduate educational programme) to prescribe medications and other medicinal products that are specific to their clinical practice (Wilson et al., 2018).

Nonmedical prescribing is also established outside Europe. In New Zealand, nonmedical prescribing is legally granted to different categories of health professionals, ranging from dentists to midwives (Raghunandan, Tordoff & Smith, 2017). Instead, in the USA, pharmacists in the majority of states are allowed to perform dependent prescribing (that is, within a supervised setting), while fewer states allow collaborative prescribing of controlled medicines. In Canada, prescribing rights for pharmacists vary by jurisdiction, but legislation is in place in the majority of provinces and the legislated prescribing authority of pharmacists is expected to expand further (Faruquee & Guirguis, 2015).

time through the delegation model under the supervision of a licensed physician (Canadian Association of Physician Assistants website, n.d).

In the USA, regulation and licensure of health professionals are defined by state-based laws and subject to state-to-state variation. In some cases, health professionals are recognized only in certain states, like dental therapists who are licensed to practice in Minnesota, but are not recognized in neighbouring North Dakota (Dower, Moore & Langelier, 2013). Similarly, in the case of midwives the regulations and scopes-of-practice vary significantly across all states. For example, Alabama allows both direct entry midwives and nurse midwives to practice and be licensed; the same is allowed in Washington State, and additionally both are eligible for Medicaid reimbursement. However, in West Virginia and many other states direct-entry midwives are not regulated (Midwives Association of North America website, n.d). In Europe, midwifery is regulated in different ways, for example through an autonomous regulatory body, a joint ministerial and midwifery or nursing and midwifery regulatory body, or a joint responsibility of a ministry and a midwifery professional association (Nursing and Midwifery Council, 2010).

Financing and payment mechanisms: key contributors to facilitating or hindering skill-mix implementation

In addition to the discussion in Section 10.2 on the role of financing and payment mechanisms, this section will expand on the topic and further include examples from the USA, Australia, the United Kingdom, Estonia and Lithuania.

One article (Brooten et al., 2012) mentions lack of adequate funding as one of the principal limiting factors for nurse practitioners in the USA to "practice to the full scope of their education and training". In Australia in 2010, nurse practitioners were granted legislated access to the Medical Benefits Scheme and Pharmaceutical Benefits Scheme, the federal schemes for third-party reimbursement for health care services and medications, as providers (Cashin, 2014). At the same time, physician assistants in Australia are not recognized under the Medical Benefits Scheme and Pharmaceutical Benefits Scheme, and as such, there are no rebates for patients who see a physician assistant and patients would pay more for medication prescribed by a physician assistant.

In the United Kingdom, the reform to strengthen primary care also makes available additional funds via a contract for GPs, which was introduced in January 2019. The contract seeks to increase capacity in primary care with more GPs and significant growth in other health professions. Overall, the aim is for general practice to employ 20 000 additional staff from a range of health care professions including pharmacists, physiotherapists and paramedics. It does this through increased capitation rates, makes available optional funding for new staff (£900 million), via an additional £2.8 billion funding to be used exclusively for primary care (Department of Health and Social Care, 2019).

Similarly, Estonia and Lithuania used financial incentives (increase in payments for GP practices employing a second family nurse) and disincentives (reduction in capitation payments for GP practices not employing at least one family nurse working in advanced roles) to promote the employment of nurses in primary care. This strategy also helps in addressing potential resistance from physicians. Further, since 2013 the Estonian Health Insurance Fund is paying for a second family nurse in a GP practice. From the experience in these two Baltic countries, financial incentives appear to help promote a greater integration of new nursing roles into primary care (OECD/European Observatory on Health Systems and Policies, 2019a, 2019b).

However, the caveat is that health financing reforms alone are not sufficient to ensure successful skill-mix implementation. Other policy levers, notably those designed to alter status quo organizational and governance arrangements, are key to facilitating the success of financing reforms. Pearce et al. (2011) underline this point, showing that the funding incentives given through the Enhanced Primary Care Programme to general practices in Australia had the greatest effect on skill-mix innovation if the leadership and climate of the general practice was collaborative and not hierarchical. Practices whose organizational arrangements did not fulfil these criteria "were unable to capitalize on the enhanced skill set of the nurse, because they continued to provide little opportunity for the nurse to have autonomy within the team", which inherently leads to wrong (and wasteful) allocation of resources without the expected staffing change (Pearce et al., 2011).

One way to recognize and incentivize the novel skill-mix is through bundled payment mechanisms such as group practices or pay-for-coordination schemes. Bundled payments not only seem to incentivize the uptake of new roles and professions, they can also stimulate a move towards care integration and teamwork, more so than fee-for-service payments. Indeed, payment systems focused on individual payments (rather than team payments) can disincentivize care integration and provider collaboration.

There is some evidence that when the reimbursement is too low, the attractiveness of the new roles may be reduced, leading to decreased uptake; when it is too high (vis-à-vis physicians especially), there may be reduced cost saving (Maier, Aiken & Busse, 2017). This is because the assumption is that care provided by a physician is more expensive than care provided by a nurse, but this might not be the case if financing mechanisms reimburse nurses at the same level as physicians and, especially in the case of the USA, if nurses need the same medical malpractice insurance to work independently. Hence, the level of reimbursement for a health service provided through a new skill-mix intervention matters, and must be crafted carefully to country context to avoid unintended consequences.

10.4   Conclusions

This chapter analysed several aspects of policy and financing that can facilitate or hinder the implementation of skill-mix changes. It should be noted that the reviews dealt with mostly high-income, Anglophone countries, hence transferability of findings may be limited.

The broader literature clearly shows that financing is potentially a powerful policy lever to incentivize or disincentivize uptake and integration of skill-mix innovation into routine health service delivery. It should be noted that different measures are necessary to address lack of reimbursement (especially in the context of some states in the USA), compared with actual funding for primary care practices, for example to employ more nurses. Further, payment mechanisms are an important policy instrument and can encourage multiple providers to work together and some will allow task delegation, while other mechanisms that pay individual providers separately (fee-for-service) can block effective collaboration and task shifts. At the same time, health financing reforms as stand-alone interventions may have limited impact, and country-specific context must be considered.

Five main factors emerged as critical to an effective policy process and reforms: (i) a clear vision and mandate for the reforms (such as in Austria, the Netherlands, Ireland and Finland); (ii) evidence of proven effectiveness of the reforms (for example, through pilots – as in Finland and Ireland); (iii) early involvement and communication with all relevant stakeholders (such as in Austria, Finland and Ireland) and flexibility and readiness to address stakeholder concerns; (iv) leadership from the government (for example, Austria, Finland, Ireland); and (v) sufficient funding and financing mechanisms for implementation (for example, in Austria, Estonia, Slovenia and the United Kingdom).

In conclusion, the limited number of studies does not allow discussion of the impact of reforms at population level, and it is difficult to discern trends, despite some promising examples that emerge from experience in different countries. While more research is certainly necessary, there is an important need, when reforms are introduced, to consistently perform evaluation to inform future policy. More focus should be placed on identifying and fostering different types of evidence, for example from pilots and local innovations. Finally, the value brought by the overview of reviews should be highlighted as it identified some key themes and aggregated the available evidence. This is despite the limitations, since this chapter identifies and deals with barriers on an individual basis, which does not fully portray the complexity of multiple barriers co-existing and possibly interacting with each other. Limitations related to the latter are addressed in the companion volume (Wismar, Glinos & Sagan, forthcoming) with in-depth case studies by country.

References

Baron RJ (2015). Professional self-regulation in a changing world: old problems need new approaches. JAMA, 313(18):1807–1808.

Bauchner H, Fontanarosa PB, Thompson AE (2015). Professionalism, governance, and self-regulation of medicine. JAMA,. 313(18):1831–1836.

Brooten D, Youngblut JAM, Hannan J et al. (2012). The impact of interprofessional collaboration on the effectiveness, significance, and future of advanced practice registered nurses. Nurs Clin North Am, 47(2):283–294. doi:10.1016/j.cnur.2012.02.005.

Bundesministerium für Arbeit, Soziales, Gesundheit und Konsumentenschutz (BMASGK) (2019). The Austrian Health Care System, Key Facts Updated edition 2019. (https://www.google.com/url?sa=t&rct=j&q=&esrc=s&source=web&cd=&ved=2ahUKEwjtj_3gk5HtAhVQ-6QKHQvzDsoQFjAAegQIAhAC&url=https%3A%2F%2Fwww.sozialministerium.at%2Fdam%2Fjcr%3A6102a229-7b92-44fd-af1f-3aa

691900296%2FBMASGK_The-Austrian_Health-Care-System__KeyFacts__
WEB.PDF&usg=AOvVaw25XagVhZv0Cg9txaHd_IzQ, 20 November
2020).

Canadian Association of Physician Assistants – Association canadienne des
adjoints au médecin website (n.d) (https://capa-acam.ca/pa-employers/
legislation/, 20 November 2020).

Carter R, Riverin B, Levesque JF et al. (2016). The impact of primary care
reform on health system performance in Canada: A systematic review. BMC
Health Serv Res, 16(1). doi:10.1186/s12913-016-1571-7.

Cashin, A. (2014). Collaborative arrangements for Australian nurse
practitioners: a policy analysis. J Am Assoc Nurse Practitioners, 26: 550–
554.

Colvin CJ, de Heer J, Winterton L et al. (2013). A systematic review of
qualitative evidence on barriers and facilitators to the implementation
of task-shifting in midwifery services. Midwifery, 29(10):1211–1221.
doi:10.1016/j.midw.2013.05.001.

Department of Health and Social Care (2019). The Government's revised
mandate to NHS England for 2018-19. 2019. (https://assets.publishing
.service.gov.uk/government/uploads/system/uploads/attachment_data/
file/803111/revised-mandate-to-nhs-england-2018-to-2019.pdf, 20
November 2020).

Dower C, Moore J, Langelier M (2013). It is time to restructure health
professions scope-of-practice regulations to remove barriers to care.
Health Affairs, 32:11. (https://www.healthaffairs.org/doi/full/10.1377/
hlthaff.2013.0537).

Farris K, Ashwood D, McIntosh J et al. (2010). Preventing unintended
pregnancy: pharmacists' roles in practice and policy via partnerships. J Am
Pharm Assoc. 50(5):604–612. doi:10.1331/JAPhA.2010.09195.

Faruquee F, Guirguis M (2015). A scoping review of research on the
prescribing practice of Canadian pharmacists. Can Pharm J / Rev Pharm
Can, 148(6):325–348. https://doi.org/10.1177/1715163515608399

Joo JY, Huber DL (2017). Barriers in case managers' roles: a
qualitative systematic review. West J Nurs Res, 40(10):1522–1542.
doi:10.1177/0193945917728689.

Karam M, Brault I, Van Durme T et al. (2018). Comparing interprofessional
and interorganizational collaboration in healthcare: a systematic review
of the qualitative research. Int J Nurs Stud, 2018;79:70–83. doi:10.1016/j
.ijnurstu.2017.11.002.

Kroezen M, Van Dijk L, Groenewegen PP et al. (2011). Nurse prescribing of
medicines in Western European and Anglo-Saxon countries: a systematic
review of the literature. BMC Health Serv Res, 11. doi:10.1186/1472-
6963-11-127.

Maier CB (2015). The role of governance in implementing task-shifting from physicians to nurses in advanced roles in Europe, U.S., Canada, New Zealand and Australia. Health Policy, 119:1627–35.

Maier CB, Aiken LH, Busse R (2017). Nurses in advanced roles in primary care: Policy levers for implementation. OECD Health Work Pap, (98):1–71. doi:http://dx.doi.org/10.1787/a8756593-en.

Mapp F, Hutchinson J, Estcourt C (2015). A systematic review of contemporary models of shared HIV care and HIV in primary care in high-income settings. Int J STD AIDS, 26(14):991–997. doi:10.1177/0956462415577496.

Midwives Association of North America website (n.d) (https://mana.org/, 20 November 2020).

NHS England (Wesbsite) (2019). News: Army of workers to support family doctors. 2019. (https://www.england.nhs.uk/2019/01/army-of-workers-to-support-family-doctors/).

Nursing and Midwifery Council (2010). Survey of European midwifery regulators. 2010. (http://www.ordre-sages-femmes.fr/wp-content/uploads/2015/10/Etude-NEMIR-de-2009.pdf, 20 November 2020).

OECD/European Observatory on Health Systems and Policies (2017). Austria: Country Health Profile 2017, State of Health in the EU. Paris, OECD Publishing /Copenhagen, WHO Regional Office for Europe.

OECD/European Observatory on Health Systems and Policies (2019a). Estonia: Country Health Profile 2019, State of Health in the EU. Paris, OECD Publishing /Copenhagen, WHO Regional Office for Europe.

OECD/European Observatory on Health Systems and Policies (2019b). Lithuania: Country Health Profile 2019, State of Health in the EU. Paris, OECD Publishing /Copenhagen, WHO Regional Office for Europe.

OECD/European Observatory on Health Systems and Policies (2019c). Slovenia: Country Health Profile 2019, State of Health in the EU. Paris, OECD Publishing / Copenhagen, WHO Regional Office for Europe.

Pearce C, Phillips C, Hall S et al. (2011). Following the funding trail: financing, nurses and teamwork in Australian general practice. BMC Health Serv Res 2011;11:38. doi:10.1186/1472-6963-11-38.

Public Health England. (2019). Guidance, social prescribing: applying All Our Health. 2019. (https://www.gov.uk/government/publications/social-prescribing-applying-all-our-health/social-prescribing-applying-all-our-health, 20 November 2020).

Raghunandan R, Tordoff J, Smith A (2017). Non-medical prescribing in New Zealand: an overview of prescribing rights, service delivery models and training. Ther Adv Drug Safety, 8(11):349–360. doi:10.1177/2042098617723312

Struckmann V, Quentin W, Busse R et al. (2016). How to strengthen financing mechanisms to promote care for people with multimorbidity in Europe?

Policy brief, NIVEL and TU Berlin 2016. (http://www.euro.who.int/__data/assets/pdf_file/0006/337587/PB_24.pdf?ua=1, 20 November 2020).

University of Westminster. Making sense of social prescribing. n.d. (https://docs.wixstatic.com/ugd/14f499_816dc79e160a4e77991599a74236d0d4.pdf, 20 November 2020).

Wilson M, Murphy J, Nam M et al. (2018). Nurse and midwifery prescribing in Ireland: a scope-of-practice development for worldwide consideration. Nurs Health Sci, 20(2):264–270. http://dx.doi.org/10.1111/nhs.12408.

Wismar M, Glinos I, Sagan A (forthcoming). Skill-mix innovation in primary and chronic care. Mobilizing patients, peers, professionals. Copenhagen, WHO Regional Office for Europe on behalf of the European Observatory on Health Systems and Policies.

World Health Organization (n.d) Health policy. (https://www.who.int/topics/health_policy/en/, 20 November 2020).

World Health Organization (2000). The World health report, 2000. Health systems: improving performance. Geneva, WHO.

11 Change management in health care settings: organizational strategies to foster skill-mix changes

MARIEKE KROEZEN, ELLEN KUHLMANN,
CHRISTIAN GERICKE, GILLES DUSSAULT

11.1 Introduction

The implementation of innovations in health care organizations is a complex process that is affected by many factors, positively or negatively (Fleuren, Wiefferink & Paulussen, 2004). Skill-mix innovation is particularly challenging, conceptually, technically and politically (Kernick & Scott, 2002). It is essential to identify the factors and strategies that influence the uptake of skill-mix interventions in organizations, in order to better inform policy and decision-making. In theory, stimulating or enabling factors give (in)direct but unintended encouragement to a skill-mix intervention, whereas drivers are objective-oriented. Barriers, on the other hand, are passive factors to be overcome, whereas impeding factors deliberately attempt to stop a skill-mix intervention. In practice, this division is hard to make, and the terms are used interchangeably. In this chapter, where a factor stimulates or expands skill-mix change in health care settings (whether intended or not), we speak of a facilitator. Any factor that limits or restricts skill-mix change in health care settings (whether intended or not), is considered a barrier. In keeping with the literature, this chapter applies the following framework in analysing the most important factors influencing the implementation of skill-mix innovations in health care settings:

- characteristics of the skill-mix innovation, such as whether the skill-mix is perceived to be imposed or not, whether there is evidence that it is safe and effective;
- institutional factors, such as the legal framework, the policy and regulatory environment, financing strategies, the influence of stakeholders such as professional councils, unions, population needs;

- organizational factors, such as organization structure and culture, remuneration mechanisms, incentives, staff volume and composition;
- individual factors, such as staff knowledge and beliefs, relationships and collaboration;
- process factors, such as the planning of the skill-mix before implementation, monitoring and evaluation.

The evidence from 21 systematic reviews, identified by an overview of systematic reviews presented in Chapter 1, shows that organizational factors and individual factors are often discussed in the literature on the implementation of skill-mix interventions at organizational level. Process factors and characteristics of the skill-mix intervention seem to play a less important role, while the institutional environment mainly seems to have a hampering effect. In most cases, the identified barriers are the 'mirror opposite' of facilitators. A final observation is that very little attention is paid to more structural approaches – such as models or frameworks for organizational change – in relation to skill-mix implementation.

When looking at the trends of the last years in how organizations try to overcome the barriers to the implementation of skill-mix innovations, and how they attempt to strengthen and implement facilitating factors, common strategies are presented in Section 11.3 and illustrated by four case studies. By providing insight into factors that may facilitate or impede implementation, the chapter concludes with recommendations on an appropriate strategy for implementing skill innovations at the organizational level (Fleuren, Wiefferink & Paulussen, 2004).

11.2   Overview of the evidence on implementation at organizational level

Characteristics of systematic reviews

The overview of systematic reviews identified 21 reviews on organizational-level factors related to the implementation of skill-mix innovations (Table 11.1). In terms of types of intervention, 11 reviews focused on the introduction of new teamwork modalities (Aquino et al., 2016; Carmont et al., 2017; Gardiner, Gott & Ingleton, 2012; Hoeft et al., 2018; Mapp, Hutchinson & Estcourt, 2015; Sangaleti et al., 2017; Savic et al., 2017; Schadewaldt et al., 2013; Supper et al., 2015; Wood, Ohlsen & Ricketts, 2017), seven focused on re-allocation of

Table 11.1 *Characteristics of the 21 systematic reviews on implementation at organizational level*

Authors	Year	Skill-mix intervention type	Description of intervention	Country coverage	No. of studies included
Dennis et al. (2012)	2012	Adding new tasks	Primary care providers developing patients' health literacy	USA, UK, AU, NZ, SE, CH, NL, CA, JP	52
Gardiner et al. (2012)	2012	(Newly) introducing teamwork	Collaborative working in palliative care	UK, AU, CA, NZ	22
Hillis et al. (2016)	2016	Adding new tasks	Role of care coordinator	USA, UK, AU, CA, IT	37
Mapp et al. (2015)	2015	(Newly) introducing teamwork	HIV shared care	AU, CH, DE, CA, UK	8
Savic et al. (2017)	2017	(Newly) introducing teamwork	Coordination in alcohol and other drug (AOD) and non-AOD services	USA, AU, CA, BE	14
Schadewaldt et al. (2013)	2013	(Newly) introducing teamwork	Collaborative practice between nurse practitioners and medical practitioners	USA, CA, UK, NL, SE, IE, NZ	27
Supper et al. (2015)	2015	(Newly) introducing teamwork	Interprofessional collaboration in primary care	UK, AU, USA, NZ, ES, CA, NL, BR	44
Wood et al. (2017)	2017	(Newly) introducing teamwork	Collaborative depression care	USA, UK, DE, CA	18

Table 11.1 (cont.)

Authors	Year	Skill-mix intervention type	Description of intervention	Country coverage	No. of studies included
Joo and Huber (2017)	2017	Adding new tasks	Case management	USA, SE, UK, AU, DK, BE	10
Hoeft et al. (2018)	2018	(Newly) introducing teamwork	Teamwork in mental health care	USA, AU, UK, NZ	55
Halter et al. (2013)	2013	Re-allocating tasks	Physician assistants in primary care	USA, UK, NL, AU	49
Farris et al. (2010)	2010	Re-allocating tasks	Pharmacists' roles in reducing unintended pregnancy	USA	38
Colvin et al. (2013)	2013	Re-allocating tasks	Task-shifting involving midwives	AU, CA, USA, SE, UK, AO, DO, GT, JO, KE, ID, MX, ZA	37
Aquino et al. (2016)	2016	(Newly) introducing teamwork	Collaboration between midwives and health visitors	AU, UK, SE, NO, CA	16
Abuzour et al. (2017)	2017	Re-allocating tasks	Non-medical independent prescribing by (student) nurses and pharmacists	UK	34
Carmont et al. (2017)	2017	(Newly) introducing teamwork	GP engagement in integrated palliative care	AU, CA, DK, NZ, UK, NL, no country reported	17

Sangaleti et al. (2017)	2017	(Newly) introducing teamwork / changing teamwork	Teamwork and interprofessional collaboration in primary care	BR, Canada, USA, IE, NZ, SE, LT, AU	21
Andregård and Jangland (2015)	2015	(Newly) introducing teamwork	Interprofessional collaboration with the introduction of the nurse practitioner	Seven countries (not specified which)	26
Meiklejohn et al. (2016)	2016	Adding new tasks	GP role in treatment, follow up or palliative cancer care	AU (7), CA (7), Europe (19), Middle East (1), UK (9), USA (15)	58
Overbeck et al. (2016)	2016	(Newly) introducing teamwork	Collaborative care for anxiety and depression	CA (1), UK (5), USA (11)	17
Khanassov et al. (2014)	2014	(Newly) introducing teamwork	Case management for dementia in primary health care	AU (1), BE (1), CN (1), IN (1), NL (4), UK (5), USA (10)	23

Abbreviations: GP: general practitioner.

Country abbreviations: AO: Angola; AU: Australia; BE: Belgium; BR: Brazil; CA: Canada; CH: Switzerland; CN: China; DE: Germany; DK: Denmark; DO: Dominican Republic; GT: Guatemala; IE: Ireland; ID: Indonesia; IN: India; IT: Italy; JO: Jordan; JP: Japan; KE: Kenya; LT: Lithuania; MX: Mexico; NL: the Netherlands; NO: Norway; NZ: New Zealand; SE: Sweden; UK: the United Kingdom; USA: the United States of America; ZA: South Africa.

Sources: Abuzour, Lewis & Tully (2017); Andregård & Jangland (2015); Aquino et al. (2016); Carmont et al. (2017); Colvin et al. (2013); Dennis et al. (2012); Farris et al. (2010); Gardiner, Gott & Ingleton (2012); Halter et al. (2013); Hillis et al. (2016); Hoeft et al. (2018); Joo & Huber (2017); Khanassov, Vefel & Pluye (2014); Mapp, Hutchinson & Estcourt (2015); Meiklejohn et al. (2016); Overbeck, Davidsen & Kousgaard (2016); Sangaleti et al. (2017); Savic et al. (2017); Schadewaldt et al. (2013); Supper et al. (2015); Wood, Ohlsen & Ricketts (2017).

tasks (Colvin et al., 2013; Farris et al., 2010; Halter et al., 2013) or the introduction of new tasks (Dennis et al., 2012; Hillis et al., 2016; Joo & Huber, 2017) and one review additionally paid attention to changing existing teamwork approaches (Sangaleti et al., 2017). Some interventions were broad and focused on general interprofessional collaboration in primary care (Supper et al., 2015), whereas others were confined to specific health professionals and conditions, such as pharmacists' role in reducing unintended pregnancy (Farris et al., 2010). Most reviews included a majority of studies from Anglophone OECD countries and northern and western European countries.

Evidence on implementation at the organizational level

In most reviews, the implementation of skill-mix interventions at organizational level was approached by focusing on specific facilitators and barriers to introduce an intervention. In many cases, the barriers were the mirror opposite of facilitators. Little attention was paid to structural approaches such as models or frameworks for organizational change. In line with the reviews, we discuss the evidence on implementation at organizational level by focusing on facilitators and barriers. The evidence is categorized according to the five categories of the framework introduced in Section 11.1: organizational factors, as they are of most importance for this chapter, followed by individual factors, characteristics of the skill-mix intervention, process and institutional factors. Organizational and individual factors are more often discussed in the systematic reviews than the other three categories (Table 11.2). This does not necessarily reflect the relative importance of each of these factors in the implementation process, but may (partly) be an indication of the convenience or the difficulty with which these aspects can be measured. Finally, it should be noted that because of the relatively small number of included reviews, the evidence for the facilitators and barriers is often limited, which has implications for generalizability.

Organizational factors

Organizations can fulfil an important facilitating role in the implementation of skill-mix interventions by making sure that practical issues are optimally addressed, such as the co-location or physical proximity of services involved in the skill-mix (Aquino et al., 2016; Overbeck, Davidsen & Kousgaard, 2016; Sangaleti et al., 2017; Savic et al., 2017;

Table 11.2 *Overview of conclusions on factors related to skill-mix implementation at organizational level in systematic reviews included*

Factor	Facilitators	Barriers
Organizational factors	• Co-location of services / proximity (Aquino et al., 2016; Overbeck et al., 2016; Sangaleti et al., 2017; Savic et al., 2017; Schadewaldt et al., 2013; Supper et al., 2015; Wood et al., 2017) • Information systems (including telemedicine) (Dennis et al., 2012; Hoeft et al., 2018; Meiklejohn et al., 2016; Schadewaldt et al., 2013; Wood et al., 2017) • Clear definition and recognition of roles and responsibilities (Carmont et al., 2017, Gardiner et al., 2012; Khanassov et al., 2014; Schadewaldt et al., 2013; Wood et al., 2017) • Practice-based education and training (Gardiner et al., 2012; Hoeft et al., 2018; Supper et al., 2015) • Strong leadership / management support (Hillis et al., 2016; Sangaleti et al., 2017; Supper et al., 2015) • Good communication (Khanassov et al., 2014; Mapp et al., 2015; Meiklejohn et al., 2016; Sangaleti et al., 2017; Schadewaldt et al., 2013) • Regular meetings (Abuzour et al., 2017; Khanassov et al., 2014; Sangaleti et al., 2017; Schadewaldt et al., 2013)	• Lack of time and financial resources (Aquino et al., 2016; Farris et al., 2010; Hoeft et al., 2018; Khanassov et al., 2014; Meiklejohn et al., 2016; Overbeck et al., 2016; Sangaleti et al., 2017; Supper et al., 2015; Wood et al., 2017) • Lack of clarity over roles and responsibilities (Andregård & Jangland, 2015; Carmont et al., 2017; Colvin et al., 2013; Gardiner et al., 2012; Joo & Huber, 2017; Meiklejohn et al., 2016; Schadewaldt et al., 2013) • Lack of clarity over scope of practice (Abuzour et al., 2017; Joo & Huber, 2017; Schadewaldt et al., 2013) • Professional territorialism / silos (Carmont et al., 2017; Colvin et al., 2013; Gardiner et al., 2012; Hoeft et al., 2018; Sangaleti et al., 2017) • Divergent models of care (Aquino et al., 2016; Colvin et al., 2013) • Inadequate information transfer (Abuzour et al., 2017; Aquino et al., 2016, Carmont et al., 2017; Overbeck et al., 2016) • Lack of communication (Colvin et al., 2013; Gardiner et al., 2012; Wood et al., 2017)

Table 11.2 *(cont.)*

Factor	Facilitators	Barriers
	• Partnership working (Mapp et al., 2015) / strong interagency relationships (Farris et al., 2010; Savic et al., 2017) / joint working (Aquino et al., 2016) • Shared organizational goals and values (Savic et al., 2017) • Culture receptive to change (Wood et al., 2017) • 'Age' of the organization in which intervention is implemented (Hillis et al., 2016)	• Organizational culture not receptive to change (Abuzour et al., 2017; Wood et al., 2017) • Little involvement with leadership (Joo and Huber, 2017) • Increased administration (Halter et al., 2013) • Physical distance (Aquino et al., 2016; Khanassov et al., 2014; Overbeck et al., 2016)
Individual factors	• Having the necessary knowledge and skills (Abuzour et al., 2017; Dennis et al., 2012; Hillis et al., 2016; Khanassov et al., 2014; Wood et al., 2017) • Good communication (Andregård & Jangland, 2015; Aquino et al., 2016; Carmont et al., 2017; Dennis et al., 2012; Gardiner et al., 2012) • Positive attitude (Andregård & Jangland, 2015; Farris et al., 2010; Overbeck et al., 2016; Schadewaldt et al., 2013) • Mutual trust and respect (Aquino et al., 2016; Schadewaldt et al., 2013) • Recognition of each other's role (Sangaleti et al., 2017; Supper et al., 2015) • Peer learning (Wood et al., 2017)	• Variable or lack of skills (Abuzour et al., 2017; Supper et al., 2015; Wood et al., 2017) • Poor communication (Aquino et al., 2016; Carmont et al., 2017; Sangaleti et al., 2017) • Attitudes (Colvin et al., 2013; Dennis et al., 2012; Farris et al., 2010; Khanassov et al., 2014) • Lack of confidence, trust and respect (Andregård & Jangland, 2015; Colvin et al., 2013; Hoeft et al., 2018; Schadewaldt et al., 2013; Supper et al., 2015) • Feeling threatened (Colvin et al., 2013; Schadewaldt et al., 2013) • Professional turf issues / divergent ideologies (Hoeft et al., 2018; Overbeck et al., 2016; Schadewaldt et al., 2013)
Intervention characteristics	• Perceived benefits for professional (Andregård & Jangland, 2015; Halter et al., 2013; Schadewaldt et al., 2013; Supper et al., 2015)	• Complexity (Joo & Huber, 2017; Wood et al., 2017) • Perceived disadvantages for patients (Dennis et al., 2012; Halter et al., 2013)

	Facilitators	Barriers
	• Perceived benefits for patients (Halter et al., 2013; Khanassov et al., 2014; Overbeck et al., 2016; Wood et al., 2017) • Strong evidence for positive outcomes intervention (Wood et al., 2017) • Sufficient duration of intervention (Khanassov et al., 2014)	• Expected challenges in patient relationship (Halter et al., 2013; Joo & Huber, 2017) • Lack of clarity of purpose (Carmont et al., 2017)
Process factors	• Access to ongoing support (Abuzour et al., 2017; Gardiner et al., 2012; Hoeft et al., 2018; Savic et al., 2017; Supper et al., 2015; Wood et al., 2017) • Formalized relationships (Hoeft et al., 2018; Savic et al., 2017) • Care protocols and guidelines (Abuzour et al., 2017; Mapp et al., 2015) • Clear expectations and goals at outset (Savic et al., 2017) • Compatible IT infrastructures between partners (Savic et al., 2017) • Engagement period (Khanassov et al., 2014)	• Lack of support (Abuzour et al., 2017; Colvin et al., 2013; Wood et al., 2017) • Lack of monitoring (Supper et al., 2015) • Participants being unprepared (Carmont et al., 2017) • Lack of guidelines (Joo & Huber, 2017)
Institutional factors	• Appropriate staff training (Dennis et al., 2012; Khanassov et al., 2014; Mapp et al., 2015; Overbeck et al., 2016; Sangaleti et al., 2017) • Supportive policies and laws (Dennis et al., 2012; Farris et al., 2010) • Funding for education (Dennis et al., 2012)	• No reimbursement model for skill-mix innovation (Carmont et al., 2017; Farris et al., 2010; Halter et al., 2013; Hoeft et al., 2018; Meiklejohn et al., 2016; Supper et al., 2015) • Lack of (long-term) funding (Mapp et al., 2015; Schadewaldt et al., 2013; Supper et al., 2015; Wood et al., 2017) • Legal liability / licensing (Colvin et al., 2013; Farris et al., 2010; Hoeft et al., 2018; Schadewaldt et al., 2013) • Insufficient training / lack of staff skills (Joo & Huber, 2017; Khanassov et al., 2014; Mapp et al., 2015; Meiklejohn et al., 2016; Sangaleti et al., 2017; Wood et al., 2017) • Federal regulations / laws / policies (Farris et al., 2010; Halter et al., 2013) • Bureaucratic processes / administration (Carmont et al., 2017)

Schadewaldt et al., 2013; Supper et al., 2015; Wood, Ohlsen & Ricketts, 2017), which offers increased opportunities for face-to-face contact, and having well-functioning information systems in place (Dennis et al., 2012; Hoeft et al., 2018; Meiklejohn et al., 2016; Schadewaldt et al., 2013; Wood, Ohlsen & Ricketts, 2017). While these relatively 'simple' practical issues can be highly beneficial, the evidence suggests that more structural issues, such as lack of time and financial resources (Aquino et al., 2016; Farris et al., 2010; Hoeft et al., 2018; Sangaleti et al., 2017; Supper et al., 2015; Wood, Ohlsen & Ricketts, 2017) and professional silos (Carmont et al., 2017; Colvin et al., 2013; Gardiner, Gott & Ingleton, 2012; Hoeft et al., 2018; Sangaleti et al., 2017) are important hampering factors. Two other important factors, acting as both facilitator and barrier, are the (lack of) clarity over roles, responsibilities and scope of practice (Abuzour, Lewis & Tully, 2017; Andregård & Jangland, 2015; Carmont et al., 2017; Colvin et al., 2013; Gardiner, Gott & Ingleton, 2012; Joo & Huber, 2017; Meiklejohn et al., 2016; Schadewaldt et al., 2013; Wood, Ohlsen & Ricketts, 2017) and the (lack of adequate) communication, including for example (no) involvement in multidisciplinary meetings or a lack of processes to establish communication between different providers (Colvin et al., 2013; Gardiner, Gott & Ingleton, 2012; Mapp, Hutchinson & Estcourt, 2015; Sangaleti et al., 2017; Schadewaldt et al., 2013; Wood, Ohlsen & Ricketts, 2017).

Individual factors
Almost all individual factors that influence the implementation of skill-mix interventions in health care organizations mirror each other, acting both as barrier and facilitator. This is the case for (a lack of) required knowledge and skills (Abuzour, Lewis & Tully, 2017; Dennis et al., 2012; Hillis et al., 2016; Khanassov, Vedel & Pluye, 2014; Supper et al., 2015; Wood, Ohlsen & Ricketts, 2017), a (lack of good) communication (Andregård & Jangland, 2015; Aquino et al., 2016; Carmont et al., 2017; Dennis et al., 2012; Gardiner, Gott & Ingleton, 2012; Khanassov, Vedel & Pluye, 2014; Sangaleti et al., 2017), attitudes, such as (lack of) a pioneering spirit (Andregård & Jangland, 2015; Colvin et al., 2013; Dennis et al., 2012; Farris et al., 2010; Overbeck, Davidsen & Kousgaard, 2016; Schadewaldt et al., 2013), and (a lack of) trust and respect, for example where one profession feels it is controlled too much, whereas the other profession feels supervision takes too much of its time (Andregård & Jangland, 2015; Aquino et al., 2016; Colvin

et al., 2013; Hoeft et al., 2018; Overbeck, Davidsen & Kousgaard, 2016; Schadewaldt et al., 2013; Supper et al., 2015).

Characteristics of skill-mix interventions
The evidence suggests that interventions can be facilitators to skill-mix changes if they are perceived as having benefits for professionals, including the promise of reduced workloads, using one's skills to the fullest, developing complementary skills and increased continuity in clinical work (Andregård & Jangland, 2015; Halter et al., 2013; Schadewaldt et al., 2013; Supper et al., 2015). The expected effects on patients also influence its uptake at organizational level, especially if a change in the quality of care is expected, either positive (Halter et al., 2013; Overbeck, Davidsen & Kousgaard, 2016; Wood, Ohlsen & Ricketts, 2017) or negative (Halter et al., 2013), or if the quality of the patient-relationship is perceived to be at risk (Halter et al., 2013; Joo & Huber, 2017).

Process factors
To facilitate the uptake of skill-mix innovations at organizational level, the evidence suggests that it may be beneficial to formalize the intervention to the extent possible, among others by formalizing relationships (Hoeft et al., 2018; Savic et al., 2017) and by using protocols and guidelines (Abuzour, Lewis & Tully, 2017; Mapp, Hutchinson & Estcourt, 2015). This gives people something to hold on to. In addition, investments in ongoing coaching and support to the professionals involved seem to facilitate the implementation process as well (Gardiner, Gott & Ingleton, 2012; Hoeft et al., 2018; Savic et al., 2017; Supper et al., 2015; Wood, Ohlsen & Ricketts, 2017).

Institutional factors
Institutional factors seem to act more as barriers for skill-mix interventions than as facilitators. The positive influence of institutional factors occurs in two main ways: through appropriate staff training (for example, teamwork being part of undergraduate training) and via supportive policies and regulations (Dennis et al., 2012; Farris et al., 2010; Mapp, Hutchinson & Estcourt, 2015; Overbeck, Davidsen & Kousgaard, 2016; Sangaleti et al., 2017), both of which can also act as barriers (Farris et al., 2010; Halter et al., 2013; Joo & Huber, 2017; Mapp, Hutchinson & Estcourt, 2015; Meiklejohn et al., 2016; Sangaleti et al., 2017; Wood, Ohlsen & Ricketts, 2017). Yet the most important

barrier is related to financing. Often, no reimbursement is available for skill-mix innovations (Carmont et al., 2017; Farris et al., 2010; Halter et al., 2013; Hoeft et al., 2018; Meiklejohn et al., 2016; Supper et al., 2015) or there is a general lack of funding (Mapp, Hutchinson & Estcourt, 2015; Schadewaldt et al., 2013; Supper et al., 2015; Wood et al., 2017). Another important barrier is related to concrete or perceived fears of liability and to licensing issues, for example in the USA where new tasks may post a challenge as roles vary widely among states of licensure (Colvin et al., 2013; Farris et al., 2010; Hoeft et al., 2018; Schadewaldt et al., 2013).

11.3   Trends in implementation at the organizational level

The evidence from the systematic reviews provides a good overview of the factors that commonly play a role in the implementation of skill-mix interventions at organizational level, acting either as barrier or facilitator. To enhance the understanding of *how* these factors influence the implementation at organizational level, the next section discusses some of the strategies that organizations can apply to overcome the most commonly identified barriers and what approaches can be taken to strengthen the identified facilitators. Subsequently, four case studies are presented, which exemplify the influence of these factors, and the complex interactions between them, in everyday health care practice.

Overcoming barriers and strengthening facilitators

Organizational factors

The overview of reviews showed that a lack of financial resources is one of the main barriers for the implementation of skill-mix innovations at organizational level. Among the organizational adjustments that the introduction of skill-mix innovations requires, payment methods of individual providers are often ignored even though their influence can be a key facilitator for the success or failure of the implementation of skill-mix interventions. Various payment methods have different impacts on the behaviour of providers and must therefore be designed in a way to facilitate the adoption of skill-mix changes.

Fee-for-service payment is known as an incentive to increase clinical activity and to induce demand for the most remunerating services. It is not likely to encourage the delegation of tasks which correspond to a source of income. However, this depends on how fee-for-service payments are structured. Even in the classic fee-for-service system, there are numerous examples of delegation of tasks to nurses or other health professionals who work under medical supervision, and so allow the doctor to charge a fee-for-service. Capitation payments can have the reverse effect by encouraging providers to delegate tasks in order to keep their workload lighter and eventually to limit their costs. This is often feared to have a negative impact on the quality of care provision, but there is no good evidence that this is an issue in practice.

More recently, linking payment to performance has been adopted by a number of countries in some form, like add-on payments in France and Germany, or pay-for-performance in Norway, Portugal and the United Kingdom (OECD, 2016). Pay-for-performance is typically used to complement other methods of remuneration, is normally an organizationally based or unit-based contract approach, and is principally used in primary care. It is usually designed to encourage teamwork – which is being promoted at all levels of care to improve effectiveness and efficiency of services – and to reward the achievement of predefined objectives such as a better follow up of (chronic) patients and more cost-effective use of medicines, such as in Family Health Units in Portugal (World Health Organization, 2018) (see also Box 11.1). Even though pay-for-performance is not explicitly used to facilitate

---

Box 11.1 Skill-mix in primary care services in Portugal: barriers to change and potential facilitators

In Portugal, since 2005, self-managed Family Health Units (FHUs), composed on average of 20 professionals (family physicians and nurses in equal numbers, plus administrative officers), serve a geographically defined population of 1500–1900 persons per physician, with service coverage and performance objectives. FHUs are characterized by teamwork, community orientation, administrative autonomy and flexibility, and evaluation of performance. Decisions are made collectively. The delivery of services is linked to **pay-for-performance**, and a mix of individual and institutional incentives. Indicators of accessibility, quality of care, user satisfaction and efficiency determine the amount of these incentives. This creates a favourable environment for reviewing the skill-mix for the provision of primary care, for instance through the expansion of the role of nurses. This has not happened, due mostly to important **institutional barriers**.

Box 11.1 (cont.)

Barriers to changing the skill-mix

- Legal definitions of scopes of practice are vague, and the Medical Council has historically claimed authority over what other health professionals are legally authorized to do, an example of **professional territorialism,** by including in its Code of Ethics a prohibition to delegate any act relating to diagnosis, prescription and clinical management (**Temido & Dussault, 2014**). Any significant change in the scopes-of-practice therefore requires amendment of existing laws, a highly demanding process.
- This position is not seriously challenged by the nursing profession, which is divided on the issue of expanded scopes-of-practice. In 2014, the Nursing Council formally adopted a statement in favour on this issue. Trade unions however did not support it, arguing that task-shifting would add to already heavy workloads and a negative perception of **characteristics of skill-mix interventions,** without the guarantee of better pay.
- Other professional groups have little voice in the political debate: nutritionists, pharmacists and psychologists mostly work in the private sector. Hence, from the perspective of **individual factors,** there is a lack of strong advocates who could influence public opinion and bring the issue to the policy agenda.
- As a result, there is little political willingness for making the skill-mix more efficient in primary care.

However, there are factors that can facilitate the process of change in the near future. There is already recognition that the present division of labour is not efficient (**World Health Organization, 2010**).

- Informal delegation by family doctors to nurses is happening, even if only informally: in some Family Health Units, nurses monitor normal pregnancies or perform cytology tests (**Temido**, Craveiro & Dussault, **2015**). Even though their professional council opposes any form of delegation, many individual practitioners are open to this (Buchan et al., 2013, Temido & Dussault, 2014).
- In FHUs, an **organizational culture** of teamwork and of results-oriented management, including rewards for good performance, is a positive environment for developing a more efficient skill-mix. The dominant payment mechanisms, for example salary plus performance-based incentives are an incentive to delegation.
- Finally, nursing education institutions and programmes are of high quality and can respond rapidly to prepare nurses to perform expanded functions.

the adoption of skill-mix innovations, it can have this effect when well designed. Moreover, it is usually accepted by providers. When applied to teams, pay-for-performance should apply to the whole team and the distribution of rewards must be transparent and acceptable to all. If applied to individuals, it may generate individualistic behaviours and competition, in which case the introduction of skill-mix innovations will likely be resisted.

Individual factors

Many factors at the individual level are related to opinions and attitudes, and less so to individuals' knowledge, skills or experiences. Opinions and attitudes can be tribal and be strongly linked to the health profession and education of an individual. This is in line with earlier findings; psychological professional barriers among health care professionals have been reported as one of the most persistent barriers to the uptake of skill-mix changes in practice (Kroezen et al., 2014a; Niezen & Mathijssen, 2014), whereas more supportive views among health care professionals have been shown to positively influence the uptake of skill-mix innovations (French, Bilton & Camplbell, 2003; Jones, Edwards & While, 2011; Travers, 2005). In other words, the barriers often result from a lack of confidence and trust in other professionals involved in the skill-mix, feelings of being threatened, for example in terms of professional autonomy, and related to that, professional turf issues. However, there are many examples where these barriers were overcome. In the Netherlands and the United Kingdom, it was observed that the more experience people have with nurse prescribing, which is being introduced in an increasing number of countries (Fernández-Ortega et al., 2016), the more positive their views become (Latter et al., 2011) (see also Box 11.2). Similar results were found in comparative studies in Europe (Köppen et al., 2018, Kuhlmann et al., 2018). Hence, for hospitals or other health care institutions thinking about introducing nurse prescribing, it is beneficial to start with a pilot project. In this way, experience can be gained, and a workable mode can be found by all health care professionals involved, before the final introduction of nurses' prescriptive authority (Kroezen et al., 2014b). Naturally, to secure change, the skill-mix intervention will subsequently have to be implemented system-wide. Another proven successful approach to overcome professional barriers is by organizing information sessions

Box 11.2 The implementation of prescribing by nurse specialists in the Netherlands

In the Netherlands, nurse specialists – registered nurses who have successfully completed a 2-year Master's programme in Advanced Nursing Practice and have subsequently registered themselves in the national Nurse Specialists Register – are legally allowed to prescribe medicines. In January 2012, they received independent prescriptive authority for any medicine within their competence and specialist area. One year after the introduction, however, a great variation was visible in the extent to which and way in which nurse specialists' legal prescriptive authority had been implemented in primary care (**Laurant et al., 2018**) as well as across hospitals (**Kroezen et al., 2014a**). This variation could be explained to a large extent by individual factors, such as the attitude of the physician with whom nurse specialists worked daily. Although some nurse specialists prescribed for up to 16 patients a day, others only wrote a prescription three times a week on average. Also, while most nurse specialists could independently prescribe both initial and repeat prescriptions, some were required to check their initial prescriptions with their medical specialist. In terms of the medicines that nurse specialists prescribed at hospital ward level, it was found that they hardly ever independently prescribed all medicines within their specialism and competence, as their legal authority allowed them to do. They were often only allowed to prescribe a relatively limited number of medicines, as set out in ward-level protocols or (personal) formularies drawn up in collaboration with physicians (**Kroezen et al., 2014a**). In general, the less familiar physicians were with nurse specialists, the less the support for their prescriptive authority (**de Bruijn-Geraets et al., 2015**). Apart from individual factors, there were also process factors, which acted as a barrier for nurse specialists to use their prescriptive authority. For example, on some hospital wards nurse specialists' prescriptive authority was not fully institutionalized. Nurse specialists would still be waiting for their own personal prescription paper or access to the digital prescription system. This prevented them from (independently) prescribing (**Kroezen et al., 2014a**). Finally, at organizational level the extent to which higher management levels were (un)aware of the role of nurse specialists and their prescriptive authority strongly influenced the way nurse specialists could work in practice, for example by (not) having a specific policy for nurse specialists in place (de Bruijn-Geraets et al., 2015).

with all actors expected to be involved in a skill-mix intervention. For example, in South-East England, when there was the possibility of support workers starting to use ionizing radiation, initial reservations by other health workers concerning professional boundaries were only overcome after meetings about the legislative, professional and practical implications took place (Ford, 2004).

The implementation of skill-mix interventions at organizational level may also be facilitated by a shared goal among health professions of providing good care for patients. For example, in Denmark gynaecologists, midwives and nurses involved in reorganized stroke rehabilitation shared a positive view on this intervention. This was driven by a shared goal of providing needs-based care for patients. In this particular skill-mix intervention, individual team members for example screened patients on behalf of members from the other professions, driven by the feeling of working independently as well as on behalf of the team (Burau et al., 2017). In a similar vein, a shared goal of improving women's health facilitated skill-mix change and collaboration between gynaecologists, midwives and nurses (Kuhlmann, 2006). Thus, people-centred care and skill-mix changes may create new forms of more integrated professionalism/professional ethics and culture (Kuhlmann, 2006; Strategic Advisory Board Well-being Health Family, 2015), which in turn facilitate implementation and sustainability of skill-mix changes.

Skill-mix intervention characteristics

When examining skill-mix innovations, which are successfully implemented into routine practice, a number of common characteristics stand out. The (perceived) improvement that a skill-mix innovation will offer, in terms of accessibility and quality of care and of responding to unmet care needs, is an important characteristic that enables its uptake in practice (Halter et al., 2013; Wood, Ohlsen & Ricketts, 2017) (see also Box 11.3). Changes in scopes of practice, for example, are more widely accepted when the health professionals transferring tasks accept that their profession does not have the capacity to continue to provide these tasks, while the skill-mix innovation makes it possible (Leggat, 2015). A study from the Netherlands showed that a high workload and increasing demand for glaucoma care, made glaucoma specialists highly interested in delegating some of their tasks. However, once care needs were fulfilled

Box 11.3 Community specialist nurses in neurology in the United Kingdom

With one neurologist per 233 600 inhabitants in 1995, the United Kingdom had one of the lowest numbers of neurologists per population in Europe (**Stevens, 1997**). This led to long waiting times for patients, shortcomings in the provision of care and proved an incentive to develop alternative solutions, including a skill-mix intervention using specialist nurses. Developed for the first time in Edinburgh in the 1990s, the advantages of a new epilepsy specialist nurse service were soon evident to all involved; the pressure on consultant-led specialist clinics was reduced and the gap between primary and tertiary services became smaller (Hosking, Duncan & Sander, 2002). So the characteristics of the skill-mix intervention acted as a facilitator for its implementation, and the model has since been adopted by several hospital trusts in the NHS and has been widened to other chronic neurological conditions (Lloyd & Evans, 2016). Looking more closely at the process of the implementation at organizational level, the following barriers and facilitators can be discerned:

Barriers to implementation of the skill-mix intervention

- Lack of streamlined NHS funding: probably the most important barrier **at institutional level** to a system-wide implementation of the neurology specialist nurse model. As this is a truly integrated care service between primary and tertiary care, in theory such a service requires co-funding between hospitals and clinical commissioning groups. Currently, most neurology specialist nurse services are funded by hospital trusts alone.
- Lack of standardized training for specialist nurses: this means varying standards from one hospital to another and reduced transferable skills for specialist nurses compared with an ideal training with clearly defined roles and standardized training curricula throughout the country.
- Perception of inferior quality care: substitution of medical specialist clinic appointments by nurse-led clinic appointments is seen by some medical specialists as inferior to the traditional model of care, a hampering **individual factor**.

Facilitators of implementation

- Dearth of neurologists: there is still a relative scarcity of neurologists compared with the burden of neurological disorders, which has

Box 11.3 (cont.)

been and still is a key factor for the use of the neurology specialist nurse model.

- Clinical champions: because of the lack of streamlined funding, the implementation of a neurology specialist nurse service is often due to **individual factors,** such as the commitment of an individual neurologist or a neurology department.
- National guidelines: in 2004, the national guideline for epilepsy in children and adolescents for the first time included the recommendation, that "epilepsy specialist nurses should be an integral part of the network of care of individuals with epilepsy" (**National Institute for Clinical Excellence, 2012**). This recommendation can now be used by neurology departments to negotiate funding for a specialist nurse service in their hospitals.

and workloads became more acceptable, there was a strong reduction in specialists' interest for task delegation (Holtzer-Goor et al., 2013). It has also been reported that one of the main reasons for GPs to employ a physician assistant or a nurse practitioner was the expectation that this would improve the quality of care provided within their practice, in particular by ensuring continuity of care. Also, some GPs considered this particular skill-mix innovation as an opportunity to expand the supply of new services (Van der Biezen et al., 2017).

Another factor that influences the uptake of a skill-mix innovation in practice is the extent to which it is perceived as a disruption of routine care. For example, in the delegation of tasks from dentists to dental hygiene therapists, it was found that tasks and patient groups that fitted closely with the accepted and traditional role of the dental hygiene therapist were more often delegated than tasks and patient groups whose delegation would bring about a larger change to usual care provision and division of labour (Wanyonyi, Radford & Gallagher, 2014).

Process factors

A lack of support for staff involved in skill-mix change can severely hamper its implementation at organizational level. Hence, access to ongoing support is one of the most important facilitators for effective skill-mix implementation. There are various ways in which health care organizations can facilitate this. Supervision or mentorship programmes seem to be one of the most frequently used instruments, and are deemed helpful by professionals in terms of peer learning (Deller et al., 2015; Supper et al., 2015; Wood, Ohlsen & Ricketts, 2017). However, if mentorship schemes are to be effective, sufficient time and resources need to be made available for this and there needs to be financial, logistical and educational support and incentives for mentors or supervisors. Another way in which organizations can support professionals involved in a skill-mix intervention, is by formalizing the newly created relationships. One example of this is by introducing explicit policies that encompass a demarcation of the new roles. This has repeatedly been found to facilitate task reallocation from doctors to nurse practitioners (Niezen & Mathijssen, 2014; Schadewaldt et al., 2016).

Institutional factors

If organizations are able to optimize staff training and can use policies and regulations to their benefit, this may contribute to the successful introduction of skill-mix innovations in health care practice. Research suggests that health professionals who have trained together have a better understanding of each other's scope of practice and are therefore better equipped for teamwork (Wanyonyi, Radford & Gallagher, 2014). Hence, where there is a lack of training integration in regular curricula, offering training in teamwork can improve staff abilities to participate in skill-mix interventions. Training in a particular health care setting can make this learning even more applicable to the local context (Lemer, Allwood & Foley, 2012).

In Germany, the establishment of dental hygienists provides an example of how regulations can act as a key facilitator for skill-mix implementation at organizational level. Changes in the legal reimbursement schemes of sickness funds supported the establishment of dental hygienists (Theobald, 2004). Since the provision of preventive/hygiene services by a dentist or a hygienist (the latter costing less) became a legal requirement for reimbursement in Germany, dentists welcomed task-shifting and training of dental hygienists to increase the economic efficiency of their surgeries. This catalysed the establishment of new training programmes for dental hygienists and the improvement of employment conditions for this professional group. It is important to emphasize in this regard, that different health care systems and contexts may have different pay systems, pay outcomes and pay differentials. This has consequences for skill-mix implementation. For example, where pay differences between professions are bigger, the scope for task substitution on cost criteria is greater (at least in theory).

Box 11.4 Health workforce change in Germany in the shadow of organizational reform

The 'organizational path' of workforce transformations in Germany, including skill-mix innovations, must be seen in the context of its **institutional conditions**. The German health care system can be characterized as a corporatist governance model, with the medical associations and sickness funds as the two key stakeholders, and an overall marginality of other health care providers in the regulatory bodies (**Blank, Burau & Kuhlmann, 2018; Busse et al., 2017**). Hence, transformations in the health workforce and skill-mix innovations must inevitably be negotiated with the medical profession. Organizational change, however, does not directly intervene in these professional silo politics and in the hierarchical order of professions. As a result, in this specific national context, the processes of skill-mix change become more incremental, focus more on lower-qualified groups of the health workforce (rather than on the professional development of nurses) and become more diverse and local, shaped by the *Länder* politics. Health workforce transformations and skill-mix innovations are primarily targeted at medical providers – integration of generalist and specialist care – and aimed at an expansion of the role of health care assistants (in a few cases also of community nurses).

The processes of workforce change and skill-mix innovations can be illustrated when looking at pilot projects that have flagship character in the German context: the new organizational model of Integrated Care Healthy Kinzigtal (*Integrierte Versorgung Gesundes Kinzigtal*) as an example of integrated primary care provision (**Groene et al., 2016**), a directive on piloting task-shifting from physicians to nurses (Federal Joint Committee, 2011) and several pilot and small-scale programmes to expand the tasks of health care assistants (*Medizinische Assistenten*) (Advisory Council on the Assessment of Developments in the Health Care System, 2014) (for a European overview, see (Kroezen et al., 2018 (forthcoming))). The most prominent example is AGnES (*Arztentlastende, Gemeindenahe, E-Health-gestützte, Systemische Intervention*), a pilot project to train medical assistants (also open to nurses) for new tasks in four formerly eastern German federal states between 2005 and 2008.

Box 11.4 (cont.)

Following successful evaluation, AGnES has been integrated into routine care and renamed as nonmedical surgery assistant. These reforms have created positive individual attitudes among health professionals. As a result, other federal states established similar programmes and a number of training programmes are now provided by Physician Chambers or the organizations of family physicians. Recently, Rhineland Palatine has introduced a further pilot programme called Community Nurse Plus (*Gemeindeschwester*PLUS), exclusively for nurses. This programme aims to fill the gap between existing social care services, rather than providing classic nursing care or taking over medical tasks (MSAGD, 2015).

11.4 Conclusions

In this chapter, we identified factors and strategies that facilitate or impede the uptake of skill-mix interventions in organizations. Based on a conceptual framework that analyses the most important factors that influence implementation, and on evidence from an overview of 21 systematic reviews, we identified various factors that foster or impede the implementation of skill-mix changes. In many cases, the barriers for implementing skill-mix interventions in organizations turned out to be the mirror opposite of facilitators. Organizational and individual factors were most often mentioned – most notably (a lack of) time and financial resources, clarity over roles and responsibilities, information systems, knowledge and skills, good communication and professional and personal attitudes. Characteristics of the skill-mix intervention, institutional factors and process factors were mentioned less frequently. Yet (a lack of) perceived benefits for health care professionals and patients, supportive laws and regulations, reimbursement and institutional support also play an important role in the implementation of skill-mix innovations in organizations. Because of the relatively small amount of identified reviews, and the fact that the majority of included studies in the reviews was from Anglophone OECD countries and northern and western European countries, the generalizability of these findings is somewhat restricted.

Skill-mix change in practice is a complex challenge, involving interdependent changes in a number of factors, as illustrated by the mini case studies presented in the previous sections. This means that there is no single appropriate strategy for implementing skill innovations that will fit all organizations. Managers must adopt an optimal strategy when implementing skill-mix, usually involving a combination of approaches best suited to local factors, to their organization and to individuals involved (Antwi & Kale, 2014). Which factors are decisive, and which change management model is most suitable, is to a large extent dependent on the specific organizational context. For example, to answer the question of which is the best payment method to optimize the utilization of all skills within an organization – an important factor when implementing a skill-mix innovation – each organization must find its own answer. What can be said is that changing the skill-mix entails changing the method of remuneration, and both are very sensitive: engaging stakeholders from the start of the process and keeping them engaged is the best advice that can be given to managers and policy-makers.

In general, the technical aspects of skill-mix analysis are more easily transferable than their application in context. Based on a comparison of change management models that are applicable to – or specifically emerged from – a health care context, Antwi & Kale (2014) have established important basic principles that are useful to all managers and policy-makers who aim to implement skill-mix changes in their organization. First, managers need to be aware of the various stages of an implementation process, and that each stage requires specific actions: from preparing for change, to implementing change and finally sustaining change. Furthermore, Antwi & Kale (2014) were able to show that the following components should always be taken into account when implementing skill-mix innovations: governance and leadership, stakeholder engagement, communication, workflow analysis and integration, education, and monitoring and evaluation. Apart from these, environmental circumstances, organizational harmony, organizational capacity, power dynamics, the nature of change and process for change can play an important facilitating or inhibiting role.

Overall, the results presented in this chapter underline the complexity of factors that either support or constrain the implementation of skill-mix innovation at the organizational level. Combined with the variety of change management models available and the complex challenge to align actions to a specific organizational context, this highlights the need for more comprehensive research on this topic.

References

Abuzour AS, Lewis PJ, Tully MP (2017). Practice makes perfect: a systematic review of the expertise development of pharmacist and nurse independent prescribers in the United Kingdom. Res Social Admin Pharmacy, 14:6–17.

Advisory Council on the Assessment of Developments in the Health Care System (2014). Needs-based health care: opportunities for rural regions and selected health care sectors. Bonn, Advisory Council on the Assessment of Developments in the Health Care System.

Andregård AC, Jangland E (2015). The tortuous journey of introducing the Nurse Practitioner as a new member of the healthcare team: a meta-synthesis. Scand J Caring Sci, 29:3–14.

Antwi M, Kale M (2014). Change management in healthcare: literature review. Kingston, ONT, Monieson Centre for Business Research in Healthcare, Queen's University.

Aquino MRJRV, Olander EK, Needle JJ et al. (2016). Midwives' and health visitors' collaborative relationships: A systematic review of qualitative and quantitative studies. Int J Nurs Stud, 62:193–206.

Blank R, Burau V, Kuhlmann E (2018). Comparative health policy, 5th edn. Basingstoke, Palgrave.

Buchan J, Temido M, Fronteira I et al. (2013). Nurses in advanced roles: a review of acceptability in Portugal. Rev Latino-Am Enferm, 21:38–46.

Burau V, Carstensen K, Fleron SL et al. (2017). Professional groups driving innovation in healthcare: interprofessional working in stroke rehabilitation in Denmark. BMC Health Serv Res, 17:662.

Busse R, Blümel M, Knieps F et al. (2017). Statutory health insurance in Germany: a health system shaped by 135 years of solidarity, self-governance, and competition. Lancet, 390:882–897.

Carmont S-A, Mitchell G, Senior H et al. (2017). Systematic review of the effectiveness, barriers and facilitators to general practitioner engagement with specialist secondary services in integrated palliative care. BMJ Support Palliat Care, bmjspcare-2016-001125.

Colvin CJ, De Heer J, Winterton L et al. (2013). A systematic review of qualitative evidence on barriers and facilitators to the implementation of task-shifting in midwifery services. Midwifery, 29:1211–1221.

De Bruijn-Geraets D, Bessems-Beks M, Van Eijk-Hustings Y et al. (2015). VoorBIGhouden: Eindrapportage Evaluatieonderzoek Art. 36a Wet BIG met betrekking tot de inzet van de Verpleegkundig Specialist en de Physician Assistant. Maastricht, Maastricht UMC.

Deller B, Tripathi V, Stender S et al. (2015). Task shifting in maternal and newborn health care: key components from policy to implementation. Int J Gynecol Obstet, 130:S25–S31.

Dennis S, Williams A, Taggart J et al. (2012). Which providers can bridge the health literacy gap in lifestyle risk factor modification education: a systematic review and narrative synthesis. BMC Fam Pract, 13, 44.

Farris KB, Ashwood D, McIntosh J, et al. (2010). Preventing unintended pregnancy: pharmacists' roles in practice and policy via partnerships. J Am Pharm Assoc, 50:604–612.

Federal Joint Committee (2011). Directive on the establishment of medical activities for transfer to professionals of nursing and elderly for the independent practice of medicine within the framework of pilot projects; § 63 para 3c according to SGB V. Directive § 63 paragraph 3c according to SGB V. Berlin, Federal Joint Committee.

Fernández-Ortega P, Cabrera-Jaime S, Estrada-Masllorens JM (2016). The oncology nurse prescribing: a Catalonian survey. Asia-Pacific J Oncol Nurs 3:108.

Fleuren M, Wiefferink K, Paulussen T (2004). Determinants of innovation within health care organizations: literature review and Delphi study. Int J Qual Health Care, 16:107–123.

Ford P (2004). The role of support workers in the department of diagnostic imaging—service managers perspectives. Radiography, 10:259–267.

French J, Bilton D, Campbell F (2003). Nurse specialist care for bronchiectasis. The Cochrane Library.

Gardiner C, Gott M, Ingleton C (2012). Factors supporting good partnership working between generalist and specialist palliative care services: a systematic review. Br J Gen Pract, 62:e353–e362.

Groene O, Hildebrandt H, Ferrer L et al. (2016). People-centred population health management in Germany. Eurohealth, 22:7–10.

Halter M, Drennan V, Chattopadhyay K et al. (2013). The contribution of physician assistants in primary care: a systematic review. BMC Health Serv Res, 13:223.

Hillis R, Brenner M, Larkin P et al. (2016). The role of care coordinator for children with complex care needs: a systematic review. Int J Integr Care, 16:12,1–18.

Hoeft TJ, Fortney JC, Patel V et al. (2018). Task-sharing approaches to improve mental health care in rural and other low-resource settings: a systematic review. J Rural Health, 34:48–62.

Holtzer-Goor KM, Plochg T, Lemij HG et al. (2013). Why a successful task substitution in glaucoma care could not be transferred from a hospital setting to a primary care setting: a qualitative study. Implementation Science, 8:14.

Hosking PG, Duncan JS, Sander JMW (2002). The epilepsy nurse specialist at a tertiary care hospital—improving the interface between primary and tertiary care. Seizure, 11:494–499.

Jones K, Edwards M, While A (2011). Nurse prescribing roles in acute care: an evaluative case study. J Adv Nurs, 67:117–126.

Joo JY, Huber DL (2017). Barriers in case managers' roles: a qualitative systematic review. West J Nurs Res, 0193945917728689.

Kernick D, Scott A (2002). Economic approaches to doctor/nurse skill mix: problems, pitfalls, and partial solutions. Br J Gen Pract, 52:42–46.

Khanassov V, Vedel I, Pluye P (2014). Case management for dementia in primary health care: a systematic mixed studies review based on the diffusion of innovation model. Clin Intervent Aging, 9:915.

Köppen J, Maier CB, Busse R et al. (2018). What are the motivating and hindering factors for health professionals to undertake new roles in hospitals? A study among physicians, nurses and managers looking at breast cancer and acute myocardial infarction care in nine countries. Health Policy, 122:1118–1125.

Kroezen M, Mistiaen P, Van Dijk L et al. (2014a). Negotiating jurisdiction in the workplace: a multiple-case study of nurse prescribing in hospital settings. Soc Sci Med, 117:107–115.

Kroezen M, Van Dijk L, Groenewegen PP et al. (2014b). Neutral to positive views on the consequences of nurse prescribing: Results of a national survey among registered nurses, nurse specialists and physicians. Int J Nurs Stud, 51:539–548.

Kroezen M, Schäfer W, Sermeus W et al. (2018). Healthcare assistants in EU Member States: an overview. Health Policy, 122:1109–1117.

Kuhlmann E (2006). Modernising health care: reinventing professions, the state and the public. Bristol, Policy Press.

Kuhlmann E, Batenburg R, Wismar M et al. (2018). A call for action to establish a research agenda for building a future health workforce in Europe. Health Res Policy Syst, 16:52.

Latter S, Blenkinsopp A, Smith A et al. (2011). Evaluation of nurse and pharmacist independent prescribing. London, Department of Health.

Laurant M, Van Der Biezen M, Wijers N et al. (2018). Nurses as substitutes for doctors in primary care. Cochrane Database Syst Rev, 7:CD001271.

Leggat SG (2015). Changing health professionals' scope of practice: how do we continue to make progress? Deakin, Deeble Institute for Health Policy Research.

Lemer C, Allwood D, Foley T (2012). Improving NHS productivity. London, The King's Fund.

Lloyd S, Evans D (2016). Neurofibromatosis type 2 service delivery in England. Neurochirurgie, 64:375–380.

Mapp F, Hutchinson J, Estcourt C (2015). A systematic review of contemporary models of shared HIV care and HIV in primary care in high-income settings. Int J STD AIDS, 26:991–997.

Meiklejohn JA, Mimery A, Martin JH et al. (2016). The role of the GP in follow-up cancer care: a systematic literature review. J Cancer Survivorship, 10:990–1011.

MSAGD (2015). Modellprojekt Gemeindeschwesterplus – Rheinland-Pfalz ist Vorreiter für Innovationen. Mainz, Ministerium für Soziales, Arbeit, Gesundheit und Demografie.

National Institute for Health and Care Excellence (2012). The epilepsies: diagnosis and management of the epilepsies in children and young people in primary and secondary care: quick reference guide. London, National Institute for Health and Care Excellence.

Niezen MGH, Mathijssen JJP (2014). Reframing professional boundaries in healthcare: a systematic review of facilitators and barriers to task reallocation from the domain of medicine to the nursing domain. Health Policy, 117:151–169.

OECD (2016). Better ways to pay for health care. Paris, OECD Publishing.

Overbeck G, Davidsen AS, Kousgaard MB (2016). Enablers and barriers to implementing collaborative care for anxiety and depression: a systematic qualitative review. Implement Sci, 11:165.

Sangaleti C, Schveitzer MC, Peduzzi M et al. (2017). Experiences and shared meaning of teamwork and interprofessional collaboration among health care professionals in primary health care settings: a systematic review. JBI Database Syst Rev Implement Rep, 15:2723–2788.

Savic M, Best D, Manning V et al. (2017). Strategies to facilitate integrated care for people with alcohol and other drug problems: a systematic review. Substance Abuse Treatment, Prevention, and Policy, 12:19.

Schadewaldt V, McInnes E, Hiller JE et al. (2013). Views and experiences of nurse practitioners and medical practitioners with collaborative practice in primary health care – an integrative review. BMC Fam Pract, 14:132.

Schadewaldt V, McInnes E, Hiller JE et al. (2016). Experiences of nurse practitioners and medical practitioners working in collaborative practice models in primary healthcare in Australia – a multiple case study using mixed methods. BMC Fam Pract, 17:99.

Stevens DL (1997). Appendix A: Neurology in the United Kingdom – numbers of clinical neurologists and trainees. J Neurol Neurosurg Psychiat, 63:S67–S72.

Strategic Advisory Board Well-Being Health Family (2015). Vision statement. A new professionalism in care and support as a task of the future. Brussels, Strategic Advisory Board Well-Being Health Family.

Supper I, Catala O, Lustman M et al. (2015). Interprofessional collaboration in primary health care: a review of facilitators and barriers perceived by involved actors. J Public Health, 37:716–727.

Temido M, Dussault G (2014). Papéis profissionais de médicos e enfermeiros em Portugal: limites normativos à mudança. Rev Port Saúde Públ, 32:45–54.

Temido MAFB, Craveiro I, Dussault G (2015). Perceções de equipas de saúde familiar portuguesas sobre o alargamento do campo de exercício da enfermagem. Rev Enferm Ref, 6:75–85.

Theobald H (2004). Entwicklung des Qualifikationsbedarfs im Gesundheitssektor: Professionalisierungsprozesse in der Physiotherapie und Dentalhygiene im europäischen Vergleich. WZB Discussion Paper, No. SP I 2004-104. Berlin, WZB.

Travers J (2005). Professional issues for the future of nurse prescribing: a qualitative study. Nurse Prescr, 3:164–167.

Van Der Biezen M, Derckx E, Wensing M et al. (2017). Factors influencing decision of general practitioners and managers to train and employ a nurse practitioner or physician assistant in primary care: a qualitative study. BMC Fam Pract, 18:16.

Wanyonyi KL, Radford DR, Gallagher JE (2014). Dental skill mix: a cross-sectional analysis of delegation practices between dental and dental hygiene-therapy students involved in team training in the South of England. Hum Res Health, 12:65.

Wood E, Ohlsen S, Ricketts T (2017). What are the barriers and facilitators to implementing collaborative care for depression? A systematic review. J Affect Disord, 214:26–43.

World Health Organization (2010). WHO evaluation of the National Health Plan of Portugal (2004-2010). Copenhagen, WHO Regional Office for Europe.

World Health Organization (2018). Health System Review Portugal: Phase 1 Final Report. Copenhagen, WHO Regional office for Europe.

Index